Goldberger's
# Clinical
# Electrocardiography

# Goldberger's
# Clinical
# Electrocardiography
## A Simplified Approach

## Ninth Edition

**Ary L. Goldberger, MD, FACC**
Professor of Medicine
Harvard Medical School
Director, Margret and H.A. Rey Institute for Nonlinear Dynamics in Physiology and Medicine
Beth Israel Deaconess Medical Center
Boston, Massachusetts

**Zachary D. Goldberger, MD, MS, FACC, FHRS**
Associate Professor of Medicine
University of Washington School of Medicine
Director, Electrocardiography and Arrhythmia Monitoring Laboratory
Division of Cardiology
Harborview Medical Center
Seattle, Washington

**Alexei Shvilkin, MD, PhD**
Assistant Professor of Medicine
Harvard Medical School
Clinical Cardiac Electrophysiologist
Beth Israel Deaconess Medical Center
Boston, Massachusetts

ELSEVIER

# ELSEVIER

1600 John F. Kennedy Blvd.
Ste. 1800
Philadelphia, PA 19103-2899

**Library of Congress Cataloging-in-Publication Data**
Goldberger, Ary Louis, 1949-
   Goldberger's clinical electrocardiography: a simplified approach / Ary L. Goldberger,
     Zachary D. Goldberger, Alexei Shvilkin.—9th ed.
    p. ; cm.
   Clinical electrocardiography
   Includes bibliographical references and index.
   ISBN 978-0-323-08786-5 (pbk. : alk. paper)
   I. Goldberger, Zachary D.  II. Shvilkin, Alexei.  III. Title.  IV. Title: Clinical electrocardiography.
   [DNLM:  1. Electrocardiography—methods.  2. Arrhythmias, Cardiac—diagnosis. WG 140]
   616.1'207547—dc23
                                                    2012019647

*Content Strategist:* Maureen Iannuzzi/Robin Carter
*Content Development Specialist:* Carole McMurray
*Publishing Services Manager:* Patricia Tannian
*Project Manager:* Anne Collett/Ted Rodgers
*Design Direction:* Miles Hitchen
*Illustration Manager:* Amy Faith Heyden
*Illustrator:* Victoria Heim

Printed in China

Last digit is the print number:  9  8  7  6  5  4  3  2  1

**ELSEVIER** your source for books, journals and multimedia in the health sciences
**www.elsevierhealth.com**

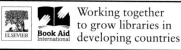

Working together to grow libraries in developing countries

www.elsevier.com • www.bookaid.org

The publisher's policy is to use paper manufactured from sustainable forests

Make everything as simple as possible, but not simpler.

*Albert Einstein*

# Contents

# Video Contents

# Introductory Remarks

## OVERVIEW

This is an introduction to electrocardiography, written especially for medical students, house officers, and nurses. The text assumes no previous instruction in reading electrocardiograms (ECGs) and has been widely deployed in entry-level electrocardiography courses. Other frontline clinicians, including hospitalists, emergency medicine physicians, emergency medical technicians, physician's assistants, and cardiology trainees wishing to review the basics, have consulted previous editions.

A high degree of ECG "literacy" is increasingly important for those involved in acute clinical care at all levels, requiring knowledge that exceeds simple pattern recognition. In a more expansive way, ECG interpretation is not only important as a focal point of clinical medicine, but as a compelling exemplar of critical thinking. The rigor demanded by competency in ECG analysis not only requires attention to the subtlest of details, but also to the subtending arcs of integrative reasoning: seeing both the trees and the forest. Furthermore, ECG analysis is one of these unique areas in clinical medicine where you literally observe physiologic and pathophysiologic dynamics "play out" over seconds to milliseconds. Not infrequently, bedside rapid-fire decisions are based on real-time ECG data. The alphabetic P–QRS–T–U sequence, much more than a flat, 2D graph, represents a dynamic map of multidimensional electrical signals literally exploding into existence (automaticity) and spreading throughout the heart (conduction) as part of fundamental processes of activation and recovery. The ECG provides some of the most compelling and fascinating connections between basic "preclinical" sciences and the recognition and treatment of potentially life-threatening problems in outpatient and inpatient settings.

This new, ninth edition follows the general format of the previous one. The material is divided into three sections. *Part I* covers the basic principles of 12-lead electrocardiography, normal ECG patterns, and the major abnormal depolarization (QRS) and repolarization (ST-T-U) patterns. *Part II* explores the mechanism of sinus rhythms, followed by a discussion of the major arrhythmias and conduction abnormalities associated with tachycardias and bradycardias. *Part III* presents more specialized material, including sudden cardiac death, pacemakers, and implantable cardioverter–defibrillators (ICDs). The final section also reviews important selected topics from different perspectives (e.g., digitalis toxicity) to enhance their clinical dimensionality. Supplementary material for review and further exploration is available online (expertconsult. inkling.com).

## ECG SKILL DEVELOPMENT AND INCREASING DEMANDS FOR ECG LITERACY

Throughout, we seek to stress the clinical applications and implications of ECG interpretation. Each time an abnormal pattern is mentioned, a clinical correlate is introduced. Although the book is not intended to be a manual of therapeutics, general principles of treatment and clinical management are briefly discussed where relevant. Whenever possible, we have tried to put ourselves in the position of the clinician who has to look at ECGs without immediate specialist back-up and make critical decisions—sometimes at 3 a.m.!

In this spirit, we have tried to approach ECGs in terms of a rational, simple differential diagnosis based on pathophysiology, rather than through the tedium of rote memorization. It is reassuring to discover that the number of possible arrhythmias that can produce a heart rate of more than 200 beats per minute is limited to just a handful of choices. Only three basic ECG patterns are found during most cardiac arrests. Similarly, only a limited number of conditions cause low-voltage patterns, abnormally wide QRS complexes, ST segment elevations, and so forth.

## ADDRESSING "THREE AND A HALF" KEY CLINICAL QUESTIONS

In approaching any ECG, readers should get in the habit of posing "three and a half" essential queries: What does the ECG show and what else could it be? What are the possible causes of the waveform pattern or patterns? What, if anything, should be done about the finding(s)?

Most basic and intermediate-level ECG books focus on the first question ("What is it?"), emphasizing pattern recognition. However, waveform analysis is only a first step, for example, in the clinical diagnosis of atrial fibrillation. The following must always be addressed as part of the other half of the initial question: What is the differential diagnosis? ("What else could it be?") Are you sure that the ECG actually shows atrial fibrillation and not another "look-alike pattern," such as multifocal atrial tachycardia, sinus rhythm with premature atrial complexes, atrial flutter with variable block, or even an artifact, for example, resulting from Parkinsonian tremor?

"What could have caused the arrhythmia?" is the question framing the next set of considerations. Is the atrial fibrillation associated with valvular or nonvalvular disease? If nonvalvular, is the tachyarrhythmia related to hypertension, cardiomyopathy, coronary disease, advanced age, hyperthyroidism, and so forth? On a deeper level are issues concerning primary electrophysiologic mechanisms. With atrial fibrillation, these mechanisms are still being worked out and involve a complex interplay of factors, including abnormal pulmonary vein automaticity, micro-reentrant loops (wavelets) in the atria, inflammation and fibrosis, and autonomic perturbations.

Finally, deciding on treatment and follow-up ("What are the therapeutic options and what is best to do [if anything] in this case?") depends in an essential way on answers to the questions posed above, with the goal of delivering the highest level of scientifically informed, compassionate care.

## ADDITIONAL NOTES ON THE NINTH EDITION

With these clinical motivations in mind, the continuing aim of this book is to present the contemporary ECG as it is used in hospital wards, office settings, outpatient clinics, emergency departments, intensive/cardiac (coronary) care units, and telemedicine, where recognition of normal and abnormal patterns is only the starting point in patient care.

This ninth edition contains updated discussions of multiple topics, including intraventricular and atrioventricular (AV) conduction disturbances, sudden cardiac arrest, myocardial ischemia and infarction, takotsubo cardiomyopathy, drug toxicities, and electronic pacemakers and ICDs. Differential diagnoses are highlighted, as are pearls and pitfalls in ECG interpretation. Familiarity with the limitations as well as the uses of the ECG is essential for novices and more seasoned clinicians. Reducing medical errors related to ECGs and maximizing the information content of these recordings are major themes.

We have also tried in this latest edition to give special emphasis to common points of confusion. Medical terminology (jargon) in general is often puzzling and filled with ambiguities. Students of electrocardiography face a barrage of challenges. Why do we call the P–QRS interval the PR interval? What is the difference between ischemia and injury? What is meant by the term "paroxysmal supraventricular tachycardia (PSVT)" and how does it differ (if it does) from "supraventricular tachycardia"? Is "complete AV heart block" synonymous with "AV dissociation"?

Finally, for this edition the supplementary online material has been updated and expanded, with the inclusion of animations designed to capture key aspects of ECG dynamics under normal and pathologic conditions.

I am delighted that the two co-authors of the previous edition, Zachary D. Goldberger, MD, and Alexei Shvilkin, MD, PhD, have continued in this role for this new edition. We thank our students and colleagues for their challenging questions, and express special gratitude to our families for their inspiration and encouragement.

This edition again honors the memory of two remarkable individuals: the late Emanuel Goldberger, MD, a pioneer in the development of electrocardiography and the inventor of the aVR, aVL, and aVF leads, who was co-author of the first five editions of this textbook, and the late Blanche Goldberger, an extraordinary artist and woman of valor.

*Ary L. Goldberger, MD*

# PART I

# Basic Principles and Patterns

# CHAPTER 1

# Essential Concepts: What Is an ECG?

The *electrocardiogram* (*ECG* or *EKG*) is a special type of graph that represents cardiac electrical activity from one instant to the next. Specifically, the ECG provides a *time-voltage chart* of the heartbeat. The ECG is a key component of clinical diagnosis and management of inpatients and outpatients because it may provide critical information. Therefore, a major focus of this book is on recognizing and understanding the "signature" ECG findings in life-threatening conditions such as acute myocardial ischemia and infarction, severe hyperkalemia or hypokalemia, hypothermia, certain types of drug toxicity that may induce cardiac arrest, pericardial (cardiac) tamponade, among many others.

The general study of ECGs, including its clinical applications, technologic aspects, and basic science underpinnings, comprises the field of electrocardiography. The device used to obtain and display the conventional (12-lead) ECG is called the *electrocardiograph*, or more informally, the *ECG machine*. It records cardiac electrical currents (voltages or potentials) by means of sensors, called *electrodes*, selectively positioned on the surface of the body.[a] Students and clinicians are often understandably confused by the basic terminology that labels the graphical recording as the electrocardio*gram* and the recording device as the electrocardio*graph*! We will point out other potentially confusing ECG semantics as we go along.

Contemporary ECGs are usually recorded with disposable paste-on (adhesive) silver–silver chloride electrodes. For the standard ECG recording, electrodes are placed on the lower arms, lower legs, and across the chest wall (precordium). In settings such as emergency departments, cardiac and intensive care units (CCUs and ICUs), and ambulatory (e.g., Holter) monitoring, only one or two "rhythm strip"

leads may be recorded, usually by means of a few chest and abdominal electrodes.

## ABCs OF CARDIAC ELECTROPHYSIOLOGY

Before the basic ECG patterns are discussed, we review a few simple-to-grasp but fundamental principles of the heart's electrical properties.

The central function of the heart is to contract rhythmically and pump blood to the lungs (pulmonary circulation) for oxygenation and then to pump this oxygen-enriched blood into the general (systemic) circulation. Furthermore, the amount of blood pumped has to be matched to meet the body's varying metabolic needs. The heart muscle and other tissues require more oxygen and nutrients when we are active compared to when we rest. An important part of these *auto-regulatory* adjustments is accomplished by changes in heart rate, which, as described below, are primarily under the control of the autonomic (involuntary) nervous system.

The signal for cardiac contraction is the spread of synchronized electrical currents through the heart muscle. These currents are produced both by *pacemaker cells* and *specialized conduction tissue* within the heart and by the working *heart muscle* itself.

Pacemaker cells are like tiny clocks (technically called *oscillators*) that automatically generate electrical stimuli in a repetitive fashion. The other heart cells, both specialized conduction tissue and working heart muscle, function like cables that transmit these electrical signals.[b]

## Electrical Signaling in the Heart

In simplest terms, therefore, the heart can be thought of as an electrically timed pump. The electrical

---

Please go to expertconsult.inkling.com for additional online material for this chapter.

[a]As discussed in Chapter 3, more precisely the ECG "leads" record the *differences* in potential between pairs or configurations of electrodes.

[b]Heart muscle cells of all types possess another important property called *refractoriness*. This term refers to fact that for a short term after they emit a stimulus or are stimulated (depolarize), the cells cannot immediately discharge again because they need to repolarize.

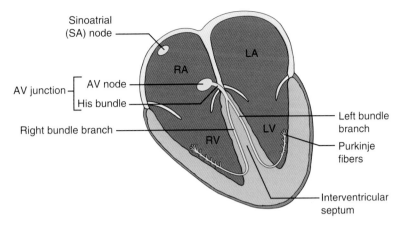

**Fig. 1.1** Normally, the cardiac stimulus (electrical signal) is generated in an automatic way by pacemaker cells in the *sinoatrial (SA)*
*node*, located in the high *right atrium (RA)*. The stimulus then spreads through the *RA* and *left atrium (LA)*. Next, it traverses the
*atrioventricular (AV)* node and the *bundle of His*, which comprise the *AV junction*. The stimulus then sweeps into the *left* and *right ventricles*
*(LV* and *RV)* by way of the *left* and *right bundle branches*, which are continuations of the *bundle of His*. The cardiac stimulus spreads
rapidly and simultaneously to the left and right ventricular muscle cells through the *Purkinje fibers*. Electrical activation of the atria
and ventricles, respectively, leads to sequential contraction of these chambers (*electromechanical coupling*).

"wiring" of this remarkable organ is outlined in
Fig. 1.1.

Normally, the signal for heartbeat initiation starts
in the pacemaker cells of the *sinus* or *sinoatrial (SA)*
*node*. This node is located in the right atrium near
the opening of the superior vena cava. The SA node
is a small, oval collection (about $2 \times 1$ cm) of specialized cells capable of automatically generating an
electrical stimulus (spark-like signal) and functions
as the normal *pacemaker* of the heart. From the sinus
node, this stimulus spreads first through the right
atrium and then into the left atrium.

Electrical stimulation of the right and left atria
signals the atria to contract and pump blood
simultaneously through the tricuspid and mitral
valves into the right and left ventricles, respectively.
The electrical stimulus then spreads through the
atria and part of this activation wave reaches specialized conduction tissues in the *atrioventricular (AV)*
*junction*.[c]

The AV junction, which acts as an electrical "relay"
connecting the atria and ventricles, is located near
the lower part of the *interatrial* septum and extends
into the *interventricular* septum (see Fig. 1.1).[d]

The upper (proximal) part of the AV junction is
the AV node. (In some texts, the terms *AV node* and
*AV junction* are used synonymously.)

The lower (distal) part of the AV junction is called
the *bundle of His*. The bundle of His then divides
into two main branches: the right bundle branch,
which distributes the stimulus to the right ventricle,
and the left bundle branch,[e] which distributes the
stimulus to the left ventricle (see Fig. 1.1).

The electrical signal spreads rapidly and simultaneously down the left and right bundle branches
into the *ventricular myocardium* (ventricular muscle)
by way of specialized conducting cells called *Purkinje*
*fibers* located in the subendocardial layer (roughly
the inside half or rim) of the ventricles. From the
final branches of the Purkinje fibers, the electrical
signal spreads through myocardial muscle toward
the epicardium (outer rim).

---

[c]Atrial stimulation is usually modeled as an advancing (radial) wave of
  excitation originating in the sinoatrial (SA) node, like the ripples
  induced by a stone dropped in a pond. The spread of activation
  waves between the SA and AV nodes may also be facilitated by
  so-called internodal "tracts." However, the anatomy and
  electrophysiology of these preferential internodal pathways, which
  are analogized as functioning a bit like "fast lanes" on the atrial
  conduction highways, remain subjects of investigation and
  controversy among experts, and do not directly impact clinical
  assessment.

[d]Note the potential confusion in terms. The muscular wall separating
  the ventricles is the *inter*ventricular septum, while a similar
  term—*intra*ventricular conduction delays (IVCDs)—is used to
  describe bundle branch blocks and related disturbances in electrical
  signaling in the ventricles, as introduced in Chapter 8.

[e]The left bundle branch has two major subdivisions called *fascicles*.
  (These conduction tracts are also discussed in Chapter 8, along
  with abnormalities called fascicular blocks or hemiblocks.)

The bundle of His, its branches, and their subdivisions collectively constitute the *His–Purkinje system*. Normally, the AV node and His–Purkinje system provide the only electrical connection between the atria and the ventricles, unless an abnormal structure called a *bypass tract* is present. This abnormality and its consequences are described in Chapter 18 on Wolff-Parkinson-White preexcitation patterns.

In contrast, impairment of conduction over these bridging structures underlies various types of AV heart block (Chapter 17). In its most severe form, electrical conduction (signaling) between atria and ventricles is completely severed, leading to third-degree (complete) heart block. The result is usually a very slow escape rhythm, leading to weakness, light-headedness or fainting, and even sudden cardiac arrest and sudden death (Chapter 21).

Just as the spread of electrical stimuli through the atria leads to atrial contraction, so the spread of stimuli through the ventricles leads to ventricular contraction, with pumping of blood to the lungs and into the general circulation.

The initiation of cardiac contraction by electrical stimulation is referred to as *electromechanical coupling*. A key part of the contractile mechanism involves the release of calcium ions inside the atrial and ventricular heart muscle cells, which is triggered by the spread of electrical activation. The calcium ion release process links electrical and mechanical function (see Bibliography).

The ECG is capable of recording only relatively large currents produced by the mass of working (pumping) heart muscle. The much smaller amplitude signals generated by the sinus node and AV node are invisible with clinical recordings generated by the surface ECG. Depolarization of the His bundle area can only be recorded from inside the heart during specialized cardiac *electrophysiologic* (EP) *studies*.

## CARDIAC AUTOMATICITY AND CONDUCTIVITY: "CLOCKS AND CABLES"

*Automaticity* refers to the capacity of certain cardiac cells to function as *pacemakers* by spontaneously generating electrical impulses, like tiny clocks. As mentioned earlier, the sinus node normally is the primary (dominant) pacemaker of the heart because of its inherent automaticity.

Under special conditions, however, other cells outside the sinus node (in the atria, AV junction, or ventricles) can also act as independent (secondary/ subsidiary) pacemakers. For example, if sinus node automaticity is depressed, the AV junction can act as a backup (escape) pacemaker. Escape rhythms generated by subsidiary pacemakers provide important physiologic redundancy (safety mechanisms) in the vital function of heartbeat generation, as described in Chapter 13.

Normally, the relatively more rapid intrinsic rate of SA node firing suppresses the automaticity of these secondary (*ectopic*) pacemakers outside the sinus node. However, sometimes, their automaticity may be abnormally increased, resulting in competition with, and even usurping the sinus node for control of, the heartbeat. For example, a rapid run of ectopic atrial beats results in *atrial tachycardia* (Chapter 14). Abnormal atrial automaticity is of central importance in the initiation of atrial fibrillation (Chapter 15). A rapid run of ectopic ventricular beats results in ventricular tachycardia (Chapter 16), a potentially life-threatening arrhythmia, which may lead to ventricular fibrillation and cardiac arrest (Chapter 21).

In addition to *automaticity*, the other major electrical property of the heart is *conductivity*. The speed with which electrical impulses are conducted through different parts of the heart varies. The conduction is *fastest* through the Purkinje fibers and *slowest* through the AV node. The relatively slow conduction speed through the AV node allows the ventricles time to fill with blood before the signal for cardiac contraction arrives. Rapid conduction through the His–Purkinje system ensures synchronous contraction of both ventricles.

The more you understand about normal physiologic stimulation of the heart, the stronger your basis for comprehending the abnormalities of heart rhythm and conduction and their distinctive ECG patterns. For example, failure of the sinus node to effectively stimulate the atria can occur because of a failure of SA automaticity or because of local conduction block that prevents the stimulus from exiting the sinus node (Chapter 13). Either pathophysiologic mechanism can result in apparent *sinus node dysfunction* and sometimes *symptomatic sick sinus syndrome* (Chapter 19). Patients may experience lightheadedness or even syncope (fainting) because of marked *bradycardia* (slow heartbeat).

In contrast, abnormal conduction within the heart can lead to various types of *tachycardia* due to *reentry*, a mechanism in which an impulse "chases its tail," short-circuiting the normal activation pathways. Reentry plays an important role in the genesis of certain paroxysmal supraventricular tachycardias (PSVTs), including those involving AV nodal *dual pathways* or an AV *bypass tract*, as well as in many variants of ventricular tachycardia (VT), as described in Part II.

As noted, blockage of the spread of stimuli through the AV node or infranodal pathways can produce various degrees of AV heart block (Chapter 17), sometimes with severe, symptomatic ventricular bradycardia or increased risk of these life-threatening complications, necessitating placement of a permanent (electronic) pacemaker (Chapter 22).

Disease of the bundle branches themselves can produce right or left bundle branch block. The latter especially is a cause of *electrical dyssynchrony*, an important contributing mechanism in many cases of heart failure (see Chapters 8 and 22).

## CONCLUDING NOTES: WHY IS THE ECG SO USEFUL?

The ECG is one of the most versatile and inexpensive clinical tests. Its utility derives from careful clinical and experimental studies over more than a century showing its essential role in:

- Diagnosing dangerous cardiac electrical disturbances causing brady- and tachyarrhythmias.
- Providing immediate information about clinically important problems, including myocardial ischemia/infarction, electrolyte disorders, and drug toxicity, as well as hypertrophy and other types of chamber overload.
- Providing clues that allow you to forecast preventable catastrophes. A major example is a very long QT(U) pattern, usually caused by a drug effect or by hypokalemia, which may herald sudden cardiac arrest due to *torsades de pointes*.

## PREVIEW: LOOKING AHEAD

The *first part* of this book is devoted to explaining the basis of the normal ECG and then examining the major conditions that cause abnormal depolarization (P and QRS) and repolarization (ST-T and U)

patterns. This alphabet of ECG terms is defined in Chapters 2 and 3.

---

### Some Reasons for the Importance of ECG "Literacy"

- Frontline medical caregivers are often required to make on-the-spot, critical decisions based on their ECG readings.
- Computer readings are often incomplete or incorrect.
- Accurate readings are essential to early diagnosis and therapy of acute coronary syndromes, including ST elevation myocardial infarction (STEMI).
- Insightful readings may also avert medical catastrophes and sudden cardiac arrest, such as those associated with the acquired long QT syndrome and torsades de pointes.
- Mistaken readings (false negatives and false positives) can have major consequences, both clinical and medico-legal (e.g., missed or mistaken diagnosis of atrial fibrillation).
- The requisite combination of attention to details and integration of these into the larger picture ("trees and forest" approach) provides a template for critical thinking essential to all of clinical practice.

---

The *second part* deals with abnormalities of cardiac rhythm generation and conduction that produce excessively fast or slow heart rates (tachycardias and bradycardias).

The *third part* provides both a review and further extension of material covered in earlier chapters, including an important focus on avoiding ECG errors.

Selected publications are cited in the Bibliography, including freely available online resources. In addition, the online supplement to this book provides extra material, including numerous case studies and practice questions with answers.

# CHAPTER 2
# ECG Basics: Waves, Intervals, and Segments

The first purpose of this chapter is to present two fundamental electrical properties of heart muscle cells: (1) depolarization (activation), and (2) repolarization (recovery). Second, in this chapter and the next we define and show how to measure the basic waveforms, segments, and intervals essential to ECG interpretation.

## DEPOLARIZATION AND REPOLARIZATION

In Chapter 1, the term *electrical activation (stimulation)* was applied to the spread of electrical signals through the atria and ventricles. The more technical term for the cardiac activation process is *depolarization.* The return of heart muscle cells to their resting state following depolarization is called *repolarization.*

These key terms are derived from the fact that normal "resting" myocardial cells are *polarized;* that is, they carry electrical charges on their surface. Fig. 2.1A shows the resting polarized state of a normal atrial or ventricular heart muscle cell. Notice that the outside of the resting cell is positive and the inside is negative (about −90 mV [millivolt] gradient between them).[a]

When a heart muscle cell (or group of cells) is stimulated, it depolarizes. As a result, the outside of the cell, in the area where the stimulation has occurred, becomes negatively charged and the inside of the cell becomes positive. This produces a difference in electrical voltage on the outside surface of the cell between the stimulated depolarized area and the unstimulated polarized area (Fig. 2.1B). Consequently, a small electrical current is formed

that spreads along the length of the cell as stimulation and depolarization occur until the entire cell is depolarized (Fig. 2.1C). The path of depolarization can be represented by an arrow, as shown in Fig. 2.1B.

*Note:* For individual myocardial cells (fibers), depolarization and repolarization proceed in the same direction. However, for the entire myocardium, depolarization normally proceeds from innermost layer (endocardium) to outermost layer (epicardium), whereas repolarization proceeds in the opposite direction. The exact mechanisms of this well-established asymmetry are not fully understood.

The depolarizing electrical current is recorded by the ECG as a *P wave* (when the atria are stimulated and depolarize) and as a *QRS complex* (when the ventricles are stimulated and depolarize).

Repolarization starts when the fully stimulated and depolarized cell begins to return to the resting state. A small area on the outside of the cell becomes positive again (Fig. 2.1D), and the repolarization spreads along the length of the cell until the entire cell is once again fully repolarized. Ventricular repolarization is recorded by the ECG as the *ST segment, T wave,* and *U wave.*

In summary, whether the ECG is normal or abnormal, it records just two basic events: (1) depolarization, the spread of a stimulus (stimuli) through the heart muscle, and (2) repolarization, the return of the stimulated heart muscle to the resting state. The basic cellular processes of depolarization and repolarization are responsible for the *waveforms, segments,* and *intervals* seen on the body surface (standard) ECG.

## FIVE BASIC ECG WAVEFORMS: P, QRS, ST, T, AND U

The ECG records the electrical activity of a myriad of atrial and ventricular cells, not just that of single fibers. The sequential and organized spread of stimuli through the atria and ventricles followed by their

---

Please go to expertconsult.inkling.com for additional online material for this chapter.

[a]Membrane polarization is due to differences in the concentration of ions inside and outside the cell. A brief review of this important topic is presented in the online material and also see the Bibliography for references that present the basic electrophysiology of the *resting membrane potential* and *cellular depolarization* and *repolarization* (the action potential) underlying the ECG waves recorded on the body surface.

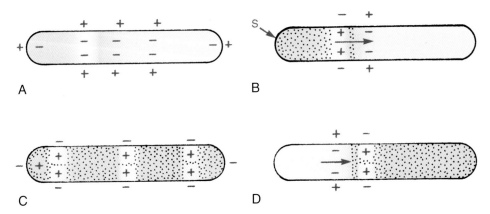

**Fig. 2.1** Depolarization and repolarization. (A) The resting heart muscle cell is polarized; that is, it carries an electrical charge, with the outside of the cell positively charged and the inside negatively charged. (B) When the cell is stimulated (*S*), it begins to depolarize (*stippled area*). (C) The fully depolarized cell is positively charged on the inside and negatively charged on the outside. (D) Repolarization occurs when the stimulated cell returns to the resting state. The directions of depolarization and repolarization are represented by arrows. Depolarization (stimulation) of the atria produces the P wave on the ECG, whereas depolarization of the ventricles produces the QRS complex. Repolarization of the ventricles produces the ST-T complex.

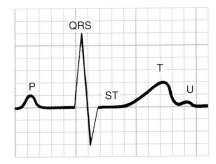

**Fig. 2.2** The P wave represents atrial depolarization. The PR interval is the time from initial stimulation of the atria to initial stimulation of the ventricles. The QRS complex represents ventricular depolarization. The ST segment, T wave, and U wave are produced by ventricular repolarization.

The P wave represents the spread of a stimulus through the atria (atrial depolarization). The QRS waveform, or *complex*, represents stimulus spread through the ventricles (ventricular depolarization). As the name implies, the QRS set of deflections (complex) includes one or more specific waves, labeled as Q, R, and S. The ST (considered both a waveform and a segment) and T wave (or grouped as the "ST-T" waveform) represent the return of stimulated ventricular muscle to the resting state (ventricular repolarization). Furthermore, the very beginning of the ST segment (where it meets the QRS complex) is called the J point. The U wave is a small deflection sometimes seen just after the T wave. It represents the final phase of ventricular repolarization, although its exact mechanism is not known.

You may be wondering why none of the listed waves or complexes represents the return of the stimulated (depolarized) atria to their resting state. The answer is that the atrial ST segment (STa) and atrial T wave (Ta) are generally not observed on the routine ECG because of their low amplitudes. An important exception is described in Chapter 12 with reference to acute pericarditis, which often causes subtle, but important deviations of the PR segment.

Similarly, the routine body surface ECG is not sensitive enough to record any electrical activity during the spread of stimuli through the atrioventricular

return to the resting state produces the electrical currents recorded on the ECG. Furthermore, each phase of cardiac electrical activity produces a specific wave or deflection. QRS waveforms are referred to as complexes (Fig. 2.2). The *five* basic ECG waveforms, labeled alphabetically, are the:

P wave – atrial depolarization
QRS complex – ventricular depolarization
ST segment ⎫
T wave     ⎬ ventricular repolarization
U wave     ⎭

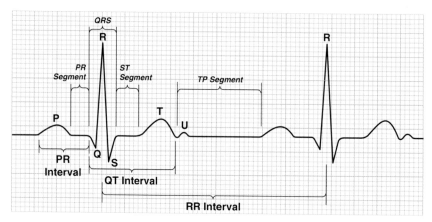

**Fig. 2.3** Summary of major components of the ECG graph. These can be grouped into 5 waveforms (P, QRS, ST, T, and U), 4 intervals (RR, PR, QRS, and QT) and 3 segments (PR, ST, and TP). Note that the ST can be considered as both a waveform and a segment. The RR interval is the same as the QRS–QRS interval. The TP segment is used as the isoelectric baseline, against which deviations in the PR segment (e.g., in acute pericarditis) and ST segment (e.g., in ischemia) are measured.

(AV) junction (AV node and bundle of His) en route to the ventricular myocardium. This key series of events, which appears on the surface ECG as a straight line, is actually not electrically "silent," but reflects the spread of electrical stimuli through the AV junction and the His–Purkinje system, just preceding the QRS complex.

In summary, the P/QRS/ST-T/U sequence represents the cycle of the electrical activity of the normal heartbeat. This physiologic signaling process begins with the spread of a stimulus through the atria (P wave), initiated by sinus node depolarization, and ends with the return of stimulated ventricular muscle to its resting state (ST-T and U waves). As shown in Fig. 2.3, the basic cardiac cycle repeats itself again and again, maintaining the rhythmic pulse of life.

## ECG SEGMENTS VS. ECG INTERVALS

ECG interpretation also requires careful assessment of the time within and between various waveforms. *Segments* are defined as the portions of the ECG bracketed by the end of one waveform and the beginning of another. *Intervals* are the portions of the ECG that include at least one entire waveform.

There are three basic segments:

1. *PR segment*: end of the P wave to beginning of the QRS complex. Atrial repolarization begins in this segment. (Atrial repolarization continues during the QRS and ends during the ST segment.)

2. *ST segment*: end of the QRS complex to beginning of the following T wave. As noted above, the ST-T complex represents ventricular repolarization. The segment is also considered as a separate waveform, as noted above. ST elevation and/or depression are major signs of ischemia, as discussed in Chapters 9 and 10.

3. *TP segment*: end of the T wave to beginning of the P wave. This interval, which represents the electrical resting state, is important because it is traditionally used as the *baseline reference* from which to assess PR and ST deviations in conditions such as acute pericarditis and acute myocardial ischemia, respectively.

In addition to these segments, *four sets of intervals* are routinely measured: PR, QRS, QT/QTc, and PP/RR.[b] The latter set (PP/RR) represents the inverse of the ventricular/atrial heart rate(s), as discussed in Chapter 3.

1. The *PR interval* is measured from the beginning of the P wave to the beginning of the QRS complex.

---

[b]The peak of the R wave is often selected. But students should be aware that any consistent points on sequential QRS complexes may be used to obtain the "RR" interval, even S waves or QS waves. Similarly, the PP interval is also measured from the same location on one P wave to that on the next. This interval gives the atrial rate. Normally, the PP interval is the same as the RR interval (see below), especially in "normal sinus rhythm." Strictly speaking, the PP interval is actually the atrial-atrial (AA) interval, since in two major arrhythmias—atrial flutter and atrial fibrillation (Chapter 15)—continuous atrial activity, rather than discrete P waves, are seen.

2. The *QRS interval* (duration) is measured from the beginning to the end of the same QRS.
3. The *QT interval* is measured from the beginning of the QRS to the end of the T wave. When this interval is corrected (adjusted for the heart rate), the designation *QTc* is used, as described in Chapter 3.
4. The *RR (QRS–QRS) interval* is measured from one point (sometimes called the *R-point*) on a given QRS complex to the corresponding point on the next. The instantaneous heart rate (beats per min)

= 60/RR interval when the RR is measured in seconds (sec). Normally, the PP interval is the same as the RR interval, especially in "normal sinus rhythm." We will discuss major arrhythmias where the PP is different from the RR, e.g., sinus rhythm with complete heart block (Chapter 17).[c]

---

[c]You may be wondering why the QRS–QRS interval is not measured from the very beginning of one QRS complex to the beginning of the next. For convenience, the peak of the R wave (or nadir of an S or QS wave) is usually used. The results are equivalent and the term RR interval is most widely used to designate this interval.

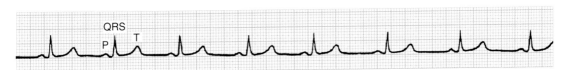

**Fig. 2.4** The basic cardiac cycle (P–QRS–T) normally repeats itself again and again.

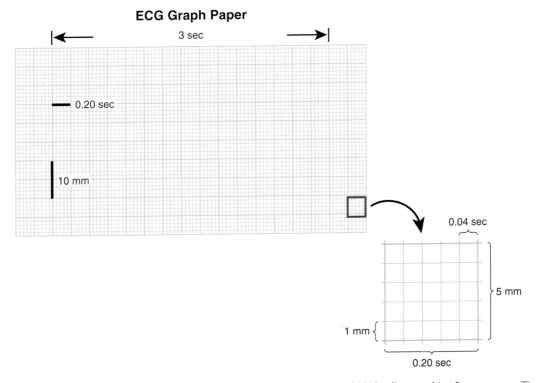

**Fig. 2.5** The ECG is recorded on graph paper divided into millimeter squares, with darker lines marking 5-mm squares. Time is measured on the horizontal (X) axis. With a paper speed of 25 mm/sec, each small (1-mm) box side equals 0.04 sec and each larger (5-mm) box side equals 0.2 sec. A 3-sec interval is denoted. The amplitude of a deflection or wave is measured in millimeters on the vertical (Y) axis.

### 5-4-3 Rule for ECG Components

To summarize, the clinical ECG graph comprises waveforms, intervals, and segments designated as follows:

5 waveforms (P, QRS, ST, T, and U)
4 sets of intervals (PR, QRS, QT/QTc, and RR/PP)
3 segments (PR, ST, and TP)

Two brief notes to avoid possible semantic confusion: (1) The ST is considered both a waveform and a segment. (2) Technically, the duration of the P wave is also an interval.

However, to avoid confusion with the PR, the interval subtending the P wave is usually referred to as the P wave *width* or *duration*, rather than the P wave interval. The P duration (interval) is also measured in units of msec or sec and is most important in the diagnosis of left atrial abnormality (Chapter 7).

The major components of the ECG are summarized in Fig. 2.3.

### ECG GRAPH PAPER

The P–QRS–T sequence is recorded on special ECG graph paper that is divided into grid-like boxes (Figs. 2.4 and 2.5). Each of the small boxes is 1 millimeter square (1 mm$^2$). The standard recording rate is equivalent to 25 mm/sec (unless otherwise specified). Therefore, horizontally, each unit represents 0.04 sec (25 mm/sec × 0.04 sec = 1 mm). Notice that the lines between every five boxes are thicker, so that each 5-mm unit horizontally corresponds to 0.2 sec (5 × 0.04 sec = 0.2 sec). All of the ECGs in this book have been calibrated using these specifications, unless otherwise indicated.

A remarkable (and sometimes taken for granted) aspect of ECG analysis is that these recordings allow you to measure events occurring over time spans as short as 40 msec or less in order to make decisions critical to patients' care. A good example is an ECG showing a QRS interval of 100 msec, which is normal, versus one with a QRS interval of 140 msec, which is markedly prolonged and might be a major clue to bundle branch block (Chapter 8), hyperkalemia (Chapter 11) or ventricular tachycardia (Chapter 16).

We continue our discussion of ECG basics in the following chapter, focusing on how to make key measurements based on ECG intervals and what their normal ranges are in adults.

# CHAPTER 3
# How to Make Basic ECG Measurements

This chapter continues the discussion of ECG basics introduced in Chapters 1 and 2. Here we focus on recognizing components of the ECG in order to make clinically important measurements from these time–voltage graphical recordings.

## STANDARDIZATION (CALIBRATION) MARK

The electrocardiograph is generally calibrated such that a 1-mV signal produces a 10-mm deflection. Modern units are electronically calibrated; older ones may have a manual calibration setting.

### ECG as a Dynamic Heart Graph

> The ECG is a real-time graph of the heartbeat. The small ticks on the horizontal axis correspond to intervals of 40 ms. The vertical axis corresponds to the magnitude (voltage) of the waves/deflections (10 mm = 1 mV)

As shown in Fig. 3.1, the standardization mark produced when the machine is routinely calibrated is a square (or rectangular) wave 10 mm tall, usually displayed at the left side of each row of the electrocardiogram. If the machine is not standardized in the expected way, the 1-mV signal produces a deflection either more or less than 10 mm and the amplitudes of the P, QRS, and T deflections will be larger or smaller than they should be.

The standardization deflection is also important because it can be varied in most electrocardiographs (see Fig. 3.1). When very large deflections are present (as occurs, for example, in some patients who have an electronic pacemaker that produces very large stimuli ["spikes"] or who have high QRS voltage

caused by hypertrophy), there may be considerable overlap between the deflections on one lead with those one above or below it. When this occurs, it may be advisable to repeat the ECG at one-half standardization to get the entire tracing on the paper. If the ECG complexes are very small, it may be advisable to double the standardization (e.g., to study a small Q wave more thoroughly, or augment a subtle pacing spike). Some electronic electrocardiographs do not display the calibration pulse. Instead, they print the paper speed and standardization at the bottom of the ECG paper ("25 mm/sec, 10 mm/mV").

Because the ECG is calibrated, any part of the P, QRS, and T deflections can be precisely described in two ways; that is, both the amplitude (voltage) and the width (duration) of a deflection can be measured. For clinical purposes, if the standardization is set at 1 mV = 10 mm, the height of a wave is usually recorded in millimeters, not millivolts. In Fig. 3.2, for example, the P wave is 1 mm in amplitude, the QRS complex is 8 mm, and the T wave is about 3.5 mm.

A wave or deflection is also described as positive or negative. By convention, an *upward* deflection or wave is called *positive*. A *downward* deflection or wave is called *negative*. A deflection or wave that rests on the baseline is said to be *isoelectric*. A deflection that is partly positive and partly negative is called *biphasic*. For example, in Fig. 3.2 the P wave is positive, the QRS complex is biphasic (initially positive, then negative), the ST segment is isoelectric (flat on the baseline), and the T wave is negative.

We now describe in more detail the ECG alphabet of P, QRS, ST, T, and U waves. The measurements of PR interval, QRS interval (width or duration), and QT/QTc intervals and RR/PP intervals are also described, with their physiologic (normative) values in adults.

Please go to expertconsult.inkling.com for additional online material for this chapter.

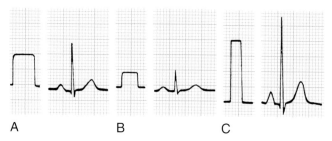

**Fig. 3.1** Before taking an ECG, the operator must check to see that the machine is properly calibrated, so that the 1-mV standardization mark is 10 mm tall. (A) Electrocardiograph set at normal standardization. (B) One-half standardization. (C) Two times normal standardization.

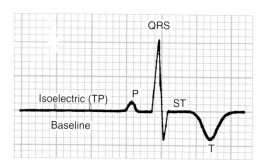

**Fig. 3.2** The P wave is positive (upward), and the T wave is negative (downward). The QRS complex is biphasic (partly positive, partly negative), and the ST segment is isoelectric (neither positive nor negative).

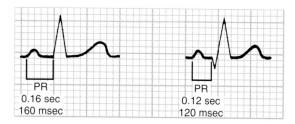

**Fig. 3.3** Measurement of the PR interval (see text).

## COMPONENTS OF THE ECG

### P Wave and PR Interval

The P wave, which represents atrial depolarization, is a small positive (or negative) deflection before the QRS complex. The normal values for P wave axis, amplitude, and width are described in Chapter 7. The PR interval is measured from the beginning of the P wave to the beginning of the QRS complex (Fig. 3.3). The PR interval may vary slightly in different leads, and the shortest PR interval should be noted when measured by hand. The PR interval represents the time it takes for the stimulus to spread through the atria and pass through the AV junction. (This physiologic delay allows the ventricles to fill fully with blood before ventricular depolarization occurs, to optimize cardiac output.) *In adults the normal PR interval is between 0.12 and 0.2 sec* (three to five small box sides). When conduction through the AV junction is impaired, the PR interval may become prolonged. As noted, prolongation of the PR interval above 0.2 sec is called *first-degree heart block (delay)* (see Chapter 17). With sinus tachycardia, AV conduction may be facilitated by increased sympathetic and decreased vagal tone modulation. Accordingly, the PR may be relatively short, e.g., about 0.10–0.12 sec, as a physiologic finding, in the absence of Wolff–Parkinson–White (WPW) preexcitation (see Chapter 18).

### QRS Complex

The QRS complex represents the spread of a stimulus through the ventricles. However, not every QRS complex contains a Q wave, an R wave, and an S wave—hence the possibility of confusion. The slightly awkward (and arbitrary) nomenclature becomes understandable if you remember three basic naming rules for the components of the QRS complex in any lead (Fig. 3.4):

1. When the initial deflection of the QRS complex is negative (below the baseline), it is called a *Q wave.*
2. The first positive deflection in the QRS complex is called an *R wave.*
3. A negative deflection following the R wave is called an *S wave.*

## How to Name the QRS Complex

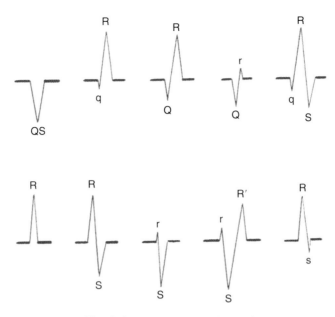

**Fig. 3.4** QRS nomenclature (see text).

Thus the following QRS complex contains a Q wave, an R wave, and an S wave:

In contrast, the following complex does not contain three waves:

If, as shown earlier, the entire QRS complex is positive, it is simply called an *R wave*. However, if the entire complex is negative, it is termed a *QS wave* (not just a Q wave as you might expect).

Occasionally the QRS complex contains more than two or three deflections. In such cases the extra waves are called *R'* (R prime) *waves* if they are positive and *S'* (S prime) *waves* if they are negative.

Fig. 3.4 shows the major possible QRS complexes and the nomenclature of the respective waves. Notice that capital letters (*QRS*) are used to designate waves

of relatively large amplitude and small letters (*qrs*) label relatively small waves. (However, no exact thresholds have been developed to say when an *s* wave qualifies as an *S* wave, for example.)

The QRS naming system does seem confusing at first. But it allows you to describe any QRS complex and evoke in the mind of the trained listener an exact mental picture of the complex named. For example, in describing an ECG you might say that lead $V_1$ showed an rS complex ("small r, capital S"):

or a QS ("capital Q, capital S"):

### QRS Interval (Width or Duration)

The QRS interval represents the time required for a stimulus to spread through the ventricles (ventricular depolarization) and is normally about

### QRS Interval

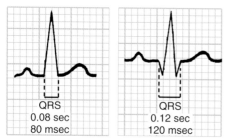

Fig. 3.5 Measurement of the QRS width (interval) (see text).

### J Point, ST Segment, and T Wave

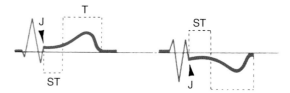

**Fig. 3.6** Characteristics of the normal ST segment and T wave. The junction (J) is the beginning of the ST segment.

≤0.10 sec (or ≤0.11 sec when measured by computer) (Fig. 3.5).[a] If the spread of a stimulus through the ventricles is slowed, for example by a block in one of the bundle branches, the QRS width will be prolonged. The differential diagnosis of a wide QRS complex is discussed in Chapters 18, 19 and 25.[b]

## ST Segment

The ST segment is that portion of the ECG cycle from the end of the QRS complex to the beginning of the T wave (Fig. 3.6). It represents the earliest phase of ventricular repolarization. The normal ST segment is usually *isoelectric* (i.e., flat on the baseline, neither positive nor negative), but it may be slightly

### ST Segments

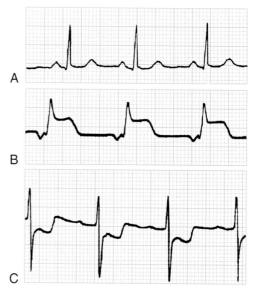

**Fig. 3.7** ST segments. (A) Normal. (B) Abnormal elevation. (C) Abnormal depression.

---

[a]You may have already noted that the QRS amplitude (height or depth) often varies slightly from one beat to the next. This variation may be due to a number of factors. One is related to breathing mechanics: as you inspire, your heart rate speeds up due to decreased cardiac vagal tone (Chapter 13) and decreases with expiration (due to increased vagal tone). Breathing may also change the QRS axis slightly due to changes in heart position and in chest impedance, which change QRS amplitude slightly. If the rhythm strip is long enough, you may even be able to estimate the patient's breathing rate. QRS changes may also occur to slight alterations in ventricular activation, as with atrial flutter and fibrillation with a rapid ventricular response (Chapter 15). Beat-to-beat QRS alternans with sinus tachycardia is a specific but not sensitive marker of pericardial effusion with tamponade pathophysiology, due to the *swinging heart phenomenon* (see Chapter 12). Beat-to-beat alternation of the QRS is also seen with certain types of paroxysmal supraventricular tachycardias (PSVTs; see Chapter 14).

[b]A subinterval of the QRS, termed the *intrinsicoid* deflection, is defined as the time between the onset of the QRS (usually in a left lateral chest lead) to the peak of the R wave in that lead. A preferred term is *R-peak time*. This interval is intended to estimate the time for the impulse to go from the endocardium of the left ventricle to the epicardium. The upper limit of normal is usually given as 0.04 sec (40 msec); with increased values seen with left ventricular hypertrophy (>0.05 sec) and left bundle branch block (>0.06 sec). However, this microinterval is hard to measure accurately and reproducibly on conventional ECGs. Therefore, it has had very limited utility in clinical practice.

elevated or depressed normally (usually by less than 1 mm). Pathologic conditions, such as myocardial infarction (MI), that produce characteristic abnormal deviations of the ST segment (see Chapters 9 and 10), are a major focus of clinical ECG diagnosis.

The very beginning of the ST segment (actually the junction between the end of the QRS complex and the beginning of the ST segment) is called the *J point*. Fig. 3.6 shows the J point and the normal shapes of the ST segment. Fig. 3.7 compares a normal isoelectric ST segment with abnormal ST segment elevation and depression.

The terms *J point elevation* and *J point depression* often cause confusion among trainees, who mistakenly think that these terms denote a specific condition. However, these terms do not indicate defined abnormalities but are only descriptive. For example, isolated J point elevation may occur as a normal variant with the *early repolarization pattern* (see Chapter 10) or as a marker of *systemic hypothermia* (where they are called Osborn or J waves; see Chapter 11). J point elevation may also be part of ST elevations with acute pericarditis, acute myocardial ischemia, left bundle branch block or left ventricular hypertrophy (leads $V_1$ to $V_3$ usually), and so forth. Similarly, J point depression may occur in a variety of contexts, both physiologic and pathologic, as discussed in subsequent chapters and summarized in Chapter 25.

### T Wave

The T wave represents the mid-latter part of ventricular repolarization. A normal T wave has an asymmetrical shape; that is, its peak is closer to the end of the wave than to the beginning (see Fig. 3.6). When the T wave is positive, it normally rises slowly and then abruptly returns to the baseline. When it is negative, it descends slowly and abruptly rises to the baseline. The *asymmetry* of the normal T wave contrasts with the symmetry of abnormal T waves in certain conditions, such as MI (see Chapters 9 and 10) and a high serum potassium level (see Chapter 11). The exact point at which the ST segment ends and the T wave begins is somewhat arbitrary and usually impossible to pinpoint precisely. However, for clinical purposes accuracy within 40 msec (0.04 sec) is usually acceptable.

### QT/QTc Intervals

The QT interval is measured from the beginning of the QRS complex to the end of the T wave (Fig. 3.8). It primarily represents the return of stimulated ventricles to their resting state (ventricular repolarization). The normal values for the QT interval depend on the heart rate. As the heart rate increases (RR interval shortens), the QT interval normally shortens; as the heart rate decreases (RR interval lengthens), the QT interval lengthens. The RR interval, as described later, is the interval between consecutive QRS complexes. (The rate-related shortening of the QT, itself, is a complex process involving direct effects of heart rate on action potential duration and of neuroautonomic factors.)

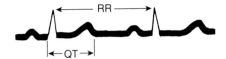

Fig. **3.8** Measurement of the QT interval. The RR interval is the interval between two consecutive QRS complexes (see text).

| TABLE 3.1 | QT Interval (Uncorrected): *Approximate* Upper Limits of Normal* | |
|---|---|---|
| **Measured RR Interval (sec)** | **Heart Rate (beats/min)** | **QT Interval Upper Normal Limit (sec)** |
| 1.20 | 50 | 0.48 |
| 1.00 | 60 | 0.44 |
| 0.86 | 70 | 0.40 |
| 0.80 | 75 | 0.38 |
| 0.75 | 80 | 0.37 |
| 0.67 | 90 | 0.35 |
| 0.60 | 100 | 0.34 |
| 0.50 | 120 | 0.31 |

*See text for two methods of computing a rate-corrected QT interval, denoted as QTc.

The QT should generally be measured in the ECG lead (or leads) showing the longest intervals. A common mistake is to limit this measurement to lead II. You can measure several intervals and use the average value. When the QT interval is long, it is often difficult to measure because the end of the T wave may merge imperceptibly with the U wave. As a result, you may be measuring the QU interval, rather than the QT interval. When reporting the QT (or related QTc) it might be helpful to cite the lead(s) use you used. Table 3.1 shows the approximate upper normal limits for the QT interval with different heart rates.

Unfortunately, there is no simple, generally accepted rule for calculating the normal limits of the QT interval. The same holds for the lower limit of the QT.

Because of these problems, a variety of indices of the QT interval have been devised, termed *rate-corrected* QT or QTc (the latter reads as "QT subscript c") intervals. A number of correction methods have been proposed, but none is ideal and no consensus has been reached on which to use. Furthermore, commonly invoked clinical "rules of thumb" (see below) are often mistakenly assumed on the wards.

---

**QT Cautions: Correcting Common Misunderstandings**

- A QT interval less than ½ the RR interval is NOT necessarily normal (especially at slower rates).
- A QT interval more than ½ the RR interval is NOT necessarily long (especially at very fast rates).

---

## QT Correction (QTc) Methods
### 1. The Square Root Method
The first, and still one of the most widely used QTc indices, is Bazett's formula. This algorithm divides the actual QT interval (in seconds) by the square root of the immediately preceding RR interval (also measured in seconds). Thus, using the "square root method" one applies the simple equation:

$$QTc = QT/\sqrt{RR}$$

Normally the QTc is between about 0.33–0.35 sec (330–350 msec) and about 0.44 sec or (440 msec).

This classic formula has the advantage of being widely recognized and used. However, it requires taking a square root, making it a bit computationally cumbersome for hand calculations. More importantly, the formula reportedly over-corrects the QT at slow rates (i.e., makes it appear too short), while it under-corrects the QT at high heart rates (i.e., makes it appear too long).[c]

### 2. A Linear Method
Not surprisingly, given the limitations of the square root method, a number of other formulas have been proposed for calculating a rate-corrected QT interval.

We present one commonly used one, called Hodges method, which is computed as follows:

$$QTc\ (msec) = QT\ (msec) \\ + 1.75\ (heart\ rate\ in\ beats/min - 60)$$

Or, equivalently, if you want to make the computation in units of seconds, not milliseconds:

$$QTc\ (sec) = QT\ (sec) \\ + 0.00175\ (heart\ rate\ in\ beats/min - 60\ beats/min)$$

The advantage here is that the equation is linear. Note also that with both of the above methods (Bazett and Hodges), the QT and the QTc (0.40 sec or 400 msec) are identical at 60 beats/min.

Multiple other formulas have been proposed for correcting or normalizing the QT to a QTc. None has received official endorsement. The reason is that no method is ideal for individual patient management. Furthermore, an inherent error/uncertainty is unavoidably present in trying to localize the beginning of the QRS complex and, especially, the end of the T wave. (You can informally test the hypothesis that substantial inter-observer and intra-observer variability of the QT exists by showing some deidentified ECGs to your colleagues and recording their QT measurements.)[d]

Note also that some texts report the upper limits of normal for the QTc as 0.45 sec (450 msec) for women and 0.44 sec (440 msec) for men. Others use 450 msec for men and 460 for women. More subtly, a substantial change in the QTc interval within the normal range (e.g., from 0.34 to 0.43 sec) may be a very early warning of progressive QT prolongation due to one of the factors below.

Many factors can abnormally prolong the QT interval (Fig. 3.9). For example, this interval can be prolonged by certain drugs used to treat cardiac arrhythmias (e.g., amiodarone, dronedarone, ibutilide, quinidine, procainamide, disopyramide, dofetilide, and sotalol), as well as a large number of other types of "non-cardiac" agents (fluoroquinolones, phenothiazines, pentamidine, macrolide

---

[c]A technical point that often escapes attention is that implementing the square root method requires that both the QT and RR be measured in seconds. The square root of the RR (sec) yield sec½. However, the QTc, itself, is always reported by clinicians in units of seconds (not awkwardly as sec/sec½ = sec½). To make the units consistent, you should measure the RR interval in seconds but record it as a unitless number (i.e., QT in sec/√RR unitless), Then, the QTc, like the QT, will be expressed in units of sec.

[d]Some references advocate drawing a tangent to the downslope of the T wave and taking the end of the T wave as the point where this tangent line and the TQ baseline intersect. However, this method is arbitrary since the slope may not be linear and the end of the T wave may not be exactly along the isoelectric baseline. A U wave may also interrupt the T wave. With atrial fibrillation, an average of multiple QT values can be used. Clinicians should be aware of which method is being employed when electronic calculations are used and always double check the reported QT.

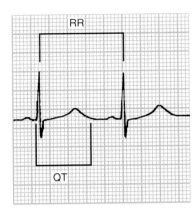

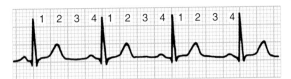

**Fig. 3.10** Heart rate (beats per minute) can be measured by counting the number of large (0.2-sec) time boxes between two successive QRS complexes and dividing 300 by this number. In this example the heart rate is calculated as 300 ÷ 4 = 75 beats/min. Alternatively (and more accurately), the number of small (0.04-sec) time boxes between successive QRS complexes can be counted (about 20 small boxes here) and divided into 1500, also yielding a rate of 75 beats/min.

**Fig. 3.9** Abnormal QT interval prolongation in a patient taking the drug quinidine. The QT interval (0.6 sec) is markedly prolonged for the heart rate (65 beats/min) (see Table 3.1). The rate-corrected QT interval (normally about 0.44–0.45 sec or less) is also prolonged.* Prolonged repolarization may predispose patients to develop *torsades de pointes*, a life-threatening ventricular arrhythmia (see Chapter 16).

*Use the methods described in this chapter to calculate the QTc.
*Answers*:
1. Using the "square root" (Bazett) method: $QTc = QT/\sqrt{RR} = 0.60 \ sec/\sqrt{0.92} = 0.63 \ sec$.
2. Using Hodges method: $QTc = QT + 1.75 \ (HR \ in \ beats/min - 60) = 0.60 + 1.75 \ (65 - 60) = 0.60 + 8.75 = 0.68 \ sec$. With both methods, the QTc is markedly prolonged, indicating a high risk of sudden cardiac arrest due to torsades de pointes (see Chapters 16 and 21).

antibiotics, haloperidol, methadone, certain selective serotonin reuptake inhibitors, to name but a sample).

Specific electrolyte disturbances (low potassium, magnesium, or calcium levels) are important causes of QT interval prolongation. Hypothermia prolongs the QT interval by slowing the repolarization of myocardial cells. The QT interval may be prolonged with myocardial ischemia and infarction (especially during the evolving phase with T wave inversions) and with subarachnoid hemorrhage. QT prolongation is important in practice because it may indicate predisposition to potentially lethal ventricular arrhythmias. (See the discussion of torsades de pointes in Chapter 16.) The differential diagnosis of a long QT interval is summarized in Chapter 25.

Table 3.1 gives (estimated) values of the upper range of the QT for healthy adults over a range of heart rates. The cut-off for the lower limits of the rate-corrected QT (QTc) in adults is variously cited as 330–350 msec. As noted, a short QT may be evidence of hypercalcemia, or of the fact that the

patient is taking digoxin (in therapeutic or toxic doses). Finally, a very rare hereditary "channelopathy" has been reported associated with short QT intervals and increased risk of sudden cardiac arrest (see Chapter 21).

### U Wave

The U wave is a small, rounded deflection sometimes seen after the T wave (see Fig. 2.2). As noted previously, its exact significance is not known. Functionally, U waves represent the last phase of ventricular repolarization. Prominent U waves are characteristic of hypokalemia (see Chapter 11). Very prominent U waves may also be seen in other settings, for example, in patients taking drugs such as sotalol, or quinidine, or one of the phenothiazines or sometimes after patients have had a cerebrovascular accident. The appearance of very prominent U waves in such settings, with or without actual QT prolongation, may also predispose patients to ventricular arrhythmias (see Chapter 16).

Normally the direction of the U wave is the same as that of the T wave. Negative U waves sometimes appear with positive T waves. This abnormal finding has been noted in left ventricular hypertrophy and in myocardial ischemia.

### RR Intervals and Calculation of Heart Rate

We conclude this section on ECG intervals by discussing the RR interval and its inverse; namely the (ventricular) heart rate. Two simple classes of methods can be used to manually measure the ventricular or atrial heart rate (reported as number of heartbeats or cycles per minute) from the ECG (Figs. 3.10 and 3.11).

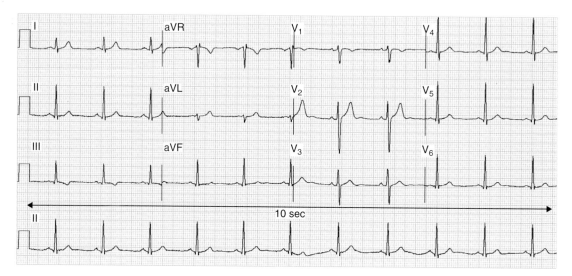

**Fig. 3.11** Quick methods to measure heart rate. Shown is a standard 12-lead ECG with a continuous rhythm strip (lead II, in this case). Method 1A: *Large box counting method* (see Fig. 3.10) shows between four and five boxes between R waves, yielding rate between 75 and 60 beats/min, where rate is 300 divided by number of large (0.2-sec) boxes. Method 1B: *Small box counting method* more accurately shows about 23 boxes between R waves, where rate is 1500 divided by number of small (0.04 sec) boxes = 65 beats/min. Method 2: *QRS counting method* shows 11 QRS complexes in 10 sec = 66 beats/60 sec or 1 min. Note: the short vertical lines here indicate a lead change, and may cause an artifactual interruption of the waveform in the preceding beat (e.g., T waves in the third beat before switch to lead aVR, aVL, and aVF).

## 1. Box Counting Methods

The easiest way, when the (ventricular) heart rate is regular, is to count the number (N) of large (0.2-sec) boxes between two successive QRS complexes and divide a constant (300) by N. (The number of large time boxes is divided into 300 because $300 \times 0.2 = 60$ and the heart rate is calculated in beats per minute, i.e., per 60 seconds.)

For example, in Fig. 3.10 the heart rate is 75 beats/min, because four large time boxes are counted between successive R waves ($300 \div 4 = 75$). Similarly, if two large time boxes are counted between successive R waves, the heart rate is 150 beats/min. With five intervening large time boxes, the heart rate will be 60 beats/min.

When the heart rate is fast or must be measured very accurately from the ECG, you can modify the box counting approach as follows: Count the number of small (0.04-sec) boxes between successive R (or S waves) waves and divide the constant (1500) by this number. In Fig. 3.10, 20 small time boxes are counted between QRS complexes. Therefore, the heart rate is $1500 \div 20 = 75$ beats/min. (The constant 1500 is used because $1500 \times 0.04 = 60$ and

the heart rate is being calculated in beats per 60 sec [beats/min].)

Note: some trainees and attending physicians have adopted a "countdown" mnemonic by which they incant: 300, 150, 100, 75, 60 ... based on ticking off the number of large (0.2-sec box sides) between QRS complexes. However, there is no need to memorize extra numbers: this countdown is simply based on dividing the number of large (0.2-sec) intervals between consecutive R (or S waves) into 300. If the rate is 30, you will be counting down for quite a while! But $300/10 = 30$/min will allow you to calculate the rate and move on with the key decisions regarding patient care.

## 2. QRS Counting Methods

If the heart rate is irregular, the first method will not be accurate because the intervals between QRS complexes vary from beat to beat. You can easily determine an average (mean) rate, whether the latter is regular or not, simply by counting the number of QRS complexes in some convenient time interval (e.g., every 10 sec, the recording length of most 12-lead clinical ECG records). Next, multiply this number by the appropriate factor (6 if you use 10-sec recordings) to obtain the rate in beats per 60 sec (see Fig. 3.11). This method is most usefully applied in arrhythmias with grossly irregular heart rates (as in atrial fibrillation or multifocal atrial tachycardia).

By definition, a heart rate exceeding 100 beats/min is termed a *tachycardia*, and a heart rate slower than 60 beats/min is called a *bradycardia*. (In Greek, *tachys* means "swift," whereas *bradys* means "slow.") Thus during exercise you probably develop a sinus tachycardia, but during sleep or relaxation your pulse rate may drop into the 50s or even lower, indicating a sinus bradycardia. (See Part III of this book for an extensive discussion of the major brady- and tachyarrhythmias.)

## HOW ARE HEART RATE AND RR INTERVALS RELATED?

The heart rate is inversely related to another interval, described earlier: the so-called *RR interval* (or QRS-to-QRS interval), which, as noted previously, is simply the temporal distance between consecutive, equivalent points on the preceding or following QRS. (Conveniently, the R wave peak is chosen, but this is arbitrary.) These measurements, when made using digital computer programs on large numbers of intervals, form the basis of *heart rate variability* (HRV) studies, an important topic that is outside our scope here but mentioned in the Bibliography and the online material.

Students should know that RR intervals can be converted to the instantaneous heart rate (IHR) by the following two simple, equivalent formulas, depending on whether you measure the RR interval in seconds (sec) or milliseconds (msec):

$$Instantaneous\ HR\ in\ beats/min = 60/RR\ (in\ sec)$$

$$Instantaneous\ HR\ in\ beats/min = 60,000/RR\ (in\ msec)$$

## PP AND RR INTERVALS: ARE THEY EQUIVALENT?

We stated in Chapter 2 that there were four basic sets of ECG intervals: PR, QRS, QT/QTc, and PP/RR. Here we refine that description by adding mention of the interval between atrial depolarizations (PP interval). The atrial rate is calculated by the same formula given above for the ventricular, based on the RR interval; namely, the atrial rate (per min) = 60/PP interval (in sec). The PP interval and RR intervals are obviously the same when sinus

rhythm is present with 1:1 AV conduction (referred to as "normal sinus rhythm"). The ratio 1:1 in this context indicates that each P wave is successfully conducted through the AV nodal/His–Purkinje system into the ventricles. In other words: each atrial depolarization signals the ventricles to depolarize.

However, as we will discuss in Parts II and III of this book, the atrial rate is not always equal to the ventricular rate. Sometimes the atrial rate is much faster (especially with second- or third-degree AV block) and sometimes it is slower (e.g., with ventricular tachycardia and AV dissociation).[e]

## ECG TERMS ARE CONFUSING!

Students and practitioners are often understandably confused by the standard ECG terms, which are arbitrary and do not always seem logical. Since this terminology is indelibly engrained in clinical usage, we have to get used to it. But, it is worth a pause to acknowledge these semantic confusions (Box 3.1).

| **BOX 3.1** | Beware: Confusing ECG Terminology! |
|---|---|

- The RR interval is really the QRS–QRS interval.
- The PR interval is really P onset to QRS onset. (Rarely, the term PQ is used; but PR is favored even if the lead does not show an R wave.)
- The QT interval is really QRS (onset) to T (end) interval.
- Not every QRS complex has a Q, R, and S wave.

## THE ECG: IMPORTANT CLINICAL PERSPECTIVES

Up to this point only the basic components of the ECG have been considered. Several general items deserve emphasis before proceeding.

1. The ECG is a recording of cardiac *electrical* activity. It does not directly measure the *mechanical* function of the heart (i.e., how well the heart is contracting and performing as a pump). Thus, a patient with acute pulmonary edema may have

---

[e]The same rule can be used to calculate the atrial rate when non-sinus (e.g., an ectopic atrial) rhythm is present. Similarly, the atrial rate with atrial flutter can be calculated by using the flutter–flutter (FF) interval (see Chapter 15). Typically, in this arrhythmia the atrial rate is about 300 cycles/min. In atrial fibrillation (AF), the atrial depolarization rate is variable and too fast to count accurately from the surface ECG. The depolarization (electrical) rate of 350–600/min rate in AF is estimated from the peak-to-peak fibrillatory oscillations.

a normal ECG. Conversely, a patient with an abnormal ECG may have normal cardiac function.

2. The ECG does *not* directly depict abnormalities in cardiac structure such as ventricular septal defects and abnormalities of the heart valves. It only records the electrical changes produced by structural defects. However, in some conditions a specific structural diagnosis such as mitral stenosis, acute pulmonary embolism, or myocardial infarction/ischemia can be inferred from the ECG because a constellation of typical electrical abnormalities develops.

3. The ECG does *not* record *all* of the heart's electrical activity. The SA node and the AV node are completely silent. Furthermore, the electrodes placed on the surface of the body record only the currents that are transmitted to the area of electrode placement. The clinical ECG records the summation of electrical potentials produced by innumerable cardiac muscle cells. Therefore, there are "silent" electrical areas of the heart that get "cancelled out" or do not show up because of low amplitude. For example, parts of the muscle

may become ischemic, and the 12-lead ECG may be entirely normal or show only nonspecific changes even while the patient is experiencing angina pectoris (chest discomfort due to myocardial ischemia).

4. The electrical activity of the AV junction can be recorded using a special apparatus and a special catheter placed in the heart (*His bundle electrogram*; see online material).

Thus, the presence of a normal ECG does not necessarily mean that all these heart muscle cells are being depolarized and repolarized in a normal way. Furthermore, some abnormalities, including life-threatening conditions such as severe myocardial ischemia, complete AV heart block, and sustained ventricular tachycardia, may occur intermittently. *For these reasons the ECG must be regarded as any other laboratory test, with proper consideration for both its uses and its limitations* (see Chapter 24).

What's next? The ECG leads, the normal ECG, and the concept of electrical axis are described in Chapters 4–6. Abnormal ECG patterns are then discussed, emphasizing clinically and physiologically important topics.

# CHAPTER 4
# ECG Leads

As discussed in Chapter 1, the heart produces electrical currents similar to the familiar dry cell battery. The strength or voltage of these currents and the way they are distributed throughout the body over time can be measured by a special recording instrument (sensor) such as an electrocardiograph.

The body acts as a conductor of electricity. Therefore, recording electrodes placed some distance from the heart, such as on the wrists, ankles, or chest wall, are able to detect the voltages of cardiac currents conducted to these locations.

The usual way of recording the electrical potentials (voltages) generated by the heart is with the 12 standard ECG leads (connections or derivations). The leads actually record and display the differences in voltages (potentials) between electrodes or electrode groups placed on the surface of the body.

Taking an ECG is like recording an event, such as a baseball game, with an array of video cameras. Multiple video angles are necessary to capture the event completely. One view will not suffice. Similarly, each ECG lead (equivalent to a different video camera angle) records a different view of cardiac electrical activity. The use of multiple ECG leads is necessitated by the requirement to generate as full a picture of the three-dimensional electrical activity of the heart as possible. Fig. 4.1 shows the ECG patterns that are obtained when electrodes are placed at various points on the chest. Notice that each lead (equivalent to a different video angle) presents a different pattern.

Fig. 4.2 is an ECG illustrating the 12 leads. The leads can be subdivided into two groups: the six *limb* (*extremity*) leads (shown in the left two columns) and the six *chest* (*precordial*) leads (shown in the right two columns).

The six limb leads—I, II, III, aVR, aVL, and aVF—record voltage differences by means of electrodes placed on the extremities. They can be further divided into two subgroups based on their historical development: three standard *bipolar* limb leads (I, II, and III) and three augmented *unipolar* limb leads (aVR, aVL, and aVF).

The six chest leads—$V_1$, $V_2$, $V_3$, $V_4$, $V_5$, and $V_6$—record voltage differences by means of electrodes placed at various positions on the chest wall.

The 12 ECG leads or connections can also be viewed as 12 "channels." However, in contrast to TV channels (which show different evens), the 12 ECG channels (leads) are all tuned to the *same* event (comprising the P-QRS-T cycle), with each lead viewing the event from a different angle.

## LIMB (EXTREMITY) LEADS
### Standard Limb Leads: I, II, and III

The extremity leads are recorded first. In connecting a patient to a standard 12-lead electrocardiograph, electrodes are placed on the arms and legs. The right leg electrode functions solely as an electrical ground. As shown in Fig. 4.3, the arm electrodes are usually attached just above the wrist and the leg electrodes are attached above the ankles.

The electrical voltages (electrical signals) generated by the working cells of the heart muscle are conducted through the torso to the extremities. Therefore, an electrode placed on the right wrist detects electrical voltages equivalent to those recorded below the right shoulder. Similarly, the voltages detected at the left wrist or anywhere else on the left arm are equivalent to those recorded below the left shoulder. Finally, voltages detected by the left leg electrode are comparable to those at the left thigh or near the groin. In clinical practice the electrodes are attached to the wrists and ankles simply for convenience.

As mentioned, the limb leads consist of standard bipolar (I, II, and III) and augmented (aVR, aVL, and aVF) leads. The bipolar leads were so named historically because they record the differences in electrical voltage between two extremities.

Please go to expertconsult.inkling.com for additional online material for this chapter.

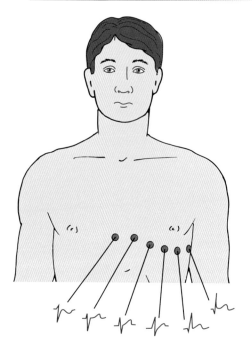

**Fig. 4.1** Chest leads give a multidimensional view of cardiac electrical activity. See Fig. 4.8 and Box 4.1 for exact electrode locations.

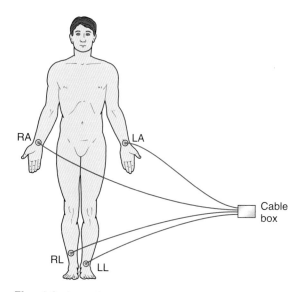

**Fig. 4.3** Electrodes (usually disposable paste-on types) are attached to the body surface to take an ECG. The right leg (*RL*) electrode functions solely as a ground to prevent alternating-current interference. *LA*, left arm; *LL*, left leg; *RA*, right arm.

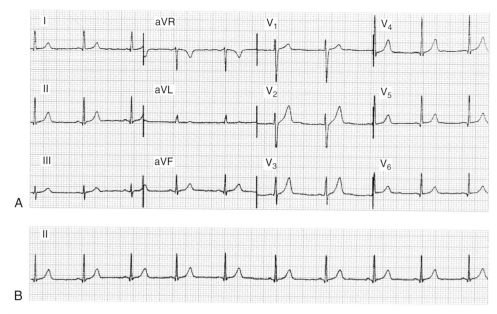

**Fig. 4.2** (A) Sample ECG showing the 12 standard leads. (B) A lead II rhythm strip. What is the approximate heart rate? (*Answer: 50–60 beats/min.*)

Lead I, for example, records the difference in voltage between the left arm (LA) and right arm (RA) electrodes:

$$Lead\ I = LA - RA$$

Lead II records the difference between the left leg (LL) and right arm (RA) electrodes:

$$Lead\ II = LL - RA$$

Lead III records the difference between the left leg (LL) and left arm (LA) electrodes:

$$Lead\ III = LL - LA$$

Consider what happens when the electrocardiograph records lead I. The LA electrode detects the electrical voltages of the heart that are transmitted to the left arm. The RA electrode detects the voltages transmitted to the right arm. Inside the electrocardiograph the RA voltages are subtracted from the LA voltages, and the difference appears at lead I. When lead II is recorded, a similar situation occurs between the voltages of LL and RA. When lead III is recorded, the same situation occurs between the voltages of LL and LA.

Leads I, II, and III can be represented schematically in terms of a triangle, called *Einthoven's triangle* after the Dutch physiologist/physicist (1860-1927) who invented the electrocardiograph. Historically, the first "generation" of ECGs consisted only of recordings from leads I, II, and III. Einthoven's triangle (Fig. 4.4) shows the spatial orientation of the three standard limb leads (I, II, and III). As you can see, lead I points horizontally. Its left pole (LA) is positive and its right pole (RA) is negative. Therefore, lead I = LA − RA. Lead II points diagonally downward. Its lower pole (LL) is positive and its upper pole (RA) is negative. Therefore, lead II = LL − RA. Lead III also points diagonally downward. Its lower pole (LL) is positive and its upper pole (LA) is negative. Therefore, lead III = LL − LA.

Einthoven, of course, could have configured the leads differently. Because of the way he arranged them, the bipolar leads are related by the following simple equation:

$$Lead\ I + Lead\ III = Lead\ II$$

In other words, add the voltage in lead I to that in lead III and you get the voltage in lead II.[a]

You can test this equation by looking at Fig. 4.2. Add the voltage of the R wave in lead I (+9 mm) to the voltage of the R wave in lead III (+4 mm) and you get +13 mm, the voltage of the R wave in lead II. You can do the same with the voltages of the P waves and T waves.

Einthoven's equation is simply the result of the way the bipolar leads are recorded; that is, the LA is positive in lead I and negative in lead III and thus cancels out when the two leads are added:

$$I = \cancel{LA} - RA$$
$$III = LL - \cancel{LA}$$
$$I + III = LL - RA = II$$

Thus, in electrocardiography, one plus three equals two.

In summary, leads I, II, and III are the standard (bipolar) limb leads, which historically were the first invented. These leads record the differences in electrical voltage among extremities.

In Fig. 4.5, Einthoven's triangle has been redrawn so that leads I, II, and III intersect at a common central point. This was done simply by sliding lead I downward, lead II rightward, and lead III leftward. The result is the *triaxial* diagram in Fig. 4.5B. This diagram, a useful way of representing the three

## Einthoven's Triangle

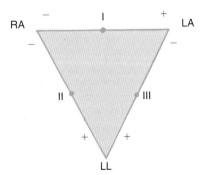

**Fig. 4.4** Orientation of leads I, II, and III. Lead I records the difference in electrical potentials between the left arm and right arm. Lead II records it between the left leg and right arm. Lead III records it between the left leg and left arm.

---

[a]*Note:* this rule of thumb is only approximate. It can be made more precise when the three standard limb leads are recorded simultaneously, as they are with contemporary multichannel electrocardiographs. The exact rule is as follows: The voltage at the peak of the R wave (or at any point) in lead II equals the sum of the voltages in leads I and III at simultaneously occurring points (since the actual R wave peaks may not occur simultaneously).

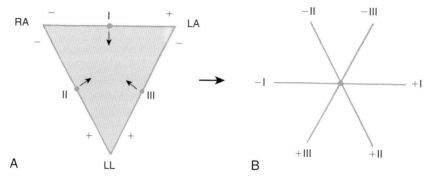

**Fig. 4.5** (A) Einthoven's triangle. (B) The triangle is converted to a triaxial diagram by shifting leads I, II, and III so that they intersect at a common point.

bipolar leads, is employed in Chapter 6 to help measure the QRS axis.

## Augmented Limb Leads: aVR, aVL, and aVF

Nine leads have been added to the original three bipolar extremity leads. In the 1930s, Dr. Frank N. Wilson and his colleagues at the University of Michigan invented the unipolar extremity leads and also introduced the six unipolar chest leads, $V_1$ through $V_6$. A short time later, Dr. Emanuel Goldberger invented the three augmented unipolar extremity leads: aVR, aVL, and aVF. The abbreviation *a* refers to *augmented*; *V* to *voltage*; and *R, L,* and *F* to *right arm*, *left arm*, and *left foot* (leg), respectively. Today 12 leads are routinely employed and consist of the six limb leads (I, II, III, aVR, aVL, and aVF) and the six precordial leads ($V_1$ to $V_6$).

A so-called unipolar lead records the electrical voltages at one location relative to an electrode with close to zero potential rather than relative to the voltages at another single extremity, as in the case of the bipolar extremity leads.[b] The near-zero potential is obtained inside the electrocardiograph by joining the three extremity leads to a central terminal. Because the sum of the voltages of RA, LA, and LL equals zero, the central terminal has a zero voltage. The aVR, aVL, and aVF leads are derived in a slightly different way because the voltages

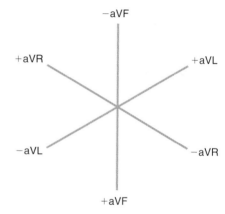

**Fig. 4.6** Triaxial lead diagram showing the relationship of the three augmented (unipolar) leads (aVR, aVL, and aVF). Notice that each lead is represented by an axis with a positive and negative pole. The term *unipolar* was used to mean that the leads record the voltage in one location relative to about zero potential, instead of relative to the voltage in one other extremity.

recorded by the electrocardiograph have been augmented 50% over the actual voltages detected at each extremity. This augmentation is also done electronically inside the electrocardiograph.[c]

Just as Einthoven's triangle represents the spatial orientation of the three standard limb leads, the diagram in Fig. 4.6 represents the spatial orientation of the three augmented extremity leads. Notice that each of these unipolar leads can also be represented by a line (axis) with a positive and negative pole.

[b]Although "unipolar leads" (like bipolar leads) are represented by axes with positive and negative poles, the historical term *unipolar* does not refer to these poles; rather it refers to the fact that unipolar leads record the voltage in one location relative to an electrodes (or set of electrodes) with close to zero potential.

[c]Augmentation was developed to make the complexes more readable.

Because the diagram has three axes, it is also called a *triaxial* diagram.

As would be expected, the positive pole of lead aVR, the right arm lead, points upward and to the patient's right arm. The positive pole of lead aVL points upward and to the patient's left arm. The positive pole of lead aVF points downward toward the patient's left foot.

Furthermore, just as leads I, II, and III are related by Einthoven's equation, so leads aVR, aVL, and aVF are related:

$$aVR + aVL + aVF = 0$$

In other words, when the three augmented limb leads are recorded, their voltages should total zero. Thus, the sum of the P wave voltages is zero, the sum of the QRS voltages is zero, and the sum of the T wave voltages is zero. Using Fig. 4.2, test this equation by adding the QRS voltages in the three unipolar extremity leads (aVR, aVL, and aVF).

You can scan leads aVR, aVL, and aVF rapidly when you first look at a mounted ECG from a single-channel ECG machine. If the sum of the waves in these three leads does not equal zero, the leads may have been mounted improperly.

## Orientation and Polarity of Leads

The 12 ECG leads have two major features, which have already been described. They all have both a specific *orientation* and a specific *polarity*.

Thus, the axis of lead I is oriented horizontally, and the axis of lead aVR is oriented diagonally, from the patient's right to left. The orientation of the three standard (bipolar) leads is shown in represented Einthoven's triangle (see Fig. 4.5), and the orientation of the three augmented (unipolar) extremity leads is diagrammed in Fig. 4.6.

The second major feature of the ECG leads is their polarity, which means that these lead axes have a positive and a negative pole. The polarity and spatial orientation of the leads are discussed further in Chapters 5 and 6 when the normal ECG patterns seen in each lead are considered and the concept of electrical axis is explored.

Do not be confused by the difference in meaning between ECG electrodes and ECG leads. An *electrode* is simply the paste-on disk or metal plate used to detect the electrical currents of the heart in any location. An ECG *lead* is the electrical connection that represents the *differences in voltage* detected by electrodes (or sets of electrodes). For example, lead I records the differences in voltage detected by the left and right arm electrodes. Therefore, a lead is a means of recording the *differences* in cardiac voltages obtained by different electrodes. To avoid confusion, we should note that for electronic pacemakers, discussed in Chapter 22, the terms lead and electrode are used interchangeably.

### Relationship of Extremity Leads

Einthoven's triangle in Fig. 4.5 shows the relationship of the three standard limb leads (I, II, and III). Similarly, the triaxial (three-axis) diagram in Fig. 4.6 shows the relationship of the three augmented limb leads (aVR, aVL, and aVF). For convenience, these two diagrams can be combined so that the axes of all six limb leads intersect at a common point. The result is the *hexaxial* (six axis) lead diagram shown in Fig. 4.7. The hexaxial diagram shows the spatial orientation of the six extremity leads (I, II, III, aVR, aVL, and aVF).

The exact relationships among the three augmented extremity leads and the three standard extremity leads can also be described mathematically. However, for present purposes, the following simple guidelines allow you to get an overall impression of the similarities between these two sets of leads.

As you might expect by looking at the hexaxial diagram, the pattern in lead aVL usually resembles that in lead I. The positive poles of lead aVR and lead II, on the other hand, point in opposite directions. Therefore, the P-QRS-T pattern recorded by lead aVR is generally the reverse of that recorded by lead II: For example, when lead II shows a qR pattern:

lead II shows an rS pattern:

Finally, the pattern shown by lead aVF usually but not always resembles that shown by lead III.

## CHEST (PRECORDIAL) LEADS

The chest leads ($V_1$ to $V_6$) show the electrical currents of the heart as detected by electrodes placed at

### Derivation of Hexaxial Lead Diagram

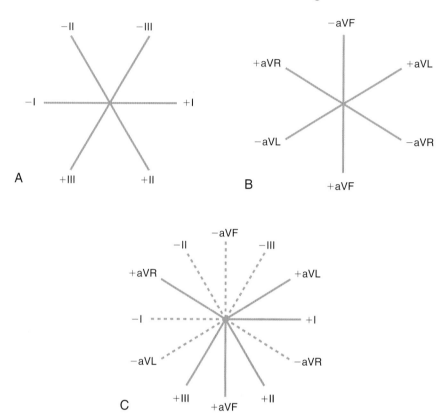

**Fig. 4.7** (A) Triaxial diagram of the so-called bipolar leads (I, II, and III). (B) Triaxial diagram of the augmented limb leads (aVR, aVL, and aVF). (C) The two triaxial diagrams can be combined into a hexaxial diagram that shows the relationship of all six limb leads. The negative pole of each lead is now indicated by a *dashed line.*

different positions on the chest wall. The precordial leads used today are also considered as unipolar leads in that they measure the voltage in any one location relative to about zero potential (Box 4.1). The chest leads are recorded simply by means of electrodes at six designated locations on the chest wall (Fig. 4.8).[d]

Two additional points are worth mentioning here:
1. The fourth intercostal space can be located by placing your finger at the top of the sternum and moving it slowly downward. After you move your finger down about 1½ inches (40 mm), you can

---

[d]Sometimes, in special circumstances (e.g., a patient with suspected right ventricular infarction or congenital heart disease), additional leads are placed on the right side of the chest. For example, lead $V_3R$ is equivalent to lead $V_3$, with the electrode placed to the right of the sternum.

| BOX 4.1 | Conventional Placement of ECG Chest Leads |

- Lead $V_1$ is recorded with the electrode in the fourth intercostal space just to the right of the sternum.
- Lead $V_2$ is recorded with the electrode in the fourth intercostal space just to the left of the sternum.
- Lead $V_3$ is recorded on a line midway between leads $V_2$ and $V_4$.
- Lead $V_4$ is recorded in the mid-clavicular line in the fifth interspace.
- Lead $V_5$ is recorded in the anterior axillary line at the same level as lead $V_4$.
- Lead $V_6$ is recorded in the mid-axillary line at the same level as lead $V_4$.

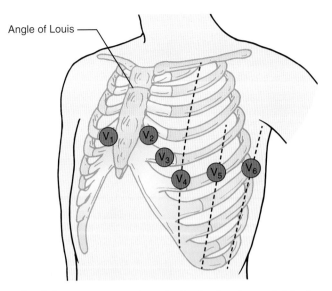

**Fig. 4.8** Locations of the electrodes for the chest (precordial) leads.

feel a slight horizontal ridge. This landmark is called the *angle of Louis*, which is located where the manubrium joins the body of the sternum (see Fig. 4.8). The second intercostal space is found just below and lateral to this point. Move down two more spaces. You are now in the fourth interspace and ready to place lead $V_4$.

2. Accurate chest lead placement may be complicated by breast tissue. To ensure accuracy and consistency, remember the following. Place the electrode *under* the breast for leads $V_3$ to $V_6$. If, as often happens, the electrode is placed *on* the breast, electrical voltages from higher interspaces are recorded. Also, avoid using the nipples to locate the position of any of the chest lead electrodes, in men or women, because nipple location varies greatly in different persons.

The chest leads, like the six extremity leads, can be represented diagrammatically (Fig. 4.9). Like the other leads, each chest lead has a positive and negative pole. The positive pole of each chest lead points anteriorly, toward the front of the chest. The negative pole of each chest lead points posteriorly, toward the back (see the dashed lines in Fig. 4.9).

## The 12-Lead ECG: Frontal and Horizontal Plane Leads

You may now be wondering why 12 leads are used in clinical electrocardiography. Why not 10 or 22

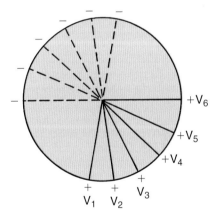

**Fig. 4.9** The positive poles of the chest leads point anteriorly, and the negative poles (*dashed lines*) point posteriorly.

leads? The reason for exactly 12 leads is partly historical, a matter of the way the ECG has evolved over the years since Dr. Willem Einthoven's original three extremity leads were developed around 1900. There is nothing sacred about the "electrocardiographer's dozen." In some situations, for example, additional leads are recorded by placing the chest electrode at different positions on the chest wall. Multiple leads are used for good reasons. The heart, after all, is a three-dimensional structure, and its electrical currents spread out in all directions across the body.

Recall that the ECG leads were described as being like video cameras by which the electrical activity of the heart can be viewed from different locations. To a certain extent, the more points that are recorded, the more accurate the representation of the heart's electrical activity.

The importance of multiple leads is illustrated in the diagnosis of myocardial infarction (MI). An MI typically affects one localized portion of either the anterior or inferior portion of the left ventricle. The ECG changes produced by an anterior MI are usually best shown by the chest leads, which are close to and face the injured anterior surface of the heart. The changes seen with an inferior MI usually appear only in leads such as II, III, and aVF, which face the injured inferior surface of the heart (see Chapters 9 and 10). The 12 leads therefore provide a three-dimensional view of the electrical activity of the heart.

Specifically, the six limb leads (I, II, III, aVR, aVL, and aVF) record electrical voltages transmitted onto the *frontal* plane of the body (Fig. 4.10). (In contrast, the six precordial leads record voltages transmitted onto the *horizontal* plane.) For example, if you walk up to and face a large window (being careful to stop!), the panel is parallel to the frontal plane of your body. Similarly, heart voltages directed upward and downward and to the right and left are recorded by the frontal plane leads.

The six chest leads ($V_1$ through $V_6$) record heart voltages transmitted onto the *horizontal* plane of the body (Fig. 4.11). The horizontal plane (figuratively) bisects your body into an upper and a lower half. Similarly, the chest leads record heart voltages directed anteriorly (front) and posteriorly (back), and to the right and left.

The 12 ECG leads are therefore divided into two sets: the six extremity leads (three unipolar and three bipolar), which record voltages on the frontal plane of the body, and the six chest (precordial) leads, which record voltages on the horizontal plane. Together these 12 leads provide a three-dimensional dynamic representation of atrial and ventricular depolarization and repolarization.[e]

---

[e]Modifications of the standard 12-lead ECG system have been developed for special purposes. For instance, the Mason–Likar system and its variants are widely employed during exercise testing. To reduce noise due to muscle movement, the extremity electrodes are placed near the shoulder areas and in the lower abdomen. These changes may produce subtle but important alterations when comparing modified ECGs with standard ones using the wrist and ankle positions.

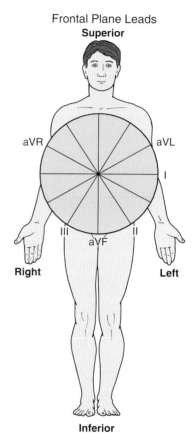

Fig. 4.10 Spatial relationships of the six limb leads, which record electrical voltages transmitted onto the frontal plane of the body.

## CARDIAC MONITORS AND MONITOR LEADS

### Bedside Cardiac Monitors

Up to now, only the standard 12-lead ECG has been considered. However, it is not always necessary or feasible to record a full 12-lead ECG. For example, many patients require continuous monitoring for a prolonged period. In such cases, special cardiac monitors are used to give a continuous beat-to-beat record of cardiac activity, usually from a single monitor lead. Continuous ECG monitors of this type are ubiquitous in emergency departments, intensive care units, operating rooms, and postoperative care units, and a variety of other inpatient settings.

Fig. 4.12 is a rhythm strip recorded from a monitor lead obtained by means of three disk electrodes on the chest wall. As shown in Fig. 4.13, one electrode (the positive one) is usually placed in the $V_1$ position. The other two are placed near the

right and left shoulders. One serves as the negative electrode and the other as the ground.

When the location of the electrodes on the chest wall is varied, the resultant ECG patterns also vary. In addition, if the polarity of the electrodes changes

Horizontal Plane Leads

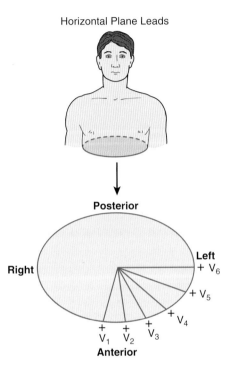

**Fig. 4.11** Spatial relationships of the six chest leads, which record electrical voltages transmitted onto the horizontal plane.

Electrode placement

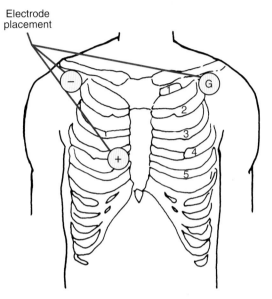

**Fig. 4.13** Monitor lead. A chest electrode (+) is placed at the lead $V_1$ position (between the fourth and fifth ribs on the right side of the sternum). The negative (–) electrode is placed near the right shoulder. A ground electrode (G) is placed near the left shoulder. This lead is therefore a modified $V_1$. Another configuration is to place the negative electrode near the left shoulder and the ground electrode near the right shoulder.

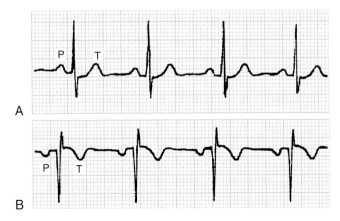

**Fig. 4.12** (A and B) Rhythm strips from a cardiac monitor taken moments apart but showing exactly opposite patterns because the polarity of the electrodes was reversed in the lower strip (B).

(e.g., the negative electrode is connected to the $V_1$ position and the positive electrode to the right shoulder), the ECG shows a completely opposite pattern (see Fig. 4.12).

## Ambulatory ECG Technology: Holter Monitors and Event Recorders

The cardiac monitors just described are useful in patients primarily confined to a bed or chair. Sometimes, however, the ECG needs to be recorded, usually to evaluate arrhythmias, in ambulatory patients over longer periods (Box 4.2). A special portable system designed in the mid-20th century by physicist Norman "Jeff" Holter records the continuous ECG of patients as they go about their daily activities (Box 4.3). The concept and the practical implementation of recording ECGs with portable systems was a technological breakthrough that helped usher in the era of modern cardiac electrophysiology.

Most of the Holter monitors currently in use consist of electrodes placed on the chest wall and lower abdomen interfaced with a special digital, portable ECG recorder. The patient can then be monitored over a sustained, continuous period (typically 24 hours; sometimes up to 48 hours). Two ECG leads are usually recorded. The digital recording can be played back, and the P-QRS-T complexes are displayed on a special screen for analysis and annotation. The recording can also be digitally archived, and selected sections can be printed out. The patient (or family member) provides a diary to record any symptoms.

A 24–48-hr Holter monitoring period (Box 4.3) is most useful for: (1) the detection or exclusion of arrhythmias associated with symptoms (especially palpitations, dizziness, or near-syncope) occurring several times a day; (2) assessing ventricular rate-control in atrial fibrillation during activities of daily living; and (3) detection of ST changes during chest discomfort or in the diagnosis of "silent ischemia."

Limitations of conventional Holter monitors in diagnosing the cause of intermittent symptoms or syncope, which are unlikely to be captured in a 24-48-hr monitoring period, have led to the ongoing development and widespread use of several additional classes of ECG monitors (Box 4.2): *external event recorders*, including patch devices, *mobile (real-time) cardiac outpatient telemetry systems (MCOTs)*, and *implanted loop recorders (ILRs)*.

*External loop recorders (ELRs)* are widely prescribed for arrhythmia analysis and detection. These devices are designed with replaceable electrodes so that patients can be monitored for prolonged periods (up to 2–4 weeks or longer) as they go about their usual activities. The ECG is continuously recorded (via a "looping mechanism") that allows for automatic erasure unless the patient (or companion)

---

**BOX 4.2    Major Types of Ambulatory ECG Monitors**

- Holter monitors
- External event monitors
  - Basic event monitor (no loop memory)
  - External loop recorders (ELRs)
  - Mobile cardiac outpatient telemetry (MCOT)
  - External patch recorders
- Implantable loop recorders (ILRs)
- Implantable pacemakers and cardioverter-defibrillators (ICDs)

---

**BOX 4.3    Some Advantages and Disadvantages of 24-Hour Holter Monitors**

**Advantages**
- Detecting very frequent, symptomatic arrhythmias or seeing if frequent symptoms (e.g., palpitations) have an arrhythmic correlate.
- Providing very accurate assessment of rate control in established atrial fibrillation.
- Detecting ST segment deviations with "silent" ischemia or more rarely in making the diagnosis of Prinzmetal's angina (see Chapter 9).
- Detecting nocturnal arrhythmias (e.g., bradycardias or atrial fibrillation with sleep apnea).
- Detecting sustained monitoring during real-world strenuous activity (e.g., certain types of "in the field" sports, especially when a graded exercise test may be of limited use).

**Disadvantages**
- Cannot capture clinically important but intermittent arrhythmias that occur less frequently than every day/other day. Such transient arrhythmias are not uncommon.
- Cannot exclude life-threatening events with a "negative" study: i.e., one with no index symptoms and/or no significant arrhythmias.

presses an event button or an auto-event trigger is electronically triggered.

When patients experience a symptom (e.g., lightheadedness, palpitations, chest discomfort), they can push a record button so that the ECG obtained around the time of the symptom is stored. The saved ECG also includes a continuous rhythm strip just (e.g., 45 sec) before the button was pressed, as well as a recording after the event mark (e.g., 15 sec). The stored ECGs can be transmitted by phone to an analysis station for immediate diagnosis. Current event recorders also have automatic settings that will record heart rates above or below preset values even if the patient is asymptomatic.

Event recorders can also be used to monitor the ECG for asymptomatic drug effects and potentially important toxicities (e.g., excessive prolongation of the QT/QTc interval with drugs such as sotalol, quinidine, or dofetilide) or to detect other potentially *proarrhythmic effects* (see Chapters 16, 20, and 21) of drugs.

Ambulatory monitoring has been extended to include *MCOT* technology. These recorders provide continuous home recording. The ECG is transmitted via wireless technology to an analysis center if the ECG rhythm exceeds predesignated rate thresholds or meets automated atrial fibrillation criteria (auto-trigger mode) or if the patient pushes a button because of symptoms (patient-trigger option). The patient's physician can then be immediately notified of the findings.

In some cases, life-threatening arrhythmias (e.g., intermittent complete heart block or sustained ventricular tachycardia) may occur so rarely that they cannot be readily detected by any of the usual ambulatory devices. In such cases, a small monitor can be surgically inserted under the skin of the upper chest (*insertable/implantable loop recorder [ILR]*) such that the device records the ECG and saves recordings when prompted by the patient (or family member if the patient faints, for example) or when activated by an automated algorithm. Such ILR devices may be used for up to 2 years.

Patch-based monitoring devices are increasingly being used in contemporary practice. These adhesive, "lead-less" recorders present an alternative to traditional ELRs, especially for 2–14 days monitoring periods. Finally, as discussed in Chapter 21, implantable pacemakers and cardioverter-defibrillators (ICDs) have arrhythmia monitoring, detection, and storage capabilities. Advances in wireless transmission, algorithm development, smartphones and recording technology are likely to accelerate progress in external and implantable ambulatory monitoring in coming years.

# CHAPTER 5

# The Normal ECG

The previous chapters reviewed the cycles of atrial and ventricular depolarization/repolarization detected by the ECG and the standard 12-lead system used to record this electrical activity. This chapter describes the appearance of the P–QRS–T patterns seen normally in the 12 leads. Fortunately, you do not have to memorize 12 or more separate patterns. Rather, understanding basic principles about the timing and orientation of cardiac depolarization and repolarization forces (vectors) will give you a good handle on actually *predicting* the normal ECG patterns in various leads. Furthermore, the same principles can be used to understand changes in conditions such as hypertrophy, bundle branch blocks, and myocardial infarction.

As the sample ECG in Fig. 4.2 showed, the lead patterns appear to be quite different, and sometimes even the opposite of each other. For example, in some leads (e.g., II, III and aVF), the P waves are normally positive (upward); in others (e.g., lead aVR) they are normally negative (downward). In some leads the QRS complexes are represented by an rS wave; in other leads they are represented by RS or qR waves. Finally, the T waves are positive in some leads and negative in others.

Two related and key questions, therefore, are: What determines this variety in the appearance of ECG complexes in the different leads, and how does the same cycle of cardiac electrical activity produce such different patterns in these leads?

## THREE BASIC "LAWS" OF ELECTROCARDIOGRAPHY

To answer these questions, you need to understand three basic ECG "laws" (Fig. 5.1):

1. A *positive (upward) deflection* appears in any lead if the mean (overall) wave of depolarization spreads toward the lead's positive pole. Thus, if the mean atrial stimulation path is directed downward and to the patient's left, toward the

positive pole of lead II, a positive (upward) P wave is seen in lead II (Figs. 5.2 and 5.3). If the mean ventricular stimulation path is directed to the left, a positive deflection (R wave) is seen in lead I (see Fig. 5.1A).

2. A *negative (downward) deflection* appears in any lead if the mean wave of depolarization spreads toward the negative pole of that lead (or away from the positive pole). Thus, if the mean atrial stimulation path spreads downward and to the left, a negative P wave is seen in lead aVR (see Figs. 5.2 and 5.3). If the mean ventricular stimulation path is directed entirely away from the positive pole of any lead, a negative QRS complex (QS deflection) is seen (see Fig. 5.1B).

3. A *biphasic deflection* (consisting of positive and negative deflections of equal size) is usually seen if the *mean* depolarization path is directed at right angles (perpendicular) to any lead axis. Thus, if the mean atrial stimulation path spreads at right angles to any lead, a biphasic P wave is seen in that lead. Similarly, if the mean ventricular stimulation path spreads at right angles to any lead, the QRS complex is biphasic (see Fig. 5.1C). A biphasic QRS complex may consist of either an RS pattern or a QR pattern.

In summary, when the mean depolarization wave spreads toward the positive pole of any lead, it produces a positive (upward) deflection. When it spreads toward the negative pole (away from the positive pole) of any lead, it produces a negative (downward) deflection. When it spreads at right angles to any lead axis, it produces a biphasic deflection.

Mention of repolarization—the return of stimulated muscle to the resting state—has deliberately been deferred until later in this chapter, in the discussion of the normal T wave.

Keeping the three ECG laws in mind, all you need to know is the general direction in which depolarization spreads through the heart at any time. Using this information, you can predict what the P waves and the QRS complexes look like in any lead.

Please go to expertconsult.inkling.com for additional online material for this chapter.

**Three Basic Laws of Electrocardiography**

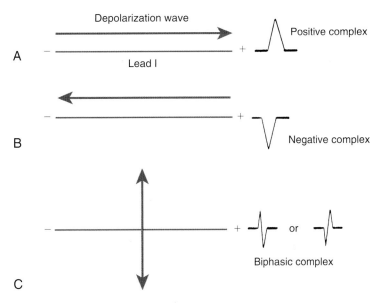

Depolarization wave

Positive complex

A

Lead I

Negative complex

B

Biphasic complex

C

**Fig. 5.1** (A) A positive complex is seen in any lead if the mean wave of depolarization spreads toward the positive pole of that lead. (B) A negative complex is seen if the depolarization wave spreads toward the negative pole (away from the positive pole) of the lead. (C) A biphasic (partly positive, partly negative) complex is seen if the mean direction of the wave is at right angles (perpendicular) to the lead. These basic "laws" apply to both the P wave (atrial depolarization) and the QRS complex (ventricular depolarization).

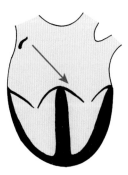

**Fig. 5.2** With sinus rhythm the atrial depolarization wave (*arrow*) spreads from the right atrium downward toward the atrioventricular (AV) junction and left leg.

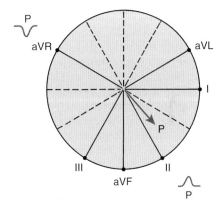

**Fig. 5.3** With sinus rhythm the normal P wave is negative (downward) in lead aVR and positive (upward) in lead II. Recall that with normal atrial depolarization the arrow points down toward the patient's left (see Fig. 5.2), away from the positive pole of lead aVR and toward the positive pole of lead II.

## PHYSIOLOGIC (NORMAL) SINUS P WAVE

The P wave, which represents atrial depolarization, is normally the first waveform seen in any cycle. Atrial depolarization is initiated by spontaneous depolarization of pacemaker cells in the sinus node in the right atrium (see Fig. 1.1). The atrial depolarization path therefore spreads from right to left and downward toward the atrioventricular (AV) junction. The spread of atrial depolarization can be represented by an arrow (*vector*) that points downward and to the patient's left (see Fig. 5.2).

Fig. 4.7C, which shows the spatial relationship of the six frontal plane (extremity) leads, is redrawn in Fig. 5.3. Notice that the positive pole of lead aVR points upward in the direction of the right shoulder. The normal path of atrial depolarization spreads downward toward the left leg (away from the positive pole of lead aVR). Therefore, with sinus rhythm lead aVR always shows a negative P wave. Conversely, lead II is oriented with its positive pole pointing downward in the direction of the left leg (see Fig. 5.3). Therefore, the normal atrial depolarization path is directed toward the positive pole of that lead (at about +60° with respect to the frontal plane. When sinus rhythm is present, lead II always records a positive (upward) P wave.[a]

In summary, when sinus rhythm is present, the P waves are always negative in lead aVR and positive in lead II. In addition, the P waves will be similar, if not identical, and the P wave rate should be appropriate to the clinical context.

Four important notes about sinus rhythm are worth keeping in mind to avoid confusion:

1. Students and clinicians, when asked to define the criteria for "normal" sinus rhythm, typically mention the requirement for a "P wave before each QRS complex and a QRS after every P wave," along with a regular rate and rhythm. However, students are often surprised to learn that these criteria are neither necessary nor sufficient. The term *sinus rhythm* answers the question: what pacemaker is controlling the atria? Therefore, you can see sinus rhythm with any degree of AV heart block, including complete heart block, and even with ventricular asystole (no QRS complexes) during cardiac arrest, because the sinus node may still be functioning normally!

2. You can see a P wave before each QRS and *not* have sinus rhythm, because an ectopic atrial mechanism is present (see Chapters 13 and 14).

3. If you state only that the rhythm is "normal sinus" and do not mention any AV node conduction abnormalities, listeners will assume that each P wave is followed by a QRS and vice versa. The more technical and physiologically rigorous way of stating this finding would be to say, "Sinus rhythm with 1:1 AV conduction and a normal PR interval." Clinically, this statement is almost never used, but if you try it out on a seasoned cardiologist you may find he or she will be astounded by your erudition!

4. Sinus rhythm does not have to be strictly regular. If you feel your own pulse, during slower breathing rates (e.g., 8–12/min) you will note increases in heart rate with inspiration and decreases with expiration. These phasic changes, called *respiratory sinus arrhythmia*, are a normal variant, and especially pronounced in young, fit people with high resting cardiac vagal tone modulation (see Chapter 13).

Using the same principles of analysis, can you also predict what the P wave looks like in leads II and aVR when the heart is being paced not by the sinus node but by the AV junction (AV junctional rhythm)? When the AV junction (or an *ectopic* pacemaker in the lower part of either atrium) is pacing the heart, atrial depolarization must spread up the atria in a *retrograde* direction, which is just the opposite of what happens with normal sinus rhythm. Therefore, an arrow representing the spread of atrial depolarization with AV junctional rhythm points upward and to the right (Fig. 5.4), just the reverse of what happens with normal sinus rhythm. The spread of atrial depolarization upward and to the right results in a positive P wave in lead aVR, because the stimulus is spreading toward the positive pole of that lead (Fig. 5.5). Conversely, lead II shows a negative P wave.

AV junctional and ectopic atrial rhythms are considered in more detail in Part II. The more advanced topic is introduced to show how the polarity of the P waves in lead aVR and lead II depends on the direction of atrial depolarization

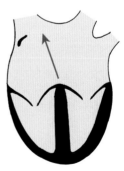

**Fig. 5.4** When the atrioventricular (AV) junction (or an ectopic pacemaker in the low atrial area) acts as the cardiac pacemaker (junctional rhythm), the atria are depolarized in a retrograde (backward) fashion. In this situation, an arrow representing atrial depolarization points upward toward the right atrium. The opposite of the pattern is seen with sinus rhythm.

---

[a]As a more advanced question, can you think of a setting where the P wave would be positive in lead II and sinus rhythm not present? One answer is an atrial tachycardia originating near but definitely outside the sinus node. A clue would be that the rhythm started and stopped abruptly and was a rate too fast for sinus in a resting subject.

and how the atrial activation patterns can be predicted using simple, basic principles.

At this point, you need not be concerned with the polarity of P waves in the other 10 leads. You can usually obtain all the clinical information you need to determine whether the sinus node is pacing the atria by simply looking at the P waves in leads II and aVR. The size and shape of these waves in other leads are important in determining whether abnormalities of the left or right atria are present (see Chapter 7).

## ▶ NORMAL QRS COMPLEX: GENERAL PRINCIPLES

The principles used to predict P waves can also be applied in deducing the appearance of the QRS

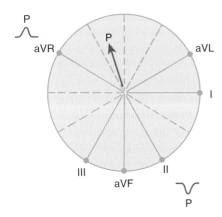

**Fig. 5.5** With atrioventricular (AV) junctional rhythm (or low atrial ectopic rhythm), the P waves are upward (positive) in lead aVR and downward (negative) in lead II.

waveform in various leads. The QRS, which represents ventricular depolarization, is somewhat more complex than the P wave, but the same basic ECG rules apply to understanding the genesis of both waves.

Anatomically, the ventricular myocardium can be grouped in two general parts: (1) the main mass of the left and right ventricles (also called the *free walls*), and (2) the *interventricular septum*. The QRS is dominated by the effects of free wall depolarization of the two ventricles. Specifically, both ventricles normally depolarize simultaneously, from the inside layer to the outside (endocardium to epicardium). These instantaneous forces can be represented by multiple arrows (vectors), as shown in Fig. 5.6A. Under normal circumstances, the electrical forces generated by the larger left ventricle predominate over those generated by the right. So an arrow representing the mean or overall direction of ventricular depolarization forces will point to the left and posteriorly (Fig. 5.6B). Based on this information, one would predict that the QRS will, normally, be relatively negative in leads placed over the right side of the chest and in aVR, and positive in leads placed over the left side of the chest and in lead II.

But, as noted above, ventricular depolarization is somewhat more complex than atrial depolarization in that the former has two sequential phases of activation (Fig. 5.7).

1. The first phase of ventricular depolarization is of relatively brief duration (shorter than 0.04 sec) and small amplitude. It results from spread of the stimulus through the interventricular septum. The septum is the first part of the ventricles to

Simultaneous Activation Forces       Overall Electrical Force

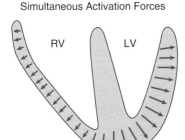
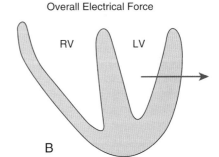

A       B

**Fig. 5.6** (A) Left and right ventricles (LV and RV) depolarize simultaneously, with activation forces (arrows or vectors) directed from inner to outer layers (endocardium to epicardium). (B) These instantaneous forces can be summarized by a single arrow (vector), representing the mean or overall direction of depolarization forces. The arrow points to the left and posteriorly due to the electrical predominance of the LV over the RV under normal condition.

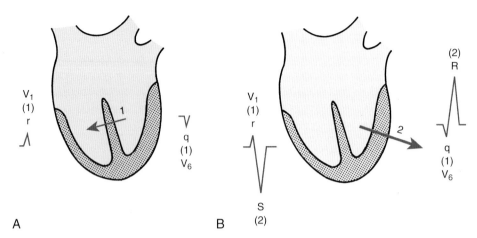

**Fig. 5.7** (A) The first phase of ventricular depolarization proceeds from the left wall of the septum to the right. An arrow representing this phase points through the septum from the left to the right side. (B) The second phase involves depolarization of the main bulk of the ventricles. The arrow points through the left ventricle because this ventricle is normally electrically predominant (see Fig. 5.6). The two phases produce an rS complex in the right chest lead (V₁) and a qR complex in the left chest lead (V₆).

be stimulated. Furthermore, the left side of the septum is stimulated first (by a branch of the left bundle of His). Thus, depolarization spreads from the left ventricle to the right across the septum. Phase one of ventricular depolarization (septal stimulation) can therefore be represented by a small arrow pointing from the left septal wall to the right (Fig. 5.7A).

2. The second phase of ventricular depolarization, already described (Fig. 5.6), involves simultaneous stimulation of the main mass of both the left and right ventricles from the endocardium to epicardium. The arrow representing phase two of ventricular stimulation points toward the more massive left ventricle (Fig. 5.7B).

In summary, the ventricular depolarization process can be divided into two main phases: stimulation of the interventricular septum (represented by a short arrow pointing through the septum into the right ventricle) and simultaneous left and right ventricular stimulation (represented by a larger arrow pointing through the left ventricle and toward the left side of the chest).

Now that the ventricular stimulation sequence has been outlined, you can begin to predict the types of QRS patterns this sequence produces in the different leads. For the moment, the discussion is limited to QRS patterns normally seen in the chest leads (the horizontal plane leads).

## The Normal QRS: Chest Leads

As discussed in Chapter 4, lead V₁ displays voltages detected by an electrode placed on the right side of the sternum (fourth intercostal space). Lead V₆, a left chest lead, shows voltages detected in the left mid-axillary line (see Fig. 4.8). What does the QRS complex look like in these leads (see Fig. 5.7)? Ventricular stimulation occurs in two phases:

1. The first phase of ventricular stimulation, septal stimulation, is represented by an arrow pointing to the right, reflecting the left-to-right spread of the depolarization stimulus through the septum (see Fig. 5.7A). This small arrow points toward the positive pole of lead V₁. Therefore, the spread of stimulation to the right during the first phase produces a small positive deflection (r wave) in lead V₁. What does lead V₆ show? The left-to-right spread of septal stimulation produces a small negative deflection (q wave) in lead V₆. Thus, the same electrical event (septal stimulation) produces a small positive deflection (r wave) in lead V₁ and a small negative deflection (q wave) in a left precordial lead, like lead V₆. (This situation is analogous to the one described for the P wave, which is normally positive in lead II but always negative in lead aVR.)

2. The second phase of ventricular stimulation is represented by an arrow pointing in the direction of the left ventricle (Fig. 5.7B). This arrow points

away from the positive pole of lead $V_1$ and toward the negative pole of lead $V_6$. Therefore, the spread of stimulation to the left during the second phase results in a negative deflection in the right precordial leads and a positive deflection in the left precordial leads. Lead $V_1$ shows a deep negative (S) wave, and lead $V_6$ displays a tall positive (R) wave.

In summary, with normal QRS patterns, lead $V_1$ shows an rS type of complex. The small initial r wave represents the left-to-right spread of septal stimulation. This wave is sometimes referred to as the *septal r wave* because it reflects septal stimulation. The negative (S) wave reflects the spread of ventricular stimulation forces during phase two, away from the right and toward the dominant left ventricle. Conversely, viewed from an electrode in the $V_6$ position, septal and ventricular stimulation produce a qR pattern. The q wave is a *septal q wave*, reflecting the left-to-right spread of the stimulus through the septum away from lead $V_6$. The positive (R) wave reflects the leftward spread of ventricular stimulation voltages through the left ventricle.

Once again, to reemphasize, the same electrical event, whether depolarization of the atria or ventricles, produces very different-looking waveforms in different leads because the spatial orientation of the leads is different.

What happens *between* leads $V_1$ and $V_6$? The answer is that as you move across the chest (in the direction of the electrically predominant left ventricle), the R wave tends to become relatively larger and the S wave becomes relatively smaller. This increase in height of the R wave, which usually reaches a maximum around lead $V_4$ or $V_5$, is called *normal R wave progression*. Fig. 5.8 shows examples of normal R wave progression.

At some point, generally around the $V_3$ or $V_4$ position, the ratio of the R wave to the S wave becomes 1. This point, where the amplitude of the R wave equals that of the S wave, is called the *transition zone* (see Fig. 5.8). In the ECGs of some normal

## Normal R Wave Progression

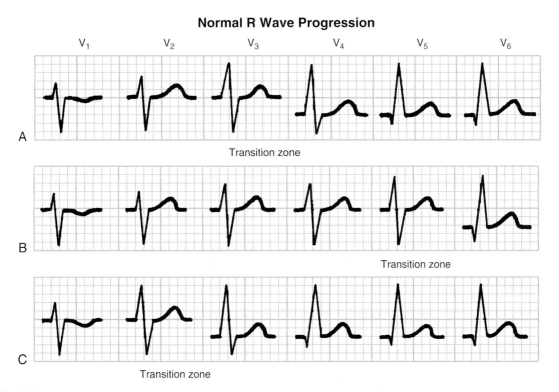

**Fig. 5.8** R waves in the chest leads normally become relatively taller from lead $V_1$ to the left chest leads. (A) Notice the transition in lead $V_3$. (B) Somewhat delayed R wave progression, with the transition in lead $V_5$. (C) Early transition in lead $V_2$.

## Normal Chest Lead ECG

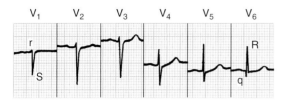

**Fig. 5.9** The transition is in lead V₄. In lead V₁, notice the normal septal r wave as part of an rS complex. In lead V₆ the normal septal q wave is part of a qR complex.

people the transition may be seen as early as lead $V_2$. This is called *early transition*. In other cases the transition zone may not appear until leads $V_5$ and $V_6$. This is called *delayed transition*.

Examine the set of normal chest leads in Fig. 5.9. Notice the rS complex in lead $V_1$ and the qR complex in lead $V_6$. The R wave tends to become gradually larger as you move toward the left chest leads. The transition zone, where the R wave and S wave are about equal, is in lead $V_4$. In normal chest leads the R wave voltage does not have to become literally larger as you go from leads $V_1$ and $V_6$. However, the overall trend should show a relative increase. In Fig. 5.9, for example, notice that the complexes in leads $V_2$ and $V_3$ are about the same and that the R wave in lead $V_5$ is taller than the R wave in lead $V_6$.

In summary, normally the precordial leads show an rS-type complex in lead $V_1$ with a steady increase in the relative size of the R wave toward the left chest and a decrease in S wave amplitude. Leads $V_5$ and $V_6$ generally show a qR-type complex.[b]

The concept of *normal R wave progression* is helpful in distinguishing normal and abnormal ECG patterns. For example, imagine the effect that an anterior wall myocardial infarction (MI) would have on normal R wave progression. Anterior wall infarction results in the death of myocardial cells and the loss of normal positive (R wave) voltages. Therefore, one major ECG sign of an anterior wall infarction is the loss of normal R wave progression in the chest leads (see Chapters 9 and 10).

---

[b]You should be aware that normal chest lead patterns may show slight variation from the patterns discussed thus far. For example, in some normal ECGs, lead $V_1$ shows a QS pattern, not an rS pattern. In other normal chest lead patterns the septal q wave in the left side of the chest leads may not be seen; thus, leads $V_5$ and $V_6$ show an R wave and not a qR complex. In other normal ECGs, leads $V_5$ and $V_6$ may show a narrow qRs complex as a normal variant (see Fig. 4.2, lead $V_4$) and lead $V_1$ may show a narrow rSr′.

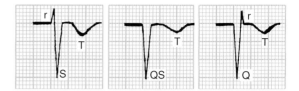

**Fig. 5.10** Lead aVR normally shows one of three basic negative patterns: an rS complex, a QS complex, or a Qr complex. The T wave also is normally negative.

An understanding of normal R wave progression in the chest leads also provides a basis for recognizing other basic ECG abnormalities. For example, consider the effect of left or right ventricular hypertrophy (enlarged muscle mass) on the chest lead patterns. As mentioned previously, the left ventricle is normally electrically predominant and left ventricular depolarization produces deep (negative) S waves in the right chest leads with tall (positive) R waves in the left chest leads. With left ventricular hypertrophy these left ventricular voltages are further increased, resulting in very tall R waves in the left chest leads and very deep S waves in the right chest leads. On the other hand, right ventricular hypertrophy shifts the balance of electrical forces to the right, producing tall positive waves (R waves) in the right chest leads (see Chapter 7).

### The Normal QRS: Limb (Extremity) Leads

Of the six limb (extremity) leads (I, II, III, aVR, aVL, and aVF), lead aVR is the easiest to visualize. The positive pole of lead aVR is oriented upward and toward the right shoulder. The ventricular stimulation forces are oriented primarily toward the left ventricle. Therefore, lead aVR normally shows a predominantly negative QRS complex. Lead aVR may display any of the QRS–T complexes shown in Fig. 5.10. In all cases the QRS is predominantly negative. The T wave in lead aVR is also normally negative.

The QRS patterns in the other five extremity leads are somewhat more complicated. The reason is that the QRS patterns in the extremity leads show considerable normal variation. For example, the extremity leads in the ECGs of some normal people may show qR-type complexes in leads I and aVL and rS-type complexes in leads III and aVF (Fig. 5.11). The ECGs of other people may show just the opposite picture, with qR complexes in leads II, III,

## Normal "Horizontal" QRS Axis

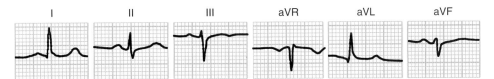

**Fig. 5.11** With a horizontal QRS position (axis), leads I and aVL show qR complexes, lead II shows an RS complex, and leads III and aVF show rS complexes.

## Normal "Vertical" QRS Axis

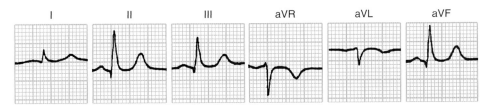

**Fig. 5.12** With a vertical QRS position (axis), leads II, III, and aVF show qR complexes, but lead aVL (and sometimes lead I) shows an RS complex. This is the reverse of the pattern that occurs with a normal horizontal axis.

and aVF and RS complexes in lead aVL and sometimes lead I (Fig. 5.12).

What accounts for this marked normal variability in the QRS patterns shown in the extremity leads? The patterns that are seen depend on the electrical orientation (position) of the heart. The term *electrical position* is virtually synonymous with *mean QRS axis*, which is described in greater detail in Chapter 6.

In simplest terms, the electrical orientation (position) of the heart may be described as either *horizontal* or *vertical*:

• When the heart is electrically horizontal (*horizontal QRS axis*), ventricular depolarization is directed mainly horizontally and to the left in the frontal plane. As the frontal plane diagram in Fig. 4.10 shows, the positive poles of leads I and aVL are oriented horizontally and to the left. Therefore, when the heart is electrically horizontal, the QRS voltages are directed toward leads I and aVL. Consequently, a tall R wave (usually as part of a qR complex) is seen in these leads.

• When the heart is electrically vertical (*vertical QRS axis*), ventricular depolarization is directed mainly downward. In the frontal plane diagram (see Fig. 4.10), the positive poles of leads II, III, and aVF are oriented downward. Therefore, when the heart is electrically vertical, the QRS voltages are directed

toward leads II, III, and aVF. This produces a relatively tall R wave (usually as part of a qR complex) in these leads.

The concepts of electrically horizontal and electrically vertical heart positions can be expressed in another way. When the heart is electrically horizontal, leads I and aVL show qR complexes similar to the qR complexes seen normally in the left chest leads ($V_5$ and $V_6$). Leads II, III, and aVF show rS or RS complexes similar to those seen in the right chest leads normally. Therefore, when the heart is electrically horizontal, the patterns in leads I and aVL resemble those in leads $V_5$ and $V_6$ whereas the patterns in leads II, III, and aVF resemble those in the right chest leads. Conversely, when the heart is electrically vertical, just the opposite patterns are seen in the extremity leads. With a vertical heart, leads II, III, and aVF show qR complexes similar to those seen in the left chest leads, and leads I and aVL show rS-type complexes resembling those in the right chest leads.

Dividing the electrical position of the heart into vertical and horizontal variants is obviously an oversimplification. In Fig. 5.13, for example, leads I, II, aVL, and aVF all show positive QRS complexes. Therefore this tracing has features of *both* the vertical and the horizontal variants. (Sometimes this pattern is referred to as an "intermediate" heart position.)

### Normal "Intermediate" QRS Axis

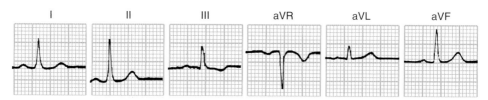

**Fig. 5.13** Extremity leads sometimes show patterns that are hybrids of vertical and horizontal variants, with R waves in leads I, II, III, aVL, and aVF. This represents an intermediate QRS axis and is also a normal variant.

For present purposes, however, you can regard the QRS patterns in the extremity leads as basically variants of either the horizontal or the vertical QRS patterns described.

In summary, the extremity leads in normal ECGs can show a variable QRS pattern. Lead aVR normally always records a predominantly negative QRS complex (Qr, QS, or rS). The QRS patterns in the other extremity leads vary depending on the electrical position (QRS axis) of the heart. With an electrically vertical axis, leads II, III, and aVF show qR-type complexes. With an electrically horizontal axis, leads I and aVL show qR complexes. Therefore, it is not possible to define a single normal ECG pattern; rather, there is a normal variability. Students and clinicians must familiarize themselves with the normal variants in both the chest leads and the extremity leads.

## NORMAL ST SEGMENT

As noted in Chapters 2 and 3, the normal ST segment, representing the early phase of ventricular repolarization, is usually isoelectric (flat on the baseline). Slight deviations (generally less than 1 mm) may be seen normally. As described in Chapter 9, the ECGs of certain normal people show more prominent ST segment elevations as a normal variant (early repolarization pattern). Finally, examine the ST segments in the right chest leads ($V_1$ to $V_3$) of Fig. 4.2. Notice that they are short and the T waves appear to take off almost from the J point (junction of the QRS complex and ST segment). This pattern, which can be considered as a variant of normal early repolarization, is not an uncommon finding in healthy individuals.

## NORMAL T WAVE

Ventricular repolarization—the return of stimulated muscle to the resting state—produces the ST segment,

T wave, and U wave. Deciding whether the T wave in any lead is normal is generally straightforward. As a rule, the T wave follows the direction of the main QRS deflection. Thus, when the main QRS deflection is positive (upright), the T wave is normally positive.

Some more specific rules about the direction of the normal T wave can be formulated. The normal T wave is always negative in lead aVR but positive in lead II. Left-sided chest leads such as $V_4$ to $V_6$ normally always show a positive T wave.

The T wave in the other leads may be variable. In the right chest leads ($V_1$ and $V_2$) the T wave may be normally negative, isoelectric, or positive but it is almost always positive by lead $V_3$ in adults. Furthermore, if the T wave is positive in any chest lead, it must remain positive in all chest leads to the left of that lead. Otherwise, it is abnormal. For example, if the T wave is negative in leads $V_1$ and $V_2$ and becomes positive in lead $V_3$, it should normally remain positive in leads $V_4$ to $V_6$.[c] The differential diagnosis of T wave inversions extending beyond $V_2$ in adults is wide and includes positional and normal variants, right ventricular cardiomyopathy, and acute right ventricular overload syndromes, as well as anterior ischemia.

The polarity of the T wave in the extremity leads depends on the electrical position of the heart. With a horizontal heart the main QRS deflection is positive in leads I and aVL and the T wave is also positive in these leads. With an electrically vertical heart the QRS is positive in leads II, III, and aVF and the T wave is also positive in these leads. However, on some normal ECGs with a vertical axis the T wave may be negative in lead III.

---

[c]In children and in some normal adults a downward T wave may extend as far left as lead $V_3$ or other leads with an rS- or RS-type complex. This normal variant is known as the juvenile T wave pattern.

# CHAPTER 6
# Electrical Axis and Axis Deviation

Normal ECG patterns in the chest and extremity leads were discussed in Chapter 5. The general terms *horizontal heart* (or *horizontal QRS axis*) and *vertical heart* (or *vertical QRS axis*) were used to describe normal, individual variations in QRS patterns seen in the extremity leads. The purpose of this chapter is to further refine the concept of electrical axis and to present methods for computing the QRS axis, quickly, simply, and in a clinically relevant way.

## MEAN QRS AXIS: A WORKING DEFINITION

The depolarization stimulus spreads through the ventricles in different directions from one instant to the next. The overall direction of the QRS complex, or *mean QRS electrical axis*, can also be described. If you draw an arrow to represent the overall, or mean, direction in which the QRS complex is pointed in the frontal plane of the body, you are representing the electrical axis of the QRS complex. The term *mean QRS axis* therefore indicates the general direction in the frontal plane toward which the QRS complex vector is predominantly pointed.

Because the QRS axis is being defined in the frontal plane, the reference is only to the six extremity leads. Therefore, the scale of reference used to measure the mean QRS axis is the diagram of the frontal plane leads (described in Chapter 4 and depicted again in Fig. 6.1). Einthoven's triangle can be readily converted into a triaxial (three-axis) lead diagram by sliding the axes of the three standard limb leads (I, II, and III) so they intersect at a central point (Fig. 6.1A). Similarly, the axes of the three augmented limb leads (aVR, aVL, and aVF) also form a triaxial lead diagram (Fig. 6.1B). These two triaxial lead diagrams can be geometrically combined to produce a hexaxial (six-axis) lead diagram (Fig. 6.1C). We use this diagram to determine the mean QRS axis and describe axis deviation.

As noted in Chapter 4, each lead has a positive and negative pole (see Fig. 6.1C). As a wave of depolarization spreads toward the positive pole, an upward (positive) deflection occurs. Conversely, as a wave spreads toward the negative pole, a downward (negative) deflection is inscribed.

Finally, a reference system is needed to determine or calculate the mean QRS axis. By convention the positive pole of lead I is located at 0°. All points below the lead I axis are positive, and all points above that axis are negative (Fig. 6.2). Thus, toward the positive pole of lead aVL (–30°), the axis becomes negative. Downward toward the positive poles of leads II, III, and aVF, the scale becomes more positive (lead II at +60°, lead aVF at +90°, and lead III at +120°).

The complete hexaxial diagram used to measure the QRS axis is shown in Fig. 6.2. By convention again, an electrical axis that points toward lead aVL is termed *leftward* or *horizontal*. An axis that points toward leads II, III, and aVF is *rightward* or *vertical*.

## MEAN QRS AXIS: CALCULATION

In calculating the mean QRS axis, you are answering this question: In what general direction or toward which lead axis is the QRS complex predominantly oriented? In Fig. 6.3, for example, notice the tall R waves in leads II, III, and aVF. These waves indicate that the heart is electrically vertical (*vertical electrical axis*). Furthermore, the R waves are equally tall in leads II and III.[a] Therefore, by simple inspection, the mean electrical QRS axis can be seen to be directed between the positive poles of leads II and III and toward the *positive pole* of lead aVF (+90°).

As a general rule, the mean QRS axis points midway between any two leads that show tall R waves of equal height.

[a]In Fig. 6.3, three leads (II, III, and aVF) have R waves of equal height. In this situation the electrical axis points toward the middle lead (i.e., toward lead aVF or at +90°).

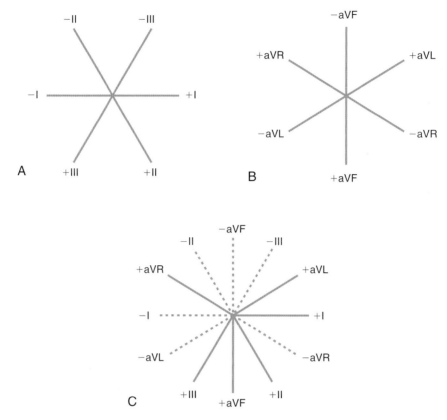

**Fig. 6.1** (A) Relationship of leads I, II, and III. (B) Relationship of leads aVR, aVL, and aVF. (C) These diagrams have been combined to form a hexaxial lead diagram. Notice that each lead has a positive and negative pole. The negative poles are designated by dashed lines.

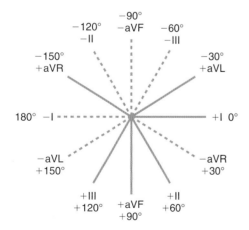

**Fig. 6.2** In the hexaxial lead diagram, notice that each lead has an angular designation, with the positive pole of lead I at 0°. All leads above lead I have negative angular values, and the leads below it have positive values.

In Fig. 6.3 the mean electrical axis can be calculated in a second way. Recall from Chapter 4 that if a wave of depolarization is oriented at right angles to any lead axis, a biphasic complex (RS or QR) is recorded in that lead. Reasoning in a reverse manner, if you find a biphasic complex in any of the extremity leads, the mean QRS axis must be directed at 90° to that lead axis. In Fig. 6.3 lead I is biphasic, showing an RS pattern. Therefore, the mean electrical axis must be directed at right angles to lead I. Because lead I on the hexaxial lead scale is at 0°, the mean electrical axis must be at right angles to 0° or at either −90° or +90°. If the axis were −90°, the depolarization forces would be oriented away from the positive pole of lead aVF and that lead would show a negative complex. In Fig. 6.3, however, lead aVF shows a positive complex (tall R wave); therefore the axis must be +90°.

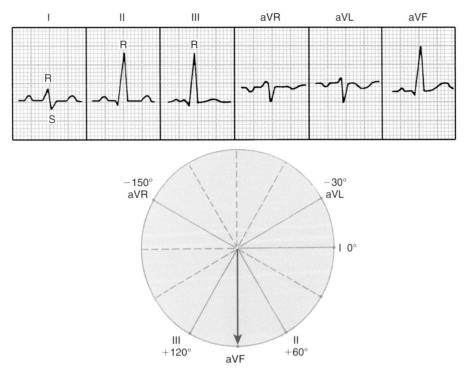

**Fig. 6.3** Mean QRS axis of +90° (see text).

Fig. 6.4 presents another example. By inspection, the mean QRS axis is horizontal, because leads I and aVL are positive and leads II, III, and aVF are predominantly negative. The precise electrical axis can be calculated by looking at lead II, which shows a biphasic RS complex. Therefore, the axis must be at right angles to lead II. Because lead II is at +60° on the hexaxial scale (see Fig. 6.2), the axis must be either –30° or +150°. If it were +150°, leads II, III, and aVF would be positive. Therefore, the axis is –30°.

Another example is given in Fig. 6.5. The QRS complex is positive in leads II, III, and aVF. Therefore the axis is relatively vertical. Because the R waves are of equal magnitude in leads I and III, the mean QRS axis must be oriented between these two leads, or at +60°.

Alternatively, in Fig. 6.5 the QRS axis can be calculated by looking at lead aVL, which shows a biphasic RS-type complex. Therefore, the mean electrical axis must be at right angles to lead aVL (–30°); that is, it must be oriented at either –120° or +60°. Since lead II shows a relatively tall R wave, the axis must be +60° in this case. Still another

example is provided in Fig. 6.6. The electrical axis is seen to be oriented away from leads II, III, and aVF and toward leads aVR and aVL, which show positive complexes. Because the R waves are of equal magnitude in leads aVR and aVL, the axis must be oriented precisely between these leads, or at –90°. Alternatively, look at lead I, which shows a biphasic RS complex. In this case the axis must be directed at right angles to lead I (0°); that is, it must be either –90° or +90°. Because the axis is oriented away from the positive pole of lead aVF and toward the negative pole of that lead, it must be –90°.

Again, look at Fig. 6.7. Because lead aVR shows a biphasic RS-type complex, the electrical axis must be at right angles to the axis of that lead. The axis of aVR is at –150°; therefore, the electrical axis in this case must be either –60° or +120°. It is –60° because lead aVL is positive and lead III shows a negative complex.[b]

---

[b]In Fig. 6.7 the QRS axis can also be calculated by looking at lead I, which shows an R wave of equal amplitude with the S wave in lead II. The mean QRS axis must be oriented between the positive pole of lead I (0°) and the negative pole of lead II (–120°). Therefore, the axis must be at –60°.

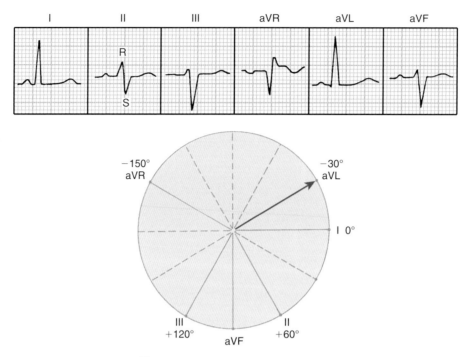

**Fig. 6.4** Mean QRS axis of −30° (see text).

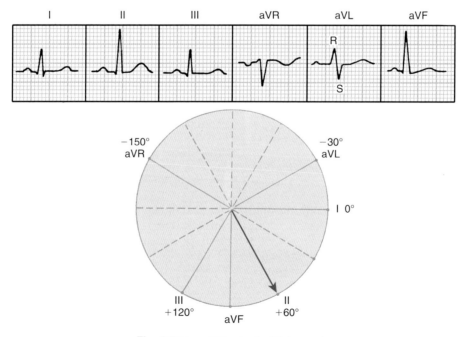

**Fig. 6.5** Mean QRS axis of +60° (see text).

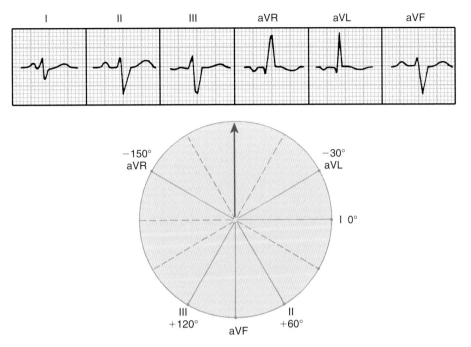

**Fig. 6.6** Mean QRS axis of −90° (see text).

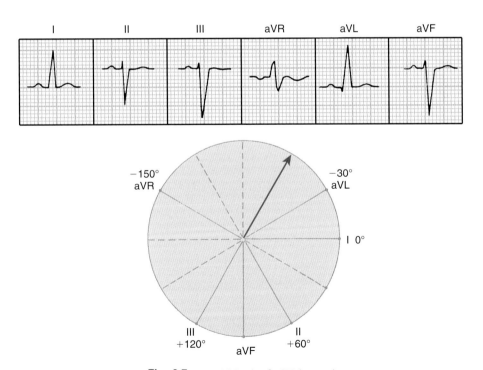

**Fig. 6.7** Mean QRS axis of −60° (see text).

These basic examples should establish the ground rules for calculating the mean QRS axis. However, such calculations are generally only an estimate or a near approximation. An error of 10° or 15° is not clinically significant. Thus it is perfectly acceptable to calculate the axis from leads in which the QRS complex is nearly biphasic or from two leads in which the R (or S) waves are of approximately equal amplitude.[c]

In summary, the mean QRS axis can be determined on the basis of one or both of the following rules:

- The mean QRS axis points midway between the axes of two extremity leads that show tall R waves of equal amplitude.
- The mean QRS axis points at 90° (right angles) to any extremity lead that shows a biphasic (QR or RS) complex and in the direction of leads that show relatively tall R waves.

## AXIS DEVIATION

The mean QRS axis is a basic measurement that should be made on every ECG. In the ECGs of most normal people this axis lies between –30° and +100°. An axis of –30° or more negative is described as *left axis deviation* (LAD), and one that is +100° or more positive is termed *right axis deviation* (RAD). In other words, LAD can be viewed as an abnormal extension of the mean QRS axis found in persons with an electrically horizontal heart orientation, and RAD as an abnormal extension of the mean QRS axis in persons with an electrically vertical heart orientation.

The mean QRS axis is determined by the anatomic position of the heart and the direction in which the stimulus spreads through the ventricles (i.e., the direction of ventricular depolarization):

- The influence of *cardiac anatomic position* on the electrical axis can be illustrated by the effects of respiration. When a person breathes in, the diaphragm descends and the heart becomes more vertical in the chest cavity. This change generally shifts the QRS electrical axis vertically (to the right). (Patients with emphysema and chronically hyperinflated lungs usually have anatomically vertical hearts and electrically vertical QRS axes.) Conversely, when the person breathes out, the diaphragm ascends and the heart assumes a more horizontal position in the chest. This generally shifts the QRS electrical axis horizontally (to the left).

- The influence of the *direction of ventricular depolarization* can be illustrated by left anterior fascicular block, in which the spread of stimuli through the more superior and leftward portions of the left ventricle is delayed and the mean QRS axis shifts to the left (see Chapter 7). By contrast, with right ventricular hypertrophy (RVH) the QRS axis shifts to the right.

Recognition of RAD and LAD is usually straightforward:

- RAD exists if the QRS axis is found to be +100° or more positive. Recall that when leads II and III show tall R waves of equal height, the QRS axis must be +90°. As an approximate rule, if leads II and III show tall R waves and the R wave in lead III exceeds the R wave in lead II, RAD is present. In addition, lead I shows an RS pattern with the S wave deeper than the R wave is tall (see Figs. 6.8 and 6.9).

- LAD exists if the QRS axis is found to be –30° or more negative. In the ECG shown in Fig. 6.4 the QRS axis is exactly –30°. Notice that lead II shows a biphasic (RS) complex. Remember that the location of lead II is aligned at +60° (see Fig. 6.2), and a biphasic complex indicates that the electrical

### Right Axis Deviation

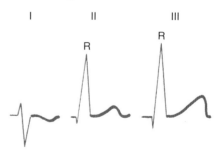

Fig. **6.8** Right axis deviation (mean QRS axis more positive than +100) can be determined by inspecting leads I, II, and III. Notice that the R wave in lead III is taller than that in lead II.

---

[c]For example, when the R (or S) waves in two leads have similar but not identical voltages, the mean QRS axis does not lie exactly between these two leads. Instead, it points more toward the lead with the larger amplitude. Similarly, if a lead shows a biphasic (RS or QR) deflection with the R and S (or Q and R) waves *not* of identical amplitude, the mean QRS axis does *not* point exactly perpendicular to that lead. If the R wave is larger than the S (or Q) wave, the axis points slightly less than 90° away from the lead. If the R wave is smaller than the S (or Q) wave, the axis points slightly more than 90° away from that lead.

## Right Axis Deviation

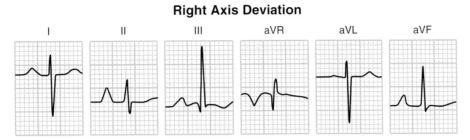

**Fig. 6.9** Notice the relatively tall R waves in the inferior leads, with R3>R2. QRS right axis deviation here was due to right ventricular hypertrophy. Note also slightly peaked P waves in lead II, which are borderline for right atrial overload (see Chapter 7). Biphasic QRS in aVR with equal Q and R waves indicates that axis is at right angles to the aVR lead axis, toward the positive pole of II (which is at −150° or +210°). Thus, the QRS axis here is +120°.

## Left Axis Deviation

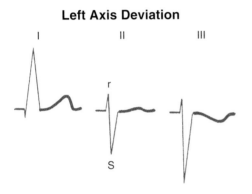

**Fig. 6.10** Left axis deviation (mean QRS axis more negative than –30°) can be determined by simple inspection of leads I, II, and III. Notice that lead II shows an rS complex (with the S wave of greater amplitude than the r wave).

axis must be at right angles to that lead (at either –30° or +150°). Thus, with an axis of –30°, lead II shows an RS complex with the R and S waves of equal amplitude. If the electrical axis is more negative than –30° (LAD), lead II shows an RS complex with the S wave deeper than the R wave is tall (Figs. 6.10 and 6.11).

The rules for recognizing QRS axis deviation can be summarized as follows:

- RAD is present if the R wave in lead III is taller than the R wave in lead II. Notice that with RAD, lead I shows an RS-type complex in which the S wave is deeper than the R wave is tall (see Figs. 6.8 and 6.9).
- LAD is present if lead I shows a tall R wave, lead III shows a deep S wave, and lead II shows either a biphasic RS complex (with the amplitude of the S wave exceeding the height of the r wave) (see

Figs. 6.10 and 6.11) or a QS complex. Leads I and aVL both show R waves.

In Chapter 5 the terms *electrically vertical* and *electrically horizontal* heart positions or orientations (mean QRS axes) were introduced. This chapter has added the terms *left axis deviation* and *right axis deviation*. What is the difference between these terms? Electrically vertical and electrically horizontal heart positions are qualitative. With an electrically vertical mean QRS axis, leads II, III, and aVF show tall R waves. Sometimes this general type of vertical axis is called *inferior*. With an electrically horizontal mean QRS axis, leads I and aVL show tall R waves. With an electrically vertical (inferior) heart axis, the actual mean QRS axis may be normal (e.g., +75°) or abnormally rightward (e.g., +120°). Similarly, with an electrically horizontal heart the actual axis may be normal (+20°) or abnormally leftward (−50°).

RAD therefore can be simply viewed as an extreme form of a vertical mean QRS axis, and LAD is an extreme form of a horizontal mean QRS axis. Saying that a patient has an electrically vertical or horizontal mean QRS axis does not tell whether actual axis deviation is present.

### Axis Deviation: Instant Recognition

For beginning students, precise calculation of the QRS axis is not as important as answering the following key related questions: Is the mean QRS axis normal, or is LAD or RAD present? The answers can be obtained by inspecting the QRS complex from leads I and II (Fig. 6.12).

If the QRS complexes in both leads are positive, the axis must be normal. If the QRS complex is predominantly positive in lead I and negative in lead II, LAD is present. If the QRS complex is

## Left Axis Deviation

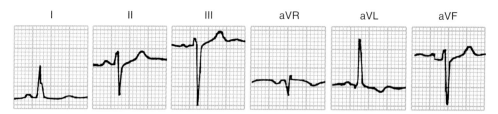

**Fig. 6.11** Notice the rS complex in lead II, from a patient with left axis deviation.

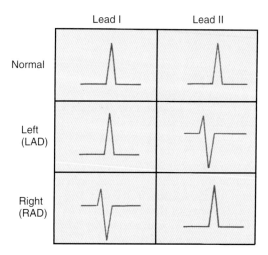

**Fig. 6.12** Simple method for telling whether the QRS axis is normal using leads I and II. (LAD, left axis deviation; RAD, right axis deviation.)

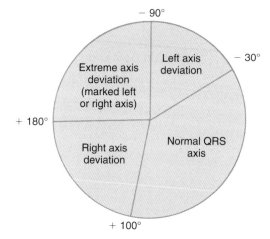

**Fig. 6.13** Normal QRS axis and axis deviation. Most ECGs show either a normal axis or left or right axis deviation. Occasionally the QRS axis is between –90° and 180°. Such an extreme shift may be caused by marked left or right axis deviation. The term extreme axis deviation is sometimes used.

predominantly negative in lead I and positive in lead II, RAD (or at least borderline RAD) is present. (Very rarely, the QRS will be predominantly negative in both leads I and II. In such unusual cases you can describe extreme right or left axis deviation.)

### Clinical Significance

Axis deviation may be encountered in a variety of settings. RAD, with a mean QRS axis +100° or more, is sometimes seen in the ECGs of normal hearts. However, RVH is an important cause of RAD (see Chapter 7). Another cause is myocardial infarction of the lateral wall of the left ventricle. In this setting, loss of the normal leftward depolarization forces may lead "by default" to a rightward axis (see Fig. 9.11). Left posterior fascicular block (hemiblock) is a much rarer cause of RAD (see Chapter 8). The ECGs of patients with chronic lung disease

(emphysema or chronic bronchitis) often show RAD. Finally, a sudden shift in the mean QRS axis to the right (not necessarily causing actual RAD) may occur with acute pulmonary embolism (see Chapters 12 and 25).

LAD, with a mean QRS axis of –30° or more, is also seen in several settings. Patients with left ventricular hypertrophy (LVH) sometimes but not always have LAD (see Chapter 7). Left anterior fascicular block (hemiblock) is a fairly common cause of marked deviation (more negative than –45°). LAD may be seen in association with left bundle branch block (see Chapter 8).

RAD or LAD is not necessarily a sign of significant underlying heart disease. Nevertheless, recognition of RAD or LAD (Figs. 6.12 and 6.13) often provides supportive evidence for LVH or RVH, ventricular

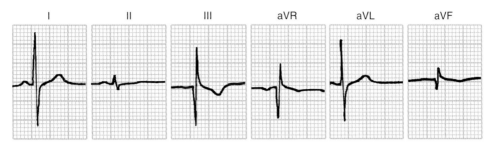

**Fig. 6.14** Indeterminate axis. Notice the biphasic complexes (RS or QR) in all six frontal plane leads. Indeterminate axis does not have a specific clinical implication.

conduction disturbance (left anterior or posterior hemiblock), or another disorder (see Chapter 25).

Finally, the limits for LAD and RAD (–30° to +100°) used in this book are necessarily arbitrary. Some authors use different criteria (e.g., 0° to +90°). These apparent discrepancies reflect the important fact that no absolute parameters have been established in clinical electrocardiography—only general criteria can be applied. The same problems will be encountered in the discussion of LVH and RVH (see Chapter 7) because different voltage criteria have been described by various authors.

On rare occasions, all six extremity leads show biphasic (QR or RS) complexes, which makes it impossible to calculate the mean frontal plane QRS axis. In such cases the term *indeterminate axis* is used (Fig. 6.14). An indeterminate QRS axis may occur as a normal variant, or it may be seen in a variety of pathologic settings.

## MEAN ELECTRICAL AXIS OF THE P WAVE AND T WAVE

To this point, only the mean electrical axis of the QRS complex in the frontal plane has been considered. The same principles can be usefully applied to the mean electrical axes of the P wave and T wave in the frontal plane.

For example, when sinus rhythm is present, the normal P wave is always negative in lead aVR and positive in lead II. Normally, therefore, the P wave is generally directed toward the positive pole of lead II (see Fig. 5.3), which makes the normal mean P wave axis approximately +60°. On the other hand, if the atrioventricular (AV) junction (and not the sinus node) is pacing the heart, the atria are stimulated in a retrograde way. When an AV junctional rhythm is present, atrial depolarization spreads upward (in a retrograde direction), toward the positive pole of lead aVR and away from the positive pole of lead II (see Fig. 5.5). In this situation, if the P wave is visible (i.e., not hidden in the QRS), the mean P wave axis must be approximately –150°.

The same principles can be used in calculating the mean electrical axis of the T wave in the frontal plane. As a rule, the mean T wave axis and the mean QRS axis normally point in the same general (but not identical) direction. In other words, when the electrical position of the heart is horizontal, T waves normally are positive in leads I and aVL, in association with tall R waves in those leads. When the electrical position is vertical, T waves are normally positive in leads II, III, and aVF, in association with tall R waves in those leads. (However, the T wave is often negative in lead III normally, regardless of the electrical position of the heart.)

In summary, the concept of mean electrical axis can be applied to the QRS complex, the P wave, or the T wave. The mean electrical axis describes the general or overall direction of depolarization or repolarization waves with respect to the frontal plane.

# CHAPTER 7
# Atrial and Ventricular Enlargement

The first six chapters have been devoted to the basics of ECGs. From this point, we focus attention primarily on the recognition and understanding of abnormal ECG patterns. This chapter discusses a major topic: the ECG manifestations of enlargement of the four cardiac chambers.

*Cardiac enlargement* describes situations in which one or more of the heart's chambers becomes bigger, either due to an increase in its cavity volume, wall thickness, or both.

When cardiac enlargement occurs, the total number of heart muscle fibers does *not* increase; rather, each individual fiber becomes larger (*hypertrophied*). With dilation, the heart muscle cells tend to become longer (termed *eccentric hypertrophy*). With enlargement due to increased wall thickness, the cells tend to become wider (termed *concentric hypertrophy*). One predictable ECG effect of advanced cardiac hypertrophy is an increase in the voltage or duration of the P wave or of the QRS complex. Not uncommonly, increased wall thickness and chamber dilation occur together, as with long-standing severe hypertension.

Chamber enlargement usually results from some type of chronic *pressure* or *volume load* on the heart muscle. Classically, pressure loads (e.g., due to systemic hypertension or aortic stenosis) cause an increase in wall thickness. In contrast, volume loads (e.g., due to valve regurgitation or dilated cardiomyopathy) are associated primarily with ventricular and atrial dilation. In rarer cases, cardiac enlargement can result from genetic abnormalities or idiopathic (as yet unknown) causes. Examples include arrhythmogenic right ventricular cardiomyopathy/dysplasia (ARVC/D; Chapter 21) and hypertrophic cardiomyopathy syndromes (Chapter 9).

Pathologic hypertrophy due to increases in wall thickness or chamber dilation are often accompanied by fibrosis (scarring) and changes in myocardial geometry (remodeling), which may both worsen myocardial function and promote arrhythmogenesis (e.g., atrial fibrillation and sustained ventricular tachycardia) and chronic heart failure (CHF). Furthermore, alterations in the autonomic nervous system, inadequate myocardial perfusion, disturbances in the nitric oxide system and the renin–angiotensin–aldosterone axis may all play roles in the complicated perturbations linking hypertrophy and fibrosis of heart muscle cells with dysfunction of other organs.

## RIGHT ATRIAL ABNORMALITY

Overload of the right atrium may increase the voltage of the P wave.

When the P wave is positive, its amplitude is measured in millimeters from the upper level of the baseline, where the P wave begins, to the peak of the wave. A negative P wave is measured from the lower level of the baseline to the lowest point of the P wave. (Measurement of the height and width of the P wave is shown in Fig. 7.1.)

Normally, at rest, the P wave in every lead is less than 2.5 mm (0.25 mV) in amplitude and less than 0.12 sec (120 msec or three small boxes) in width. (During exercise, P wave amplitude in lead II or equivalent may increase transiently as a physiological finding.)

Overload of the right atrium in pathologic conditions may produce an abnormally tall P wave (2.5 mm or more), as a sustained finding. Occasionally, right atrial abnormality (RAA) will be associated with a deep (negative) but narrow P wave in lead $V_1$, due to the relative inferior location of the right atrium relative to this lead. This finding may cause confusion with left atrial abnormality (LAA), sometimes leading to a false-positive identification of RAA.

However, because pure RAA generally does not increase the total duration of atrial depolarization, the width of the P wave is normal (less than 0.12 sec [120 msec], or three small box lengths). The abnormal P wave in RAA is sometimes referred to as

Please go to expertconsult.inkling.com for additional online material for this chapter.

*P pulmonale* because the atrial enlargement that it signifies often occurs with severe pulmonary disease (Figs. 7.2 and 7.3).

The tall, narrow P waves characteristic of RAA can usually be seen best in leads II, III, aVF, and sometimes V₁. The ECG diagnosis of P pulmonale can be made by finding a P wave exceeding 2.5 mm in any of these leads. *Echocardiographic* evidence, however, indicates that the finding of a tall, peaked P wave does not consistently correlate with RAA.

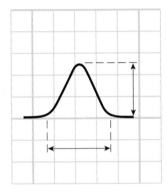

**Fig. 7.1** The normal P wave is usually less than 2.5 mm in height and less than 0.12 sec in width.

### Right Atrial Abnormality (Overload)

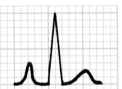

**Fig. 7.2** Tall narrow P waves may indicate right atrial abnormality or overload (formerly referred to as P pulmonale pattern).

On the other hand, patients may have actual right atrial overload and not tall P waves. In other words, tall peaked P waves are of limited sensitivity and specificity in the diagnosis of right atrial enlargement (see Chapter 24).

RAA is seen in a variety of important clinical settings. It is usually associated with right ventricular enlargement. Four of the most important are: (1) pulmonary disease; (2) congenital heart disease; (3) acquired tricuspid valve disease; and (4) cardiomyopathy such as arrhythmogenic right ventricular cardiomyopathy/dysplasia (ARVC/D). The pulmonary disease may be either acute (bronchial asthma, pulmonary embolism), chronic (emphysema, bronchitis, chronic thromboembolic pulmonary hypertension), or combined (chronic obstructive lung disease with an exacerbation due to pneumonia). Congenital heart lesions that produce RAA include pulmonary valve stenosis, atrial septal defects, Ebstein's anomaly (a malformation of the tricuspid valve), and tetralogy of Fallot. RAA may also be due to acquired disease of the tricuspid valve, including regurgitation (e.g., from endocarditis) and stenosis (e.g., with rheumatic heart disease or with carcinoid syndrome).

### LEFT ATRIAL ABNORMALITY/OVERLOAD

Enlargement of the left atrium also produces predictable changes in the P wave. Normally the left atrium depolarizes after the right atrium. Thus, left atrial enlargement should prolong the total duration of atrial depolarization, indicated by an abnormally wide P wave. Left atrial enlargement (LAE) characteristically produces a wide P wave with duration of 0.12 sec (120 msec) or more (at least three small boxes). With enlargement of the left atrium the

## Right Atrial Abnormality

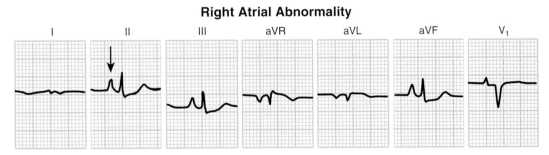

| I | II | III | aVR | aVL | aVF | V₁ |

**Fig. 7.3** Tall P waves (*arrow*) are seen in leads II, III, aVF, and V₁ from the ECG of a patient with chronic lung disease. This finding is sometimes called the P pulmonale pattern.

amplitude (height) of the P wave may be either normal or increased.

Some patients, particularly those with coronary artery disease, may have broad P waves without detectable enlargement of the left atrium on imaging studies. The abnormal P waves probably represent an atrial conduction delay in a relatively normal-sized chamber. Therefore, rather than *left atrial enlargement*, the more general term *left atrial abnormality* is recommended to describe these abnormally broad P waves.

Fig. 7.4 illustrates the characteristic P wave changes seen in LAA. As shown, the P wave sometimes has a distinctive humped or notched appearance (Fig. 7.4A). The second hump corresponds to the delayed depolarization of the left atrium. These humped P waves are usually best seen in one or more of the extremity leads (Fig. 7.5). (The older term *P mitrale* is sometimes still used to describe wide P waves seen with LAA because these waves were first observed in patients with rheumatic mitral valve disease.)

In patients with LAA, lead $V_1$ sometimes shows a distinctive biphasic P wave (see Figs. 7.4B and 7.6). This wave has a small, initial positive deflection and a prominent, wide negative deflection. The negative component is longer than 0.04 sec (40 msec) in duration or 1 mm or more in depth. The prominent negative deflection corresponds to the delayed stimulation of the enlarged left atrium. Remember that anatomically the left atrium is situated posteriorly, up against the esophagus, whereas the right atrium lies anteriorly, against the sternum. The initial positive deflection of the P wave in lead $V_1$ therefore indicates right atrial depolarization, whereas the deep negative deflection is a result of left atrial depolarization voltages directed posteriorly (away from the positive pole of lead $V_1$).

In some cases of LAA you may see both the broad, often humped, P waves in leads I and II and the biphasic P wave in lead $V_1$. In other cases, only broad, notched P waves are seen. Sometimes a biphasic P wave in lead $V_1$ is the only ECG evidence of LAA. The terminal part (vector) of the P wave may be deviated to the left in the frontal plane (i.e., toward lead aVL).

### Left Atrial Abnormality

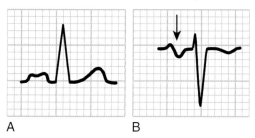

A                    B

**Fig. 7.4** Left atrial abnormality/enlargement may produce the following: (A) wide, sometimes notched P waves in one or more extremity leads (formerly referred to as *P mitrale* pattern), and (B) wide biphasic P waves (*arrow*) in lead $V_1$.

─────────── Key Point ───────────

Clinically, LAA may occur in a variety of important settings, including:
- Valvular heart disease, particularly aortic stenosis, aortic regurgitation, mitral regurgitation, and mitral stenosis*
- Hypertensive heart disease, which causes left ventricular overload and eventually LAA
- Cardiomyopathies (dilated, hypertrophic, and restrictive)
- Coronary artery disease

*With severe mitral stenosis, obstruction to emptying of the left atrial blood into the left ventricle results in a backup of pressure through the pulmonary vessels to the right ventricle. A major clue to mitral stenosis is LAA (or atrial fibrillation) with signs of right ventricular hypertrophy (RVH), as depicted in Fig. 24.1.

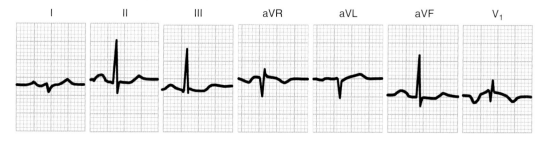

**Fig. 7.5** Broad, humped P waves from the ECG of a patient with left atrial enlargement (abnormality).

Atrial Enlargement (Abnormality)

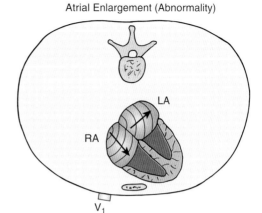

| | Normal | Right | Left |
|---|---|---|---|
| II | RA LA | RA LA | RA LA |
| $V_1$ | RA LA | RA LA | RA LA |

**Fig. 7.6** Overload of the right atrium (RA) may cause tall, peaked P waves in the extremity or chest leads. An abnormality of the left atrium (LA) may cause broad, often notched P waves in the extremity leads and a biphasic P wave in lead $V_1$ with a prominent negative component representing delayed depolarization of the left atrium. (Modified from Park MK, Guntheroth WG: How to read pediatric ECGs, 4th ed. St. Louis, Mosby/Elsevier, 2006.)

In some cases of severe LAA, the negative component of the P wave is very prolonged (80 msec or more in duration). However, the amplitude of the negative part of the P wave may not necessarily be enlarged. *The term intra-atrial conduction delay (IACD) has been used in this context.*

The increase in amplitude and/or duration of the negative portion of the P wave in lead $V_1$ is sometimes referred to as increased *P terminal forces in $V_1$* (PTFV1).

LAA by ECG, especially when marked, indicates an increased risk of atrial fibrillation; conversely, patients with a history of paroxysmal atrial fibrillation not uncommonly have ECG signs of LAA when in sinus rhythm.

The patterns of LAA and RAA are summarized schematically in Fig. 7.6.

Patients with enlargement of both atria (*biatrial enlargement or abnormality*) may show a combination of patterns (e.g., tall and wide P waves), as illustrated

in Fig. 7.7. This finding may occur, for example, with severe cardiomyopathy or valvular heart disease (e.g., combined mitral and tricuspid dysfunction).

## RIGHT VENTRICULAR HYPERTROPHY

You can predict the ECG changes produced by both right ventricular hypertrophy (RVH) and left ventricular hypertrophy (LVH) based on what you already know about normal QRS patterns. These findings are most likely to be seen with chronic pressure loads leading to increased wall thickness. Normally the left and right ventricles depolarize simultaneously, and the left ventricle is electrically predominant because it has greater mass (see Chapter 5). As a result, leads placed over the right side of the chest (e.g., $V_1$) record rS-type complexes:

r

S

## Biatrial Abnormality

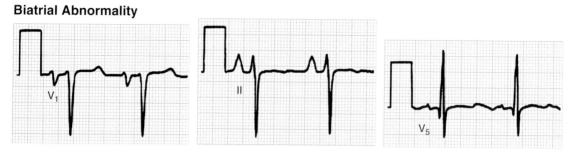

**Fig. 7.7** Biatrial enlargement (abnormality) may produce P waves that are both tall in lead II and biphasic in lead $V_1$, with a prominent, terminal negative component in that lead. The P wave is also notched here in lead $V_5$. (Reproduced from Mirvis D, Goldberger AL. Electrocardiography. In: Mann DL, Zipes DP, Libby P, Bonow RO, editors. Braunwald's heart disease: A textbook of cardiovascular medicine. 10th ed. Philadelphia: WB Saunders/Elsevier; 2015. Fig. 12.15.)

In these rS-type complexes the deep negative S wave indicates the spread of depolarization voltages away from the right and toward the left side. Conversely, leads placed over the left side of the chest (e.g., $V_5$, $V_6$) record a qR-type complex:

In this complex the tall positive R wave indicates the predominant depolarization voltages that point to the left and are generated by the left ventricle.

If sufficient hypertrophy of the right ventricle occurs, the normal electrical predominance of the left ventricle can be overcome. In this situation, what type of QRS complex might you expect to see in the right chest leads? With RVH the right chest leads show tall R waves, indicating the spread of positive voltages from the hypertrophied right ventricle toward the right (Fig. 7.8). Figs. 7.9 and 7.10 show clinical examples of RVH. Instead of the rS complex normally seen in lead $V_1$, a tall positive (R) wave indicates marked hypertrophy of the right ventricle.

How tall does an R wave in lead $V_1$ have to be to make a diagnosis of RVH? In adults the normal R wave in lead $V_1$ is generally smaller than the S wave in that lead. An R wave exceeding the S wave in lead $V_1$ is suggestive but not diagnostic of RVH. Sometimes a small q wave precedes the tall R wave in lead $V_1$ (see Fig. 7.9).

Along with tall right chest R waves, RVH often produces two additional QRS findings: right axis deviation (RAD) and T wave inversions in right to mid-precordial leads.

RVH affects both depolarization (QRS complex) and repolarization (ST-T complex). For reasons not fully understood, hypertrophy of the heart muscle alters the normal sequence of repolarization. With RVH the characteristic repolarization change is the appearance of inverted T waves in the right and middle chest leads (see Figs. 7.9 and 7.10).

These right chest T wave inversions were formerly referred to as a *right ventricular "strain" pattern.* Left precordial T wave inversions due to LVH were referred to as *left ventricular "strain."* Preferable and more contemporary designations are *T wave inversions associated with right ventricular or left ventricular overload,* respectively.

With RVH the chest leads to the left of leads showing tall R waves may display a variable pattern. Sometimes the middle and left chest leads show slow R wave progression, with rS or RS complexes all the way to lead $V_6$ (see Fig. 7.10). In other cases, normal R wave progression is preserved and the left chest leads also show R waves (see Fig. 7.9).

Factors causing RVH, such as congenital heart disease or lung disease, also often cause right atrial overload. So, not uncommonly, signs of RVH are accompanied by tall P waves. The major exception to this rule, in which signs of RVH are, paradoxically, accompanied by marked LAA is mitral stenosis, as illustrated in Fig. 24.1.

The presence of a right bundle branch block (RBBB) pattern by itself does not indicate RVH. However, a complete or incomplete RBBB pattern with RAD should raise strong consideration of a right ventricular enlargement syndrome.

**QRS in hypertrophy**

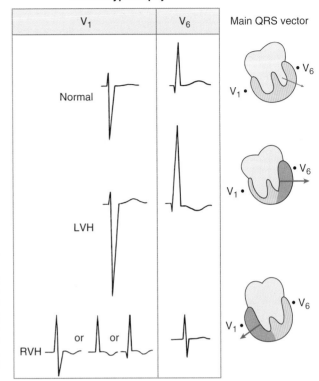

**Fig. 7.8** The QRS patterns with left ventricular hypertrophy (LVH) and right ventricular hypertrophy (RVH) can be anticipated based on the abnormal physiology. Notice that LVH exaggerates the normal pattern, causing deeper right precordial S waves and taller left precordial R waves. By contrast, RVH shifts the QRS vector to the right, causing increased right precordial R waves. (Reproduced from Mirvis D, Goldberger AL. Electrocardiography. In: Mann DL, Zipes DP, Libby P, Bonow RO, editors. Braunwald's heart disease: A textbook of cardiovascular medicine. 10th ed. Philadelphia: WB Saunders/Elsevier; 2015. Fig. 12.16.)

In summary, with RVH the ECG may show tall R waves in the right chest leads and the R wave may be taller than the S wave in lead aVR or $V_1$. In addition, RAD and right precordial T wave inversions are often present. Tall P waves due to right atrial overload are not uncommon (unless the underlying cause is mitral stenosis). Some cases of RVH are more subtle, and the ECG may show only one of these patterns, or none of all (limited sensitivity).

RVH may occur in a variety of clinical settings. An important cause is congenital heart disease, such as pulmonary stenosis, atrial septal defect,[a] tetralogy of Fallot, or Eisenmenger's syndrome. Patients with long-standing severe pulmonary disease may have pulmonary artery hypertension and RVH. As noted, mitral stenosis can produce a combination of LAA

and RVH. T wave inversions in leads $V_1$ to $V_3$ due to right ventricular overload may also occur without other ECG signs of RVH, as in acute pulmonary embolism (see Chapter 12).

═══════════════ Key Point ═══════════════

The following QRS triad (in adults) strongly points to marked RVH due to a pressure load (pulmonary hypertension or pulmonic stenosis):
1. Tall right precordial R waves (as Rs, pure R, or qR morphologies)
2. Right axis deviation (RAD), especially 100° or more positive in adults
3. Right-mid precordial T wave inversions (e.g., $V_1$ to $V_3$ or $V_4$)

*Note:* Tall P waves consistent with right atrial abnormality (RAA), in concert with these findings, make RVH even more likely. However, this constellation of findings, while highly specific, has very low sensitivity.

---

[a]Patients with right ventricular enlargement from the most common form of atrial septal defect (*secundum type*) typically exhibit a right bundle branch block-type pattern (RSR' in lead $V_1$) with a vertical or rightward QRS axis.

## Severe Right Ventricular Hypertrophy

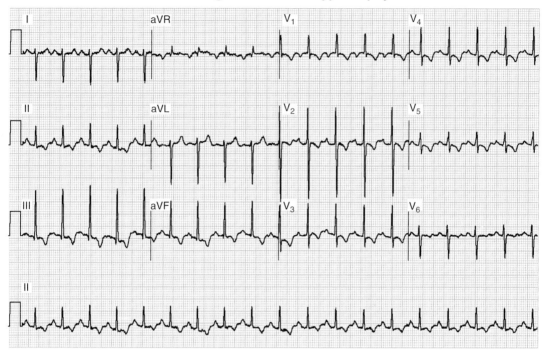

**Fig. 7.9** A tall R wave (as part of an Rs complex) with an inverted T wave caused by right ventricular overload is seen in leads $V_1$ to $V_5$ (also in II, III, and aVF) from a patient with right ventricular hypertrophy (RVH) that was multifactorial. Marked right axis deviation is also present because the R wave in lead III is much taller than the R wave in lead II. In fact, the RVH is so severe that the R wave progression pattern is actually reversed (rS in $V_6$). The negative but prominent P wave in $V_1$ is probably due to right atrial overload, with slightly peaked P waves in leads II, III, and aVF.

In patients who have right ventricular overload associated with emphysema, the ECG may not show any of the patterns just described. Instead of tall R waves in the right precordial leads, very slow R wave progression is seen. RAD is also commonly present, along with low voltage QRS complexes (see Fig. 12.6). These findings may simulate anterior wall infarction.

## LEFT VENTRICULAR HYPERTROPHY

The major ECG changes produced by LVH, like those from RVH, are predictable (see Fig. 7.8). Normally, the left ventricle, because of its relatively larger mass, is electrically predominant over the right ventricle. As a result, prominent negative (S) waves are produced in the right chest leads, and tall positive (R) waves are seen in the left chest leads. When LVH is present, the balance of electrical forces is shifted even further to the left and posteriorly. Thus, with LVH, abnormally

tall, positive (R) waves are usually seen in the left chest leads, and abnormally deep negative (S) waves are present in the right chest leads.

*Important note:* the voltage criteria used to diagnose LVH in the chest and limb leads are by no means absolute. In fact, many different ECG indexes have been proposed, reflecting the imperfection of the ECG in providing findings with both high sensitivity and specificity.

Clinicians should recognize that LVH can affect at least five ECG features: QRS voltages, repolarization (ST-T) changes, QRS axis and duration, and P wave characteristics.

Commonly used guidelines for the ECG diagnosis of LVH include the following considerations and caveats:

1. Consider LVH if the sum of the depth of the S wave in lead $V_1$ ($S_{V1}$) and the height of the R wave in either lead $V_5$ or $V_6$ ($R_{V5}$ or $R_{V6}$) exceeds 35 mm

## Right Ventricular Hypertrophy

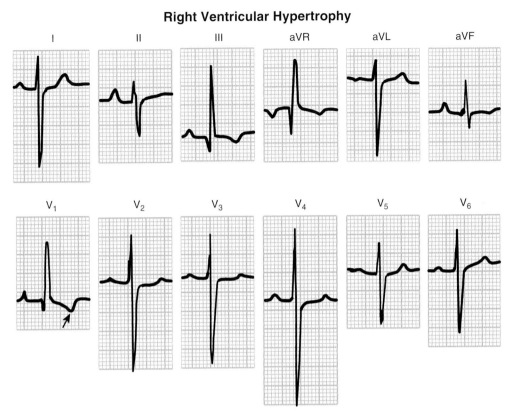

**Fig. 7.10** With right ventricular hypertrophy, lead $V_1$ sometimes shows a tall R wave as part of the qR complex. Because of right atrial enlargement, peaked P waves are seen in leads II, III, and $V_1$. The T wave inversion in lead $V_1$ and the ST segment depressions in leads $V_2$ and $V_3$ are due to right ventricular overload. The PR interval is also prolonged (0.24 sec).

(3.5 mV) (Fig. 7.11), especially in middle-aged or older adults. *However, high voltage in the chest leads is a common normal finding, particularly in athletic or thin young adults.* Consequently, high voltage in the chest leads ($S_{V1}$ + $R_{V5}$ or $R_{V6}$ >35 mm) is not a *specific* LVH indicator (Fig. 7.12).

2. Another proposed set of LVH criteria (the Cornell voltage indexes) are based by summing components of the QRS voltages in leads $V_3$ and aVL: for men, $S_{V3}$ + $R_{aVL}$ >28 mm; for women, $S_{V3}$ + $R_{aVL}$ >20 mm.

3. Sometimes LVH produces tall R waves in lead aVL. An R wave of 11–13 mm (1.1 to 1.3 mV) or more in lead aVL is another sign of LVH (see Fig. 7.10). A tall R wave in lead aVL may be the only ECG sign of LVH, and the voltage in the chest leads may be normal. In other cases the chest voltages are abnormally high, with a normal R wave seen in lead aVL.

4. Just as RVH is sometimes associated with repolarization abnormalities due to ventricular overload, so ST-T changes are often seen in LVH. Fig. 7.13 illustrates the characteristic shape of the ST-T complex with LVH. Notice that the complex usually has a distinctively asymmetrical appearance, with a slight ST segment depression followed by a broadly inverted T wave. In some cases these T wave inversions are very deep. This LV overload-related repolarization abnormality (formerly called LV "strain") is usually best seen in leads with tall R waves (see Fig. 7.11).

5. With LVH the electrical axis is usually horizontal. Actual left axis deviation (i.e., an axis −30° or more negative) may also be seen. In addition, the

## Left Ventricular Hypertrophy

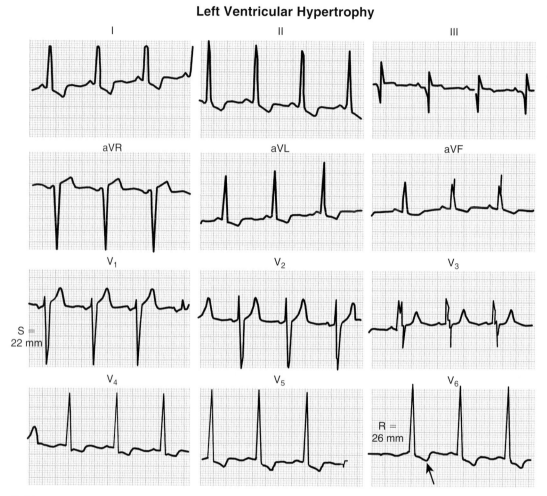

**Fig. 7.11** Pattern of left ventricular hypertrophy in a patient with severe hypertension. Tall voltages are seen in the chest leads and lead aVL (R = 17 mm). A repolarization (ST-T) abnormality, formerly referred to as a "strain" pattern, is also present in these leads. In addition, enlargement of the left atrium is indicated by a biphasic P wave in lead V₁.

QRS complex may become wider. Not uncommonly, patients with LVH eventually develop an incomplete or complete left bundle branch block (LBBB) pattern. Indeed, most patients with LBBB have underlying LVH (see Chapter 8). LVH is a common cause of an intraventricular conduction delay (IVCD) with features of LBBB.

6. Finally, signs of LAA (broad P waves in the extremity leads or biphasic P waves in lead V₁, with a prominent negative, terminal wave) are often seen in patients with ECG evidence of LVH. Most conditions that lead to LVH ultimately produce left atrial overload as well.

In summary, the diagnosis of LVH can be made with a high degree of specificity, but only modest sensitivity from the ECG if you find high QRS voltages (tall R waves in left-sided leads and deep S waves in right-sided ones), associated ST-T changes with well-defined signs of LAA. Because high voltage in the chest or extremity leads can routinely be seen in healthy people, especially athletes and young adults, the diagnosis of LVH should not be made based on this finding alone. Occasionally, ST-T changes resulting from left ventricular overload can also occur without voltage criteria for LVH.

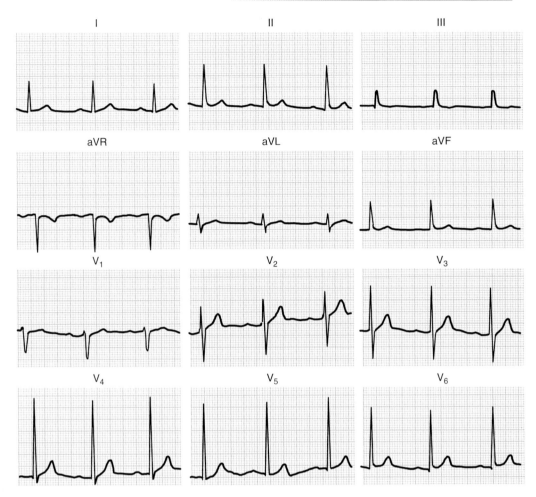

**Fig. 7.12** Tall voltages in the chest leads ($S_{V1}$ + $R_{V5}$ = 36 mm) from a 20-year-old man represent a common normal ECG variant, particularly in athletic or thin young adults. The ST-T complexes are normal, without evidence of repolarization (ST-T) abnormalities or left atrial abnormality.

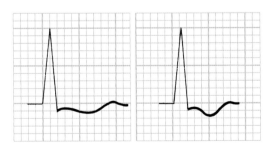

**Fig. 7.13** Repolarization abnormalities associated with left ventricular hypertrophy were formerly referred to as the "strain" pattern, an imprecise but still sometimes used term. Notice the characteristic slight ST segment depression with T wave inversion in the leads that show tall R waves. These repolarization changes can be referred to as "LVH-related ST-T changes" or "ST-T changes due to LV overload."

## THE ECG IN LVH: A CLINICAL PERSPECTIVE

═══════════ Key Points ═══════════

The recognition of LVH is clinically important for two major reasons:

1. *Diagnostically*, LVH is a clue to the presence of a potentially life-threatening *pressure* or *volume* overload state. The two most common and important pressure overload states are systemic hypertension and aortic stenosis. The three major clinical conditions associated with left ventricular volume overload are aortic regurgitation, mitral regurgitation, and dilated cardiomyopathy

of multiple causes. LVH patterns may also occur with hypertrophic cardiomyopathies.

2. *Prognostically*, patients with LVH from any cause are at increased risk for major cardiovascular complications, including *chronic heart failure* and serious atrial or ventricular arrhythmias, including atrial fibrillation, and ventricular tachyarrhythmias that may lead to sudden cardiac arrest. As noted, the myocardial fibrosis and neurochemical abnormalities often accompanying hypertrophy may potentiate both the mechanical decompensation and electrical instability.

---

If hypertrophy is present in both ventricles, the ECG usually shows mainly evidence of LVH. Another pattern that may provide an important clue to *biventricular hypertrophy* is LVH with rightward axis deviation. Biventricular hypertrophy may be present, for example, in some cases of severe dilated cardiomyopathy from a variety of causes or rheumatic valvular disease.

Finally, it is worth reemphasizing that in the assessment of cardiac size, the ECG is only an indirect assessment. A person may have underlying cardiac enlargement that does not show up on the ECG. Conversely, the ECG may show high voltage in the healthiest of individuals (young athletes) who do not have cardiac pathology. When the presence or degree of cardiac chamber enlargement must be determined with more precision, an *echocardiogram* should be obtained. For some suspected conditions, such as arrhythmogenic right ventricular cardiomyopathy/dysplasia (ARVC/D) or apical hypertrophic cardiomyopathy, a cardiac *magnetic resonance imaging* (MRI) study may be indicated.

# CHAPTER 8

# Ventricular Conduction Disturbances: Bundle Branch Blocks and Related Abnormalities

Recall that in the normal process of ventricular activation the electrical stimulus (signal) reaches the ventricles from the atria by way of the atrioventricular (AV) node and His–Purkinje system (Chapters 1 and 5). The first part of the ventricles to be stimulated (depolarized) is the left side of the ventricular septum. Soon after, the depolarization spreads simultaneously to the main mass of the left and right ventricles by way of the left and right bundle branches. Normally the entire process of ventricular depolarization in adults is completed within approximately 0.1 sec (100 msec). This is the reason the normal width of the QRS complex from all 12 leads is less than or equal to 110 msec by electronic measurements (or visually approximated at about 2.5 small boxes on the ECG graph paper). Any perturbation that interferes with the physiologic, near simultaneous stimulation of the ventricles through the His–Purkinje system may prolong the QRS width or change the QRS axis. This chapter primarily focuses on a major topic: the effects of blocks or delays within the bundle branch system on the QRS complex and ST-T waves. The clinical implications of these findings are also described.

## ECG IN VENTRICULAR CONDUCTION DISTURBANCES: GENERAL PRINCIPLES

A unifying principle in predicting what the ECG will show with a bundle branch or fascicular block is:

*The last (and usually dominant) component of the QRS vector will be shifted in the direction of the last part of the ventricles to be depolarized. In other words, the major QRS vector (arrow) shifts toward the regions of the heart that are most delayed in being stimulated (Box 8.1).*

Please go to expertconsult.inkling.com for additional online material for this chapter.

## RIGHT BUNDLE BRANCH BLOCK

Let's first consider the effect of cutting the right bundle branch, or slowing conduction in this structure relative to the left bundle. Right ventricular stimulation will be delayed and the QRS complex will be widened. The shape of the QRS with a right bundle branch block (RBBB) can be predicted on the basis of some familiar principles.

Normally, the first part of the ventricles to be depolarized is the left side of the interventricular septum (see Fig. 5.6A). On the normal ECG, this septal depolarization produces a small septal r wave in lead $V_1$ and a small septal q wave in lead $V_6$ (Fig. 8.1A). Because the left side of the septum is stimulated by a branch of the *left* bundle, RBBB will not affect septal depolarization.

The *second* phase of ventricular stimulation is the simultaneous depolarization of the left and right ventricles (see Fig. 6.6B). RBBB should not affect this phase much either, because the left ventricle is normally so electrically predominant, producing deep S waves in the right chest leads and tall R waves in the left chest leads (Fig. 8.1B). The change in the QRS complex produced by RBBB is a result of the delay in the total time needed for stimulation of the right ventricle. This means that after the left ventricle has completely depolarized, the right ventricle continues to depolarize.

This delayed right ventricular depolarization produces a *third* phase of ventricular stimulation. The electrical voltages in the third phase are directed to the right, reflecting the delayed depolarization and slow spread of the depolarization wave outward through the right ventricle. Therefore, a lead placed over the right side of the chest (e.g., lead $V_1$) records this phase of ventricular stimulation as a positive wide deflection (R′ wave). The rightward spread of

**61**

the delayed and slow right ventricular depolarization voltages produces a wide negative (S wave) deflection in the left chest leads (e.g., lead $V_6$) (Fig. 8.1C).

Based on an understanding of this step-by-step process, the pattern seen in the chest leads with RBBB can be derived. With RBBB, lead $V_1$ typically shows an rSR′ complex with a broad R′ wave. Lead $V_6$ shows a qRS-type complex with a broad S wave. The wide, tall R′ wave in the right chest leads and the deep terminal S wave in the left chest leads represent the same event viewed from opposite sides of the chest—the slow spread of delayed depolarization voltages through the right ventricle.

To make the initial diagnosis of RBBB, look at leads $V_1$ and $V_6$ in particular. The characteristic appearance of QRS complexes in these leads makes the diagnosis simple. (Fig. 8.1 shows how the delay in ventricular depolarization with RBBB produces the characteristic ECG patterns.)

In summary, the ventricular stimulation process in RBBB can be divided into three phases. The first two phases are normal septal and left ventricular depolarization. The third phase is delayed stimulation of the right ventricle. These three phases of ventricular stimulation with RBBB are represented on the ECG by the triphasic complexes seen in the chest leads:

- Lead $V_1$ shows an rSR′ complex with a wide R′ wave.
- Lead $V_6$ shows a qRS pattern with a wide S wave.

With RBBB pattern the QRS complex in lead $V_1$ generally shows an rSR′ pattern (Fig. 8.2). Occasionally, however, the S wave does not "make its way" below the baseline. Consequently, the complex in lead $V_1$ has the appearance of a wide, notched R wave, with largest amplitude at the end of the complex (Fig. 8.3).

Figs. 8.2 and 8.3 are typical examples of RBBB. Do you notice anything abnormal about the ST-T complexes in these tracings? If you look carefully, you can see that the T waves in the right chest leads are inverted. T wave inversions in the right chest leads are a characteristic finding with RBBB.

## Right Bundle Branch Block

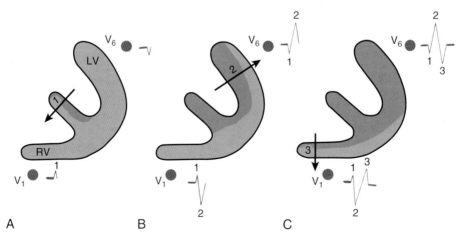

**Fig. 8.1** Step-by-step sequence of ventricular depolarization in right bundle branch block (see text).

## Right Bundle Branch Block

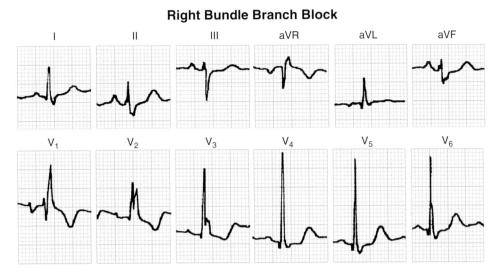

**Fig. 8.2** Notice the wide rSR′ complex in lead $V_1$ and the qRS complex in lead $V_6$. Inverted T waves in the right precordial leads (in this case $V_1$ to $V_3$) are common with right bundle branch block and are called *secondary* T wave inversions. Note also the left atrial abnormality pattern (biphasic P in $V_1$ with prominent negative component) and prominent R waves in $V_5$, consistent with underlying left ventricular hypertrophy.

### Right Bundle Branch Block Variant

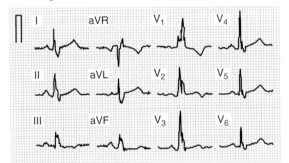

**Fig. 8.3** Instead of the classic rSR′ pattern with right bundle branch block, the right precordial leads sometimes show a wide notched R wave (seen here in leads $V_1$ to $V_3$). Notice the *secondary* T wave inversions in leads $V_1$ to $V_2$.

Slight-moderate ST depressions also may be seen, sometimes simulating ischemia. These alterations are referred to as *secondary changes* because they reflect just the delay in ventricular stimulation. By contrast, *primary ST-T wave abnormalities* reflect alterations in repolarization, independent of any QRS change. Examples of primary T wave abnormalities include T wave inversions resulting from ischemia (Chapters 9 and 10), selected electrolyte abnormalities (e.g.,

hypokalemia, hyperkalemia) (Chapter 11), and drugs (e.g., digoxin) (Chapter 20).

Of note, some ECGs show both primary and secondary ST-T changes. In Fig. 8.3 the T wave inversions in leads $V_1$ to $V_3$ and leads II, III, and aVF, can be explained solely on the basis of the RBBB because the negative T waves occur in leads with an rSR′-type complex. However, the T wave inversions or ST segment depressions in other leads ($V_4$ and $V_5$), not seen here, would represent a primary change, perhaps resulting from ischemia or a drug effect.

### Complete and Incomplete RBBB

RBBB is traditionally subdivided into complete and incomplete forms, depending on the width of the QRS complex. Complete RBBB in adults is defined by a QRS that is 0.12 sec or more in duration with an rSR′ in lead $V_1$ and a qRS in lead $V_6$. Incomplete RBBB shows the same QRS patterns, but with a waveform duration between 0.11 and 0.12 sec.

### Clinical Significance

RBBB may be caused by a number of factors. First, some people have RBBB as an incidental finding without any identifiable underlying heart disorder. Therefore RBBB, itself, as an isolated ECG abnormality does not indicate underlying heart disease. Furthermore, even under pathologic conditions,

RBBB is nonspecific. Second, it may be associated with many types of organic heart disease. It may occur with virtually any condition that affects the right side of the heart, including atrial septal defect with left-to-right shunting of blood, chronic pulmonary disease with pulmonary hypertension, and valvular lesions such as pulmonary stenosis, as well as cardiomyopathies and coronary disease. In some people (particularly older individuals), RBBB is sometimes related to chronic degenerative changes in the conduction system. RBBB may also occur transiently or permanently after cardiac surgery.

Acute pulmonary embolism, which produces acute right-sided heart overload, may cause a right ventricular conduction delay, usually associated with sinus tachycardia (see Chapter 11).

By itself, RBBB does not require any specific treatment. RBBB may be permanent or transient. Sometimes it appears only when the heart rate exceeds a certain critical value (rate-related RBBB), a non-diagnostic finding. *However, as noted later, in patients with acute ST segment elevation anterior myocardial infarction (MI), a new RBBB is of major importance because it indicates an increased risk of complete heart block, particularly when the RBBB is associated with left anterior or posterior fascicular block and a prolonged PR interval. A new RBBB in that setting is also a marker of more extensive myocardial damage, often associated with heart failure or even cardiogenic shock (see Chapter 9, Fig. 9.20).*

Chagas disease, a parasitic infection due to *Trypanosoma cruzi*, most prevalent in Latin America, may cause severe dilated cardiomyopathy, along with intraventricular and AV conduction abnormalities, including complete heart block and ventricular tachyarrhythmias. RBBB with left anterior fascicular block has been widely reported with this condition

A pattern resembling RBBB ("pseudo-RBBB") is characteristic of the *Brugada pattern*, important because it may be associated with increased risk of ventricular tachyarrhythmias (see Chapter 21; Fig. 21.9).

*Note:* An rSr′ pattern with a narrow QRS duration (100–110 msec or less in adults) and a very small (≤1–2 mm) terminal r′ wave in $V_1$ or $V_1$–$V_2$ is a common normal variant and should not be over-read as incomplete right bundle branch block.

## LEFT BUNDLE BRANCH BLOCK

Left bundle branch block (LBBB) also produces a pattern with a widened QRS complex. However, the QRS complex with LBBB is very different from that observed with RBBB. The major reason is that RBBB affects mainly the terminal phase of ventricular activation, whereas LBBB also affects the early phases.

Recall that, normally, the first phase of ventricular stimulation—depolarization of the left side of the septum—is started by a branch of the left bundle. LBBB alters the normal initial activation sequence. When LBBB is present, the septum depolarizes from *right* to *left* and not from left to right. Thus, the first major ECG change produced by LBBB is a loss of the normal septal r wave in lead $V_1$ and the normal septal q wave in lead $V_6$ (Fig. 8.4A). Furthermore, the total time for left ventricular depolarization is prolonged with LBBB. As a result, the QRS complex is abnormally wide. Lead $V_6$ shows a wide, entirely positive (R) wave (Fig. 8.4B). The right chest leads (e.g., $V_1$) record a negative QRS (QS) complex because

**Left Bundle Branch Block**

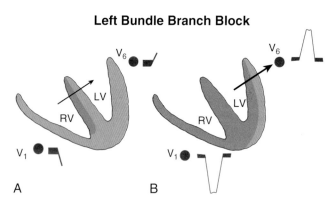

**Fig. 8.4** The sequence of early (A) and mid-late (B) ventricular depolarization in left bundle branch block (LBBB) produces a wide QS complex in lead $V_1$ and a wide R wave in lead $V_6$. (*Note:* Some authors also require that for classical LBBB, present here, the time from QRS onset to R wave peak, sometimes referred to as the *intrinsicoid deflection*, or *R wave peak time*, in leads $V_5$ and $V_6$ be greater than 60 msec; normally this subinterval is 40 msec or less.) However, this subinterval is difficult to measure, and we do not use it formally here.

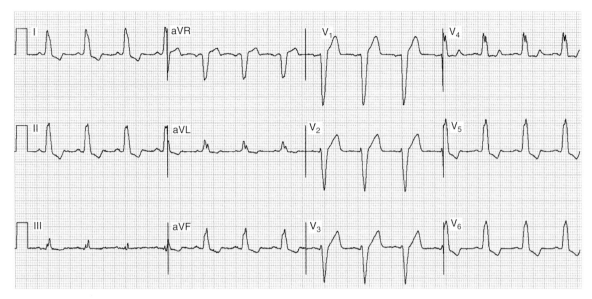

**Fig. 8.5** Classic example of complete left bundle branch block (LBBB). Underlying rhythm is sinus at rate of about 80/min. Note the wide QRS complexes in lead $V_1$ and the wide, notched R waves in leads $V_4$ to $V_6$ ("M-shape" in $V_4$). The ST depressions and T wave inversions (secondary repolarization abnormalities) in leads with predominant R waves are also characteristic of LBBB, as are the slight J point/ST elevations in leads $V_1$ to $V_3$.

the left ventricle is still electrically predominant with LBBB and therefore produces greater voltages than the right ventricle.

Thus, with LBBB the entire process of ventricular stimulation is oriented toward the left chest leads; that is, the septum depolarizes from right to left, and stimulation of the electrically predominant left ventricle is prolonged. Fig. 8.4 illustrates the sequence of ventricular activation in LBBB.[a]

With LBBB, the QS wave in lead $V_1$ sometimes shows a small notching at its nadir, giving the wave a characteristic W shape. Similarly, the broad R wave in lead $V_6$ may show a notching at its peak, giving it a distinctive M shape. An example of LBBB pattern is presented in Fig. 8.5.

Just as *secondary* T wave inversions occur with RBBB, they also occur with LBBB. As Fig. 8.5 shows, the T waves in the leads with tall R waves (e.g., the left precordial leads) are inverted; this is characteristic of LBBB. However, T wave inversions in the right precordial leads cannot be explained solely on the

basis of LBBB. If present, these T wave inversions reflect some *primary* abnormality, such as ischemia (see Fig. 9.21).

In summary, the diagnosis of complete LBBB pattern can be made with high probability when you find a wide QRS (≥0.12 sec or 120 msec) such that:

- Lead $V_1$ usually shows an entirely negative QS complex (more rarely, a wide rS complex, with a small r wave), and
- Lead $V_6$ shows a wide, tall R wave without a q wave.[b]

Usually, you should have no problem differentiating classic LBBB and RBBB patterns (Fig. 8.6). However, occasionally an ECG shows abnormally wide QRS complexes that are not typical of RBBB or LBBB pattern. In such cases the general term *intraventricular delay (IVCD)* is used (Fig. 8.7). *Cautions:*

- The term intraventricular conduction delay (IVCD) is used in two different and potentially confusing

---

[a]A variation of this pattern sometimes occurs: Lead $V_1$ may show an rS complex with a very small r wave and a wide S wave. This suggests that the septum is being stimulated normally from left to right. However, lead $V_6$ will still show an abnormally wide and notched R wave *without* an initial q wave.

[b]More refined definitions are sometimes given. For example, some authorities include an R-peak time (intrinsicoid) deflection (see Chapter 3) of >60 msec in leads $V_5$ and $V_6$. The QRS onset to R-peak time may be difficult to assess by eye. Thus, this criterion is not used in most clinical settings.

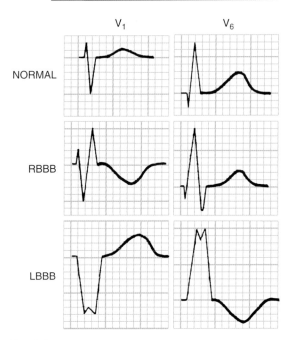

**Fig. 8.6** Comparison of patterns in leads $V_1$ and $V_6$, with normal conduction, right bundle branch block (RBBB), and left bundle branch block (LBBB). Normally lead $V_1$ shows an rS complex and lead $V_6$ shows a qR complex. With RBBB, lead $V_1$ shows a wider rSR′ complex and lead $V_6$ shows a qRS complex. With LBBB, lead $V_1$ shows a wide QS complex and lead $V_6$ shows a wide R wave.

ways clinically. First, it applies as a general term for QRS widening (especially ≥0.12 second) or more observed during a supraventricular tachycardia (e.g., sinus tachycardia, atrial fibrillation, atrial flutter, PSVT). As such, IVCD includes classic LBBB and RBBB waves, as well as more atypical morphologies.

- However, IVCD is often used to denote a wide QRS that does not have a classic LBBB or RBBB appearance (Fig. 8.7). This type of IVCD, especially resembling LBBB, is not uncommon due to severe LVH, and may progress to complete LBBB patterns. The distinction between LVH with an IVCD and LBBB is not always feasible.

## Complete and Incomplete LBBB
LBBB, like RBBB, has complete and incomplete forms. With complete LBBB, the QRS complex has the characteristic appearance described previously and is 0.12 sec or wider. With incomplete LBBB the QRS is between 0.1 and 0.12 sec wide. Incomplete

LBBB, with slow or absent r wave progression in leads $V_1$ to $V_3$, may be difficult or impossible to differentiate from actual underlying Q wave MI patterns or LVH. Sometimes, lead misplacement may contribute to the confusion. Echocardiography may be useful in looking for evidence of an actual infarction.

### Clinical Significance
Unlike RBBB, which is occasionally seen without evident cardiac disease, LBBB is usually a marker of organic heart disease. LBBB may develop in patients with long-standing hypertensive heart disease, a valvular lesion (e.g., calcification of the mitral annulus, aortic stenosis, or aortic regurgitation), or different types of cardiomyopathy (Chapter 12). It is also seen in patients with coronary artery disease and often correlates with impaired left ventricular function. Most patients with LBBB have underlying left ventricular hypertrophy (LVH) (Chapter 7). Degenerative changes in the conduction system may lead to LBBB, particularly in the elderly, as may injury or inflammation due to cardiac surgery or transcutaneous aortic value replacement (TAVR). Often, more than one contributing factor may be identified (e.g., hypertension and coronary artery disease). Rarely, otherwise normal individuals have LBBB pattern without evidence of organic heart disease by examination or even invasive studies. Echocardiograms usually show septal *dyssynchrony* due to abnormal ventricular activation patterns; other findings (e.g., valvular abnormalities, LVH, and diffuse wall motion disorders due to cardiomyopathy) are not unusual.

LBBB, like RBBB, may be permanent or transient. It also may appear only when the heart rate exceeds a certain critical value (tachycardia- or acceleration-dependent LBBB). Much less commonly, LBBB occurs only when the heart decelerates below some critical value (bradycardia or deceleration-dependent).

---
 Key Point
---

LBBB may be the first clue to four previously undiagnosed but clinically important structural abnormalities:
- Advanced coronary artery disease
- Valvular heart disease (mitral and/or aortic)
- Hypertensive heart disease
- Cardiomyopathy

---

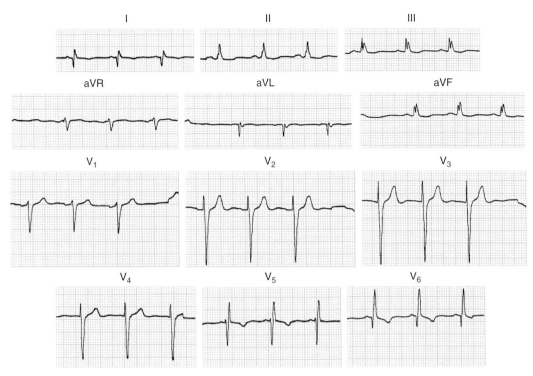

**Fig. 8.7** With a nonspecific intraventricular conduction delay (ICVD), the QRS complex is abnormally wide (≥0.12 sec). However, such a pattern is not typical of left or right bundle branch block. In this patient the pattern was caused by an anterolateral wall Q wave myocardial infarction (Chapter 9).

Finally, LBBB is often not only a marker of major underlying cardiac disease, but the *dyssynchrony* induced by this conduction abnormality may, itself, worsen cardiac function, especially in those with advanced heart disease. The use of *biventricular pacemaker* therapy to *resynchronize* ventricular contraction in patients with LBBB and heart failure is described in Chapter 22.

═══════════ Key Point ═══════════

The single most useful lead to distinguish RBBB and LBBB is V₁. With RBBB the last segment of the QRS (and sometimes the entire complex) will always be positive. With LBBB, the last segment (and usually the entire QRS) is negative.

## DIFFERENTIAL DIAGNOSIS OF BUNDLE BRANCH BLOCKS

Wide QRS complexes resembling complete bundle branch blocks and related IVCDs can be seen in other contexts, causing confusion and misdiagnosis. For example, left and right bundle branch block-appearing patterns are seen during ventricular pacing (Chapter 22). As you might predict, pacing from an endocardial lead positioned in the standard position (right ventricular apex) usually produces a QRS resembling LBBB. (Earlier activation of the right ventricle is equivalent to delayed activation of the left.) Furthermore, as you might predict, the mean frontal plane QRS vector usually points leftward and superiorly, that is, toward the positive poles of leads I and aVL and away from the positive poles of leads II, III, and aVF.

What does the QRS complex look like with biventricular pacing (for resynchronization therapy), which is usually accomplished by two electrodes

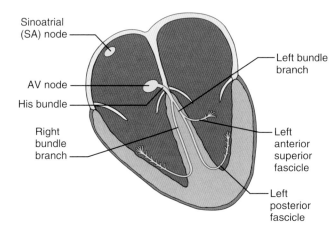

Sinoatrial
(SA) node

AV node

His bundle

Right
bundle
branch

Left bundle
branch

Left
anterior
superior
fascicle

Left
posterior
fascicle

**Fig. 8.8** Trifascicular conduction system. Notice that the left bundle branch subdivides into left anterior fascicle and left posterior fascicle. This highly schematized diagram is a revision of the original drawing of the conduction system (Fig. 1.1). In actuality, the fascicles are complex, tree-like branching structures. AV, atrioventricular.

pacing the ventricles in a near simultaneous way, one from a left ventricular lead located in the coronary sinus or a left posterolateral coronary vein, and the other in the right ventricle? Answer: If the left ventricular lead is programmed to fire milliseconds before the right, the QRS will usually resemble RBBB pattern with a wide, tall R wave in lead $V_1$ and a negative QRS complex in lead I. This pattern is consistent with a depolarization vector oriented from left to right and back to front (see also Chapter 21).

LBBB and RBBB are examples of *intrinsic* IVCDs. These patterns may be mimicked by *extrinsic* metabolic disturbances such as hyperkalemia (Chapter 11) and certain drug toxicities (e.g., flecainide) that block sodium ion influx into His–Purkinje-myocardial cells and slow conduction velocity. Paradoxically, a wide QRS may also occur with preexcitation (not delayed excitation), a hallmark of Wolff–Parkinson–White patterns and syndromes (Chapter 18). The differential diagnosis of a wide QRS is summarized in Chapter 25.

Finally, students and clinicians should be aware of the possible confusion surrounding the use of the *terms left bundle branch block or right bundle branch block morphology to describe ventricular tachycardias (VT)*. In this special context, the terms are used morphologically to describe the shape of the QRS, *not* presence of a bundle branch block per se. With VT originating from the right ventricle, the QRS usually shows a wide-complex tachycardia with LBBB morphology. With VT originating from the left ventricle or the left ventricular side of the septum, one generally sees a wide-complex tachycardia with

RBBB morphology. These important issues are discussed in Chapters 16 and 21.

## FASCICULAR BLOCKS (HEMIBLOCKS)

*Fascicular blocks*, or *hemiblocks*, are part of a slightly more complex but important topic. To this point, the left bundle branch system has been described as if it were a single pathway. Actually this system has been known for many years to be subdivided into an *anterior fascicle* and a *posterior fascicle* ("fascicle" is derived from the Latin *fasciculus*, meaning "small bundle"). The right bundle branch, by contrast, is a single pathway and consists of just one main fascicle or bundle. This revised concept of the bundle branch system as a *trifascicular* highway (one right lane and two left lanes) is illustrated in Fig. 8.8. More realistically, clinicians should recognize that the trifascicular concept, itself, is an oversimplification: the fascicles themselves are more complex in their structure, more like ramifying fans than single pathways.

However, clinically it is still useful to predict the effects of block at single or multiple locations in this trifascicular network. The ECG pattern with RBBB has already been presented (Figs. 8.2 and 8.3). The pattern of LBBB can occur in one of two ways: by a block in the left main bundle before it divides or by blocks in both subdivisions (anterior and posterior fascicles).

Now imagine that a block occurs in just the anterior or just the posterior fascicle of the left bundle. A block in either fascicle of the left bundle branch system is called a *fascicular block* or hemiblock. The recognition of fascicular blocks is intimately related to the subject of axis deviation (Chapter 6). Somewhat surprisingly, a left bundle fascicular block (or, synonymously, hemiblock), unlike a complete LBBB or RBBB, does not widen the QRS complex markedly. Experiments and clinical observations show that the main effect of slowing conduction in the fascicles of the left ventricular conduction system is a marked change in the QRS axis, with only minor increases in QRS duration. Specifically, along with some other changes, the most characteristic ECG finding from *left anterior* fascicular block (LAFB) is marked left axis deviation (about –45° or more negative); conversely, *left posterior* fascicular block (LPFB) produces marked right axis deviation (RAD) (about +120° or more positive).[c]

Complete bundle branch blocks, unlike fascicular blocks (hemiblocks), do *not always* cause a characteristic shift in the mean QRS axis. In contrast, LAFB shifts the QRS axis to the left by delaying activation of the more superior and leftward portions of the left ventricle. LPFB shifts it inferiorly and to the right by delaying activation of the more inferior and rightward portions of the left ventricle. Thus, in both cases the QRS axis is shifted *toward* the direction of delayed activation.

In summary, the major fascicular blocks are partial blocks in the left bundle branch system, involving either the anterior or posterior subdivisions. The diagnosis of a fascicular block is made primarily from the mean QRS axis in the extremity (frontal plane) leads. This situation contrasts with the diagnosis of complete (or incomplete) RBBB or LBBB, which is made primarily from the distinctive wide QRS patterns in the chest (horizontal plane) leads.

## Left Anterior Fascicular Block

Isolated (pure) LAFB is diagnosed by finding a mean QRS axis of −45° or more and a QRS width of less than 0.12 sec. As a rough but useful rule of thumb: A mean QRS axis of −45° or more can be easily recognized because the depth of the S wave in lead III is 1.4 or more times the height of the R wave in lead I or the depth of the S wave in aVF is equal to

# Left Anterior (Hemiblock) Fascicular Block

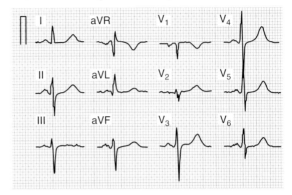

**Fig. 8.9** Left anterior (hemiblock) fascicular block. Notice the marked left axis deviation without significant widening of the QRS duration. (Left atrial abnormality is also present.) Compare this most common type of fascicular block with left posterior fascicular block (Fig. 10.8B), which produces marked right axis deviation.

or greater than the height of the R wave in lead I (Fig. 8.9). Leads I and sometimes aVL usually show a qR complex, with rS complexes in leads II, III, and aVF (or QS waves if an inferior MI is also present).

In general, the finding of isolated LAFB is a very common, nonspecific abnormality. This pattern may be seen with hypertension, aortic valve disease, coronary disease, and aging-related degenerative disease, and sometimes without identifiable cause (Fig. 8.10).

## Left Posterior Fascicular Block

Isolated LPFB is diagnosed by finding a mean QRS axis of +120° or more positive, with a QRS width of less than 0.12 sec. Usually an rS complex is seen in both leads I and aVL, in concert with a qR complex, is seen in leads II, III, and aVF. However, *the diagnosis of LPFB can be considered only after one of the other, far more common, causes of RAD have been excluded* (see Chapter 25). These factors include: normal variants, right ventricular hypertrophy (RVH), emphysema and other chronic lung diseases, lateral wall infarction (see Fig. 9.11), and acute or chronic pulmonary thromboembolism (or other causes of acute or sustained right ventricular overload, such as severe asthma or pulmonic stenosis). Of course, left–right arm electrode reversal, a spurious and not uncommon cause of right or extreme axis deviation, must be excluded (see Chapter 23).

## Bifascicular Block: Right Bundle Branch Block with Left Anterior Fascicular Block

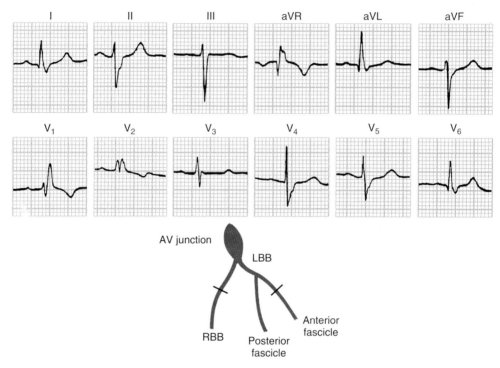

**Fig. 8.10** Right bundle branch block with left anterior fascicular block. Notice that the chest leads show a typical right bundle branch block pattern (rSR′ in lead V₁ and rS in lead V₆). The limb leads show left axis deviation (mean QRS axis about −45°), consistent with left anterior fascicular block. Thus, a bifascicular block involving the right bundle branch (RBB) and the anterior fascicle of the left bundle branch (LBB) system is present (as shown in the diagram). AV, atrioventricular.

Although LAFB is relatively common, isolated LPFB is extremely rare. Most often it occurs with RBBB, as shown in Fig. 8.11.

### Bifascicular and Trifascicular Blocks

Bifascicular block indicates blockage of any two of the three fascicles. For example, RBBB with LAFB produces a RBBB pattern with marked LAD (see Fig. 8.10); RBBB with LPFB (Fig. 8.10) produces a RBBB pattern with RAD (provided other causes of RAD, especially RVH and lateral MI, are excluded). Similarly, a complete LBBB may indicate blockage of both the anterior and posterior fascicles. Clinically, the term "bifascicular block" is usually reserved for RBBB with LAFB or LPFB. (Some authorities have recommended against using the term "bifascicular block," since it oversimplifies the patho-anatomy; but it is still widely employed.)

Bifascicular blocks of this type are potentially significant because they make ventricular conduction dependent on the single remaining fascicle. Additional damage to this third remaining fascicle may completely block AV conduction, producing third-degree heart block (the most severe form of *trifascicular block*).

The acute development of new bifascicular block, usually RBBB and LAFB (especially with a prolonged PR interval) during an acute anterior wall MI (see Chapters 9 and 10) may be an important warning signal of impending complete heart block and is considered by some an indication for a temporary pacemaker. However, chronic bifascicular blocks with normal sinus rhythm have a low rate of progression to complete heart block and are not indications by themselves for permanent pacemakers.

## Bifascicular Block: Right Bundle Branch Block with Left Posterior Fascicular Block

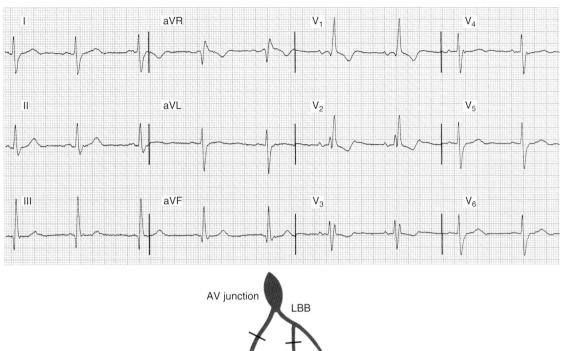

**Fig. 8.11** Bifascicular block (right bundle branch block [RBBB] with left posterior fascicular block). The chest leads show a typical RBBB pattern, while the limb leads show prominent right axis deviation (RAD). The combination of these two findings (in the absence of other more common causes of RAD such as right ventricular hypertrophy or lateral myocardial infarction [MI]) is consistent with chronic bifascicular block due to left posterior fascicular block in concert with the RBBB. This elderly patient had severe coronary artery disease. The prominent Q waves in leads III and aVF suggest underlying inferior wall MI. AV, atrioventricular.

Asymptomatic individuals (especially older ones) may have ECGs resembling the one in Fig. 8.10 showing RBBB with left axis deviation due to LAFB. Patients with chronic bifascicular block of this kind do not generally require a permanent pacemaker unless they develop second- or third-degree AV block.

*Trifascicular block with 1:1 AV conduction is rarely present on an ECG.* How can one infer trifascicular block from a 12-lead ECG without sustained or intermittent complete or advanced AV block? The answer is that sometimes patients will display alternating bundle branch block (RBBB and LBBB). Rarely, this type of alternation may occur on a beat-to-beat basis (be careful not to mistake

ventricular bigeminy for this!), or at different times during more prolonged periods of monitoring or on serial ECGs. For instance, if a patient presents with syncope and has RBBB on admission, and you note LBBB shortly afterwards, criteria for trifascicular block are met. Permanent pacemaker implantation (Chapter 22) is indicated for alternating LBBB and RBBB (trifascicular block) because of the high risk of abrupt complete AV heart block.

*Caution:* A common misconception is that bifascicular block (especially RBBB and LAFB) with a prolonged PR interval is indicative of trifascicular disease. This assumption is not correct. Indeed, a very long PR interval with RBBB and LAFB is more likely to indicate AV node disease in concert with bifascicular block. However, trifascicular disease cannot be inferred on the basis of this combination.

## DIAGNOSIS OF HYPERTROPHY IN THE PRESENCE OF BUNDLE BRANCH BLOCKS

The ECG diagnosis of hypertrophy (Chapter 7) in the presence of bundle branch blocks may pose special problems. A few general guidelines are helpful.

When RVH occurs with RBBB, RAD is often present. Tall peaked P waves with RBBB should also suggest underlying RVH.

The usual voltage criteria for LVH can be applied in the presence of RBBB. However, clinicians should recognize that RBBB may mask typical voltage increases by decreasing the size of the S wave in lead $V_1$. The presence of left atrial abnormality (LAA) with RBBB suggests underlying LVH (see Fig. 8.3).

The finding of LBBB, regardless of the QRS voltage, is highly suggestive of underlying LVH. Finding LBBB with prominent QRS voltages *and* evidence of left atrial abnormality virtually ensures the diagnosis of LVH (see Chapter 7).

Finally, it should be reemphasized that the *echocardiogram* is much more accurate than the ECG in the diagnosis of cardiac enlargement (see Chapter 7).

## DIAGNOSIS OF MYOCARDIAL INFARCTION IN THE PRESENCE OF BUNDLE BRANCH BLOCKS

The ECG diagnosis of acute and chronic MI in the presence of bundle branch blocks is discussed in Chapters 9 and 10.

# CHAPTER 9

# Myocardial Ischemia and Infarction, Part I: ST Segment Elevation and Q Wave Syndromes

This chapter and the next examine one of the most important topics in ECG analysis and clinical medicine, namely the diagnosis of myocardial ischemia and infarction (ischemic heart disease),[a] including ST segment elevation myocardial infarction (STEMI). Basic terms and concepts are briefly discussed first.

## MYOCARDIAL ISCHEMIA: GENERAL

Myocardial cells require oxygen and other nutrients to function. Oxygenated blood is supplied by the coronary arteries. If severe narrowing or complete blockage of a coronary artery causes the blood flow to become inadequate to meet demands for oxygen and nutrients, ischemia of the heart muscle develops. This intuitive notion underlies the concept of ischemia as related to a "mismatching of supply/demand" such that the denominator exceeds the numerator.

The three key factors that determine left ventricular myocardial oxygen demands are: (1) the heart rate (chronotropic state); (2) the strength of its contractions (contractility or inotropic state); and (3) the systolic pressure developed in the main pumping chamber (the variable most important in determining the wall tension).

Myocardial ischemia may occur transiently. For example, patients who experience classic angina pectoris (e.g., discomfort in the central chest area) often report this symptom with exertion, which increases all three determinants of myocardial oxygen demand. Sustained ischemia of sufficient degree is

Please go to expertconsult.inkling.com for additional online material for this chapter.
[a]The terms *infarction* and *infarct* are used interchangeably in this book and clinical practice.

the cause of necrosis (myocardial infarction) of a portion of heart muscle.

The related term *acute coronary syndrome (ACS)* refers to conditions associated with an abrupt decrease in effective coronary artery perfusion, and includes unstable angina (specially that occurring at rest or with increasing severity or duration), actual myocardial infarction (MI), and sudden cardiac arrest due to acute myocardial ischemia.

The everyday term "heart attack" refers to MI. However, keep in mind that what a patient or even another caregiver has labeled a "heart attack" may or may not have been a *bona fide* MI. Careful and critical review of available documentation, especially ECGs, serum cardiac enzyme levels, and relevant noninvasive and invasive studies, is essential to confirm this history.

Our discussion focuses primarily on ischemia and infarction of the left ventricle, the main pumping chamber of the heart. The important clinical topic of right ventricular infarction is also discussed briefly. The typical serial changes involving ST elevations and Qs wave on the ECG are examined in this chapter. Chapter 10 discusses the variability of ischemia-related ECG patterns, highlighting non-ST segment elevation ischemia/infarction and non-Q wave infarctions.

## TRANSMURAL AND SUBENDOCARDIAL ISCHEMIA

A much simplified cross-sectional diagram of the left ventricle is presented in Fig. 9.1. Notice that the left ventricle consists of an outer layer (*epicardium* or *subepicardium*) and an inner layer (*endocardium* or *subendocardium*). This distinction is important because myocardial ischemia may primarily affect

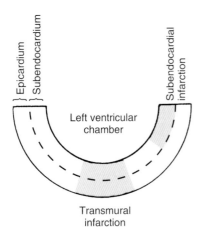

**Fig. 9.1** Schematic cross-section of the left ventricle comparing a *subendocardial* infarct, which involves the inner half of the ventricular wall, and a *transmural* infarct, which involves the full thickness (or almost the full thickness) of the wall. As discussed in the text, pathologic Q waves may be a marker of transmural infarction. However, not all transmural myocardial infarctions produce abnormal Q waves. Furthermore, in some cases, non-transmural infarctions are associated with Q waves.

part of the inner layers, or it may be severe enough to affect virtually the entire thickness of the ventricular wall: subendocardial and subepicardial. This "through and through" combination is termed *transmural ischemia*.

## MYOCARDIAL BLOOD SUPPLY

The cardiac blood supply is delivered by the three main coronary arteries and their branches (Fig. 9.2). MIs tend to be *localized* to the general region (i.e., anterior vs. inferior) of the left ventricle supplied by one of these arteries or their major tributaries The right coronary artery (RCA) supplies both the inferior (diaphragmatic) portion of the heart and the right ventricle. The left main coronary artery is short and divides into (1) the left anterior descending (LAD), which generally supplies the ventricular septum and a large part of the left ventricular free wall, and (2) the left circumflex (LCx) coronary artery, which supplies the lateral wall of the left ventricle. This circulation pattern may be quite variable from one person to the next. In most individuals the RCA

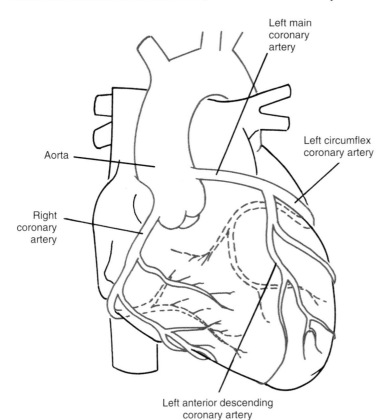

**Fig. 9.2** The major coronary arteries that supply blood to the heart muscle.

also supplies the posterior and sometimes even a section of the lateral wall. Less often the circumflex artery supplies the inferoposterior portion of the left ventricle.

## ST SEGMENT ELEVATION ISCHEMIA AND ACUTE MYOCARDIAL INFARCTION

ST elevation myocardial infarction (STEMI) is characterized by severe ischemia and ultimately necrosis of a portion of the entire (or nearly the full) thickness of a portion of the left (and sometimes right) ventricular wall. Most patients who present with acute STEMI have underlying atherosclerotic coronary artery disease. The usual pathophysiology of STEMI, sometimes evolving into a Q wave MI, relates to blockage of one of the major epicardial coronary arteries by a ruptured or eroded (ulcerated) atherosclerotic plaque, an event followed by the formation of a clot (thrombus) at this intra-coronary site. The "culprit artery" thrombus is composed of platelets and fibrin, blocking the blood flow to myocardial tissue downstream.

Multiple factors other than atherosclerotic plaque disruption may initiate or contribute to acute STEMI, including coronary artery dissections (rare events occurring post-partum, with connective tissue disease, or induced during percutaneous coronary procedures), coronary emboli, spontaneous or drug-induced (e.g., cocaine) coronary vasospasm, and the syndrome known as stress (*takotsubo*) cardiomyopathy (see page 91 and Chapter 10).

Not surprisingly, the more extensive and severe MIs are the most likely to produce changes in both myocardial repolarization (ST-T) and depolarization (QRS complex). The earliest ECG changes seen with acute transmural ischemia/infarction typically occur in the ST-T complex in the two major, sequential phases:

1. The *acute* phase is marked by the appearance of ST segment elevations and sometimes tall positive (so-called *hyperacute*) T waves in multiple (usually two or more) leads. The term "STEMI" refers specifically to MIs with new or increased elevation of the ST segment, sometimes with prominent T waves, which are usually associated with complete or near complete occlusion of an epicardial coronary artery. *Reciprocal* ST depressions may occur in leads whose positive poles are directed about 180° degrees from those showing

ST elevations. Thus, an inferior MI may be marked by ST elevations in leads II, III, and aVF, along with ST depressions in I, and aVL. ST depressions may also be present in $V_1$ to $V_3$ if there is associated lateral or posterior wall involvement.

2. The *evolving* phase occurs hours or days later and is characterized by deep T wave inversions in the leads that previously showed ST elevations.

ST elevation MIs are also described in terms of the presumed location of the infarct. *Anterior* means that the infarct involves the anterior or lateral wall of the left ventricle, whereas *inferior* indicates involvement of the lower (diaphragmatic) wall of the left ventricle (Fig. 9.3). For example, with an acute anterior wall MI, the ST segment elevations and tall hyperacute T waves appear in two or more of the anterior leads (chest leads $V_1$ to $V_6$ and extremity leads I and aVL) (Fig. 9.4). With an inferior wall MI the ST segment elevations and tall *hyperacute* T waves are seen in two or more of the inferior leads II, III, and aVF (Fig. 9.5).

The ST segment elevation pattern seen with acute MI is technically called a *current of injury* and indicates that damage involves the epicardial (outer) layer of the heart as a result of severe ischemia. The exact reasons that acute MI produces ST segment elevation are complicated and not fully known. What follows is a very brief overview of the mechanism of the injury current reflected in ST deviations.

Under normal conditions, no net current flows at the time ST segment is inscribed since the myocardial fibers all attain about the same voltage level during the corresponding (plateau) phase of the ventricular action potential. Severe ischemia, with

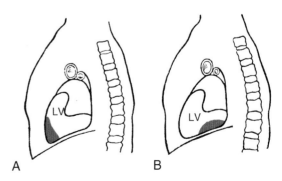

**Fig. 9.3** Myocardial infarctions are most generally localized to either the anterior portion of the left ventricle (A) or the inferior (diaphragmatic) portion of the walls of this chamber (B).

### ECG Sequence with Anterior Wall Q Wave Infarction

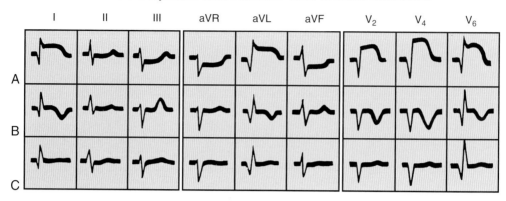

**Fig. 9.4** (A) Acute phase of an anterior wall ST elevation/Q wave infarction: ST segment elevations and new Q waves. (B) Evolving phase: deep T wave inversions. (C) Resolving phase: partial or complete regression of ST-T changes (and sometimes of Q waves). In (A) and (B), notice the reciprocal ST-T changes in the inferior leads (II, III, and aVF).

### ECG Sequence with Inferior Wall Q Wave Infarction

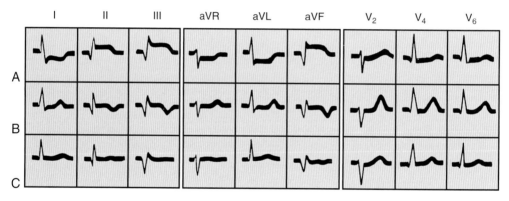

**Fig. 9.5** (A) Acute phase of an inferior wall myocardial infarction: ST segment elevations and new Q waves. (B) Evolving phase: deep T wave inversions. (C) Resolving phase: partial or complete regression of ST-T changes (and sometimes of Q waves). In (A) and (B), notice the reciprocal ST-T changes in the anterior leads (I, aVL, V$_2$, V$_4$).

or without actual infarction, alters the balance of electrical charges across the myocardial cell membranes. As a result, a voltage gradient forms between normal and ischemic cells during the plateau phase (and other phases) of their action potentials. This voltage gradient leads to current flow – the current of injury. The emergence of the ST segment deviations on the body surface ECG is related to these cellular injury currents.

The ST segment elevations seen with acute MI may have different morphologies (Fig. 9.6). Notice that the ST segment may be plateau-shaped or

dome-shaped. Sometimes it is obliquely elevated, or it may retain its concave (unsloping) appearance.[b] Furthermore, the morphology of the ST elevations may vary from one time to the next in the same individual during an STEMI.

Pathologic ST segment elevations (and reciprocal ST depressions) are the *earliest* ECG signs of infarction, and are generally seen within minutes of blood

---

[b]Marked ST elevations and tall positive T waves in the context of an STEMI are sometimes informally referred to as the "tombstone" pattern because of their appearance and ominous prognosis. The more technical term is a *monophasic current of injury* pattern.

flow occlusion. As noted, relatively tall, positive (hyperacute) T waves may also be seen at this time (Figs. 9.7 and 9.8). These T waves have the same significance as the ST elevations. In some cases, hyperacute T waves actually precede the ST elevations.

Guidelines for assessing whether ST segment (and associated J point) elevations are due to acute ischemia have been proposed. However, invoking strict criteria is of limited use because of false positives (due to normal variants, left ventricular hypertrophy, left bundle branch block, etc., as described in Chapter 10) and false negatives (e.g., T wave positivity may precede ST elevations, the ST elevations may be less than 1–2 mm in amplitude, and they may not be present in an adjacent lead).[c]

Clinicians should also be aware that ST changes in acute ischemia may evolve rapidly with a patient under observation. If the initial ECG is not diagnostic of STEMI but the patient continues to have symptoms consistent with myocardial ischemia, obtaining serial ECGs at 5- to 10-minute intervals (or continuous 12-lead ST segment monitoring) is strongly recommended.

After a variable time lag (usually hours to a few days) the elevated ST segments start to return to the baseline. At the same time the T waves become inverted (negative) in leads that previously showed ST segment elevations. This phase of T wave inversions is called the *evolving phase* of the infarction. Thus with an anterior wall infarction the T waves become inverted in one or more of the anterior leads ($V_1$ to $V_6$, I, aVL). With an *inferior* wall infarction the T waves become inverted in one or more of the inferior leads (II, III, aVF). These T wave inversions are illustrated in Figs. 9.4 and 9.5. The spontaneous sequence of evolving ST-T changes may be substantially altered by interventions designed to produce reperfusion of an occluded coronary artery.

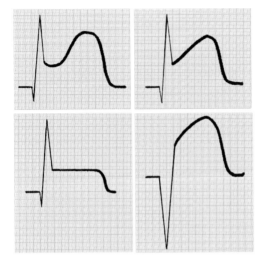

**Fig. 9.6** Variable shapes of ST segment elevations seen with acute myocardial infarctions.

---

[c] Consider an inferolateral MI with ST elevations in II, III, aVF, and $V_6$ or one involving occlusion of the left main coronary artery with primary ST elevations in leads aVR and $V_1$ (see Chapter 10). The leads here are not "contiguous."

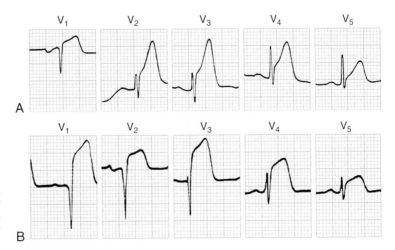

**Fig. 9.7** Chest leads from a patient with acute anterior ST segment elevation myocardial infarction (STEMI). (A) In the earliest phase of the infarction, tall, positive (hyperacute) T waves are seen in leads $V_2$ to $V_5$. (B) Several hours later, marked ST segment elevations are present in the same leads (*current of injury pattern*), and abnormal Q waves are seen in leads in $V_1$ and $V_2$.

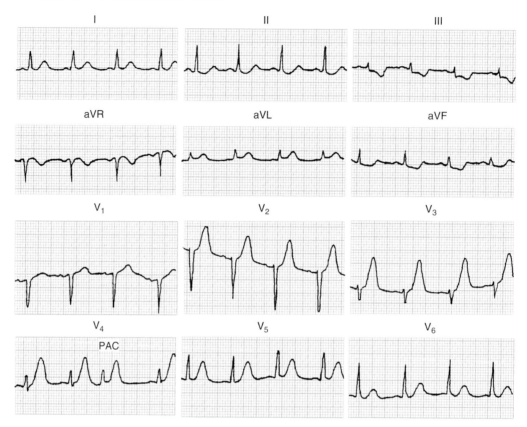

**Fig. 9.8** Hyperacute T waves with anterior ST segment elevation myocardial infarction (STEMI). This patient complained of severe chest discomfort. Notice the very tall (hyperacute) T waves in the chest leads. In addition, slight ST segment elevations are present in lead aVL and reciprocal ST depressions are seen in leads II, III, and aVF. A premature atrial complex (PAC) is present in lead $V_4$.

---

## Avoiding Semantic Confusion: Ischemia vs. Injury vs. Infarction

Confusion among students and clinicians is understandable given that these terms are used in different ways by different authors. Based on "current" evidence, we favor the following:

- Avoid the term *myocardial injury*. It is nonspecific and ambiguous.
- Use *current of injury* to refer to abnormal current flow caused by acute ischemia. A current of injury underlies the pathophysiology of both ST elevations and ST depressions caused by acute ischemia.

- Reserve stating that: "an ECG shows a *current of injury* pattern" for situations where you mean to say that the recording shows ischemic ST elevations or depressions. Then specify what leads show these changes.

Keep in mind that ECG evidence of infarction may not only relate to ST deviations (current of injury patterns), but also to T wave inversions, and sometimes to the appearance of pathologic Q waves.

- Emergency reperfusion therapies with percutaneous coronary interventions or intravenous thrombolytic medications have been shown consistently to improve mortality only for acute STEMI.
- The earlier such therapy is given after the onset of the acute STEMI the more likely it is to reduce the size of the infarct and the risk of major complications, including heart failure and death.
- The most successful reperfusion therapy for STEMI is associated with a prompt decrease in the amplitude of the ischemic ST elevations and the absence of new Q waves.

## QRS Changes: Q Waves of Infarction

MI, particularly when large and transmural, often produces distinctive changes in the QRS (depolarization) complex. The characteristic depolarization sign is the appearance of new Q waves. Why do certain MIs lead to pathologic Q waves? Recall that a Q wave is simply an initial negative deflection of the QRS complex. If the entire QRS complex is negative, it is called a *QS complex*:

A Q wave (negative initial QRS deflection) in any lead indicates that the electrical voltages are directed away from that particular lead. With a transmural infarction, necrosis of heart muscle occurs in a localized area of the ventricle. As a result the electrical voltages produced by this portion of the myocardium disappear. Instead of positive (R) waves over the infarcted area, Q waves are often recorded (either a QR or QS complex).

As discussed in the next chapter, the common clinical tendency to equate pathologic Q waves with transmural necrosis is an oversimplification. *Not all transmural infarcts lead to Q waves, and not all Q wave infarcts correlate with transmural necrosis.*

The new Q waves of an MI generally appear within the first day or so of the infarct. With an anterior wall infarction these Q waves are seen in one or more of leads $V_1$ to $V_6$, I, and aVL (see Fig. 9.4). With an inferior wall MI the new Q waves appear in leads II, III, and aVF (see Fig. 9.5).

In summary, abnormal Q waves, in the appropriate context, are characteristic markers of infarction. They signify the loss of positive electrical voltages (potential), which is caused by the death of heart muscle.

## ECG LOCALIZATION OF INFARCTIONS

As mentioned earlier, MIs are generally localized to a specific portion of the left ventricle, affecting either the anterior or the inferior wall. Anterior infarctions are often further designated by ECG readers as *anteroseptal, anterior free wall,* or *high lateral* depending on the leads that show signs of the infarction (Figs. 9.9–9.11). However, these traditional ECG-MI correlations, also including terms such *anterolateral* or *anteroapical*, are at best approximate, and often misleading or ambiguous when compared to more direct anatomic determinations of infarct location obtained with contemporary imaging (echocardiographic or magnetic resonance) studies or from post-mortem studies.

### Anterior Wall Q Wave Infarctions

The characteristic feature of an anterior wall Q wave infarct is *the loss of normal R wave progression in at least two to three of the chest leads.* Recall that normally the height of the R wave (R/S ratio) increases progressively as you move from lead $V_1$ toward lead $V_6$. An anterior infarct interrupts this progression, and the result may be pathologic Q waves in one or more of the chest leads. As noted, cardiologists often attempt to further localize anterior MIs based on the leads showing Q waves.

### Anteroseptal Infarctions

Remember from Chapter 5 that the ventricular septum is normally depolarized from left to right, and in an anterior direction, so that leads $V_1$ and $V_2$ show small positive (r) waves (septal r waves). Now consider the effect of damaging the septum. Obviously, septal depolarization voltages are lost. Thus the r waves in leads $V_1$ to $V_3$ may disappear and an entirely negative (QS) complex appears. The septum is supplied with blood by the left anterior descending coronary artery. Septal infarction generally suggests that this artery or one of its branches is occluded.

### Anterior Free Wall/Antero-Apical Infarctions

An infarction of the free wall and apex of the left ventricle usually produces changes in the more

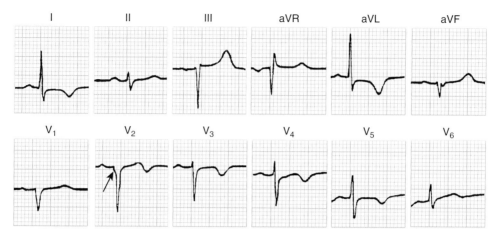

**Fig. 9.9** Anterior wall infarction. The QS complexes in leads $V_1$ and $V_2$ indicate anteroseptal infarction. A characteristic notching of the QS complex, often seen with infarcts, is present in lead $V_2$ (*arrow*). In addition, the diffuse ischemic T wave inversions in leads I, aVL, and $V_2$ to $V_5$ indicate generalized anterior wall ischemia or non-Q wave myocardial infarction.

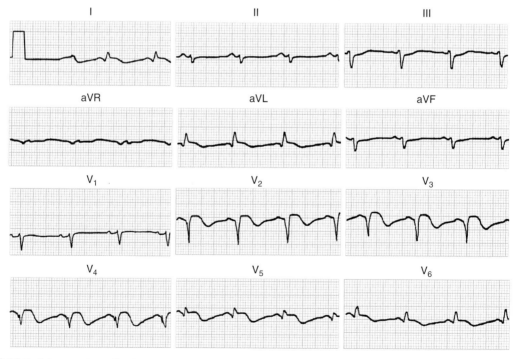

**Fig. 9.10** Evolving anterior wall infarction. The patient sustained the infarct 1 week earlier. Notice the abnormal Q waves (leads I, aVL, and $V_2$ to $V_5$) with slight ST segment elevations and deep T wave inversions. Marked left axis deviation resulting from left anterior fascicular block is also present (see Chapter 8).

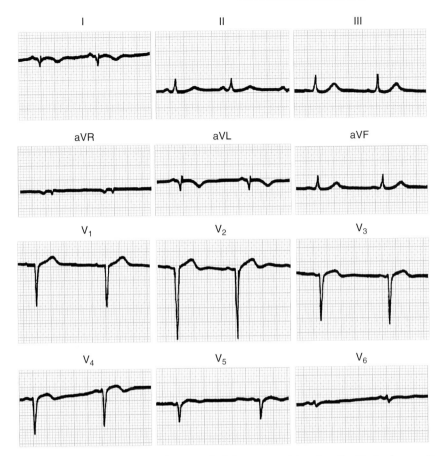

**Fig. 9.11** Evolving extensive anterior-lateral wall infarction. The infarct occurred 1 week earlier. Notice the poor R wave progression in leads $V_1$ to $V_5$ with Q waves in leads I and aVL. The T waves are slightly inverted in these leads. In this ECG, right axis deviation is the result of loss of lateral wall forces, with Q waves seen in leads I and aVL.

central and laterally situated chest leads. With such infarctions, abnormal Q waves, as part of QS or QR complexes, appear in leads $V_3$ to $V_6$ (see Fig. 8.7). The infarcts are typically caused by occlusion of the left anterior descending coronary artery, involving one or more diagonal branches.

## High Lateral Infarctions

ST elevations and pathologic Q waves localized to leads I and aVL are often ascribed to a "high lateral" MI. The "culprit artery" in such cases is usually an occluded diagonal branch of the left anterior descending or branch (ramus) of the left circumflex coronary.

## ECG Localization of Anterior Wall Infarctions: Comments and Caveats

To emphasize, the foregoing classification of anterior infarctions is not absolute, and infarct loci often overlap. To avoid ambiguity, clinicians can describe a suspected or confirmed infarct most effectively by referring to the patterns seen and giving the specific leads. For example you might say or write: "The ECG shows findings consistent with an anterior ST elevation/Q wave with primary changes in lead $V_2$ to $V_5$ and probable reciprocal ST depressions in leads II, III, and aVF." Not surprisingly, anterior infarctions associated with large Q waves in leads $V_1$ to $V_5$ or $V_6$ usually represent extensive damage and substantially reduced left ventricular (LV) function (LV ejection fraction) (see Fig. 9.11).

## Inferior Wall Infarctions

Infarction of the inferior (diaphragmatic) portion of the left ventricle is indicated by changes in leads II, III, and aVF (Figs. 9.12–9.14). These three leads, as shown in the diagram of the frontal plane axis, are oriented downward/inferiorly (see Fig. 6.1). Thus they record positive voltages originating from the inferior portion of the ventricle. Larger inferior wall infarctions are more like to produce abnormal Q waves in leads II, III, and aVF. This type of infarction is generally caused by occlusion of the right coronary artery. Less commonly inferior wall MI occurs due to occlusion of a left circumflex coronary obstruction.

## Posterior Infarctions

Infarctions can occur in the posterior (back) surface of the left ventricle. These infarctions may be difficult to diagnose because characteristic abnormal ST elevations may not appear in any of the 12 conventional leads. Instead, tall R waves and ST depressions may occur in leads $V_1$ and $V_2$ (reciprocal to the Q waves and ST segment elevations that would be recorded at the back of the heart). During the evolving phase of these infarctions, when deep T wave inversions appear in the posterior leads, the anterior chest leads show reciprocally tall positive T waves (Fig. 9.15).

An MI isolated exclusively to the posterior left ventricle ("true posterior") is relatively rare. Most cases of posterior MI, manifest with involvement of the lateral infarction (producing characteristic changes in lead $V_5/V_6$), and/ or in the context of an inferior MI, producing characteristic changes in leads II, III, and aVF (see Fig. 9.15). Because of the overlap between *inferior, lateral,* and *posterior* infarctions, the more general terms *inferoposterior* or *posterolateral* are often used, depending on which leads are involved.

## Acute Inferolateral STEMI

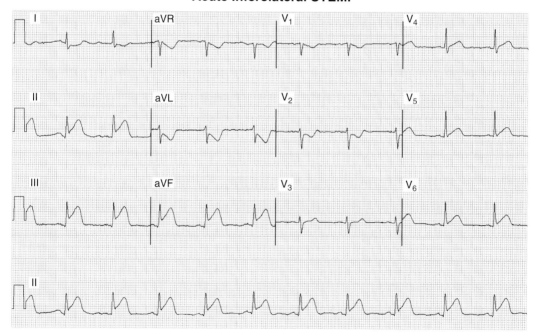

**Fig. 9.12** Acute inferolateral wall ST segment elevation myocardial infarction (STEMI). Notice the prominent ST elevations in leads II, III, and aVF, as well as, more subtly, in $V_5$ and $V_6$. The reciprocal ST depressions are in leads I and aVL, and $V_1$ to $V_2$. The latter finding may be reciprocal to lateral or posterior ischemia. (Reproduced with permission from Nathanson LA, McClennen S, Safran C, Goldberger AL. ECG wave-maven: Self-assessment program for students and clinicians. http://ecg.bidmc.harvard.edu.)

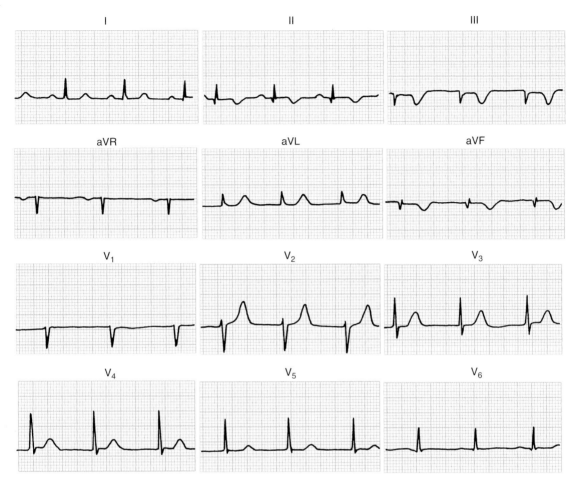

**Fig. 9.13** Inferior wall infarction. This patient sustained a myocardial infarction 1 month previously. Notice the abnormal Q waves and symmetrical T wave inversions in leads II, III, and aVF. In addition, T wave flattening is seen in lead $V_6$. After infarction, Q waves and ST-T changes may persist indefinitely or may resolve partially or completely.

Clinicians may find it useful to place additional electrodes around the patient's back to record leads $V_7$ to $V_9$ to enhance the sensitivity of the ECG in detecting ST elevations associated with acute infarctions involving the posterolateral wall (see Box 9.1).

### Right Ventricular Infarctions

Clinical imaging and post-mortem studies have shown that patients with an inferior infarct not uncommonly have associated right ventricular involvement. Right ventricular involvement may occur in as many as one-third of cases of inferior MI. Clinically, patients with a right ventricular infarct may have elevated central venous pressure (distended neck veins) because of the abnormally high diastolic

| BOX 9.1 | Additional Posterior Leads for MI Diagnosis |
|---|---|
| $V_7$ | Posterior axillary line at the same horizontal plane as for $V_4$ to $V_6$ electrodes |
| $V_8$ | Posterior scapular line at the same horizontal plane as $V_4$ to $V_6$ electrodes |
| $V_9$ | Left border of spine at the same horizontal plane as $V_4$ to $V_6$ electrodes |

filling pressures in the right side of the heart. If the damage to the right ventricle is severe, hypotension and even cardiogenic shock may result. Atrioventricular conduction disturbances are not uncommon in this setting, including AV Wenckebach and

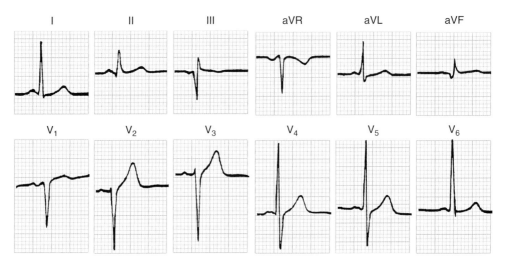

**Fig. 9.14** Prior (chronic) inferior wall infarction. Notice the prominent Q waves in leads II, III, and aVF from a patient who had a myocardial infarction 1 year previously. The ST-T changes have essentially reverted to normal.

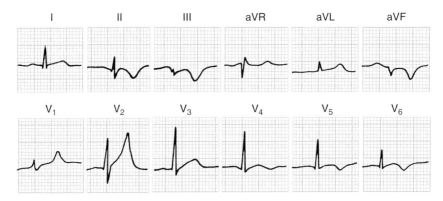

**Fig. 9.15** "Posterior" infarction. Notice the tall R waves in leads $V_1$ and $V_2$. This patient had a previous inferior infarction (Q waves in leads II, III, aVF) and probably a lateral infarction as well (T wave inversions in leads $V_4$ to $V_6$). Notice also the reciprocally tall, positive T waves in anterior precordial leads $V_1$ and $V_2$. (Reproduced from Goldberger AL. Myocardial infarction: Electrocardiographic differential diagnosis. 4th ed. St. Louis: Mosby; 1991.)

sometimes complete heart block. The presence of jugular venous distention in patients with acute inferoposterior wall MIs—or an acute drop in blood pressure after administration of nitroglycerin—should always suggest the diagnosis of associated right ventricular MI. Many of these patients also have ST segment elevations in leads reflecting the right ventricle, such as $V_1$ and $V_3R$ to $V_6R$, as shown in Fig. 9.16 (see also Chapter 4).

## CLASSIC SEQUENCE OF ST-T CHANGES AND Q WAVES WITH STEMI

To this point the ventricular depolarization (QRS complex) and repolarization (ST-T complex) changes produced by an acute MI have been discussed separately. As shown in Figs. 9.4 and 9.5, these changes often occur sequentially.

Ordinarily, the earliest sign of transmural ischemia is ST segment elevations (with reciprocal

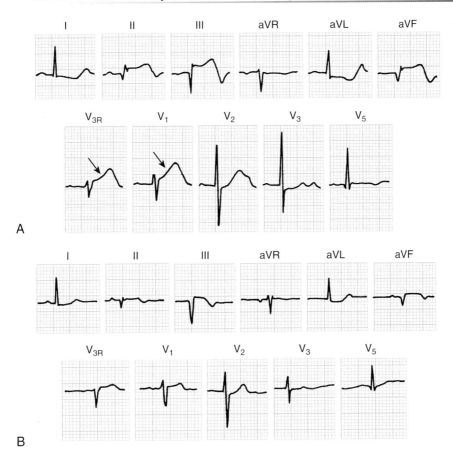

**Fig. 9.16** Acute right ventricular ischemia with inferior wall infarction. (A) Q waves and ST segment elevations in leads II, III, and aVF are accompanied by ST segment elevations (*arrows*) in the right precordial leads ($V_3R$ and $V_1$). The ST-T changes in lead $V_6$ are consistent with lateral wall ischemia. The ST segment depressions in leads I and aVL are probably reciprocal to inferior lead ST elevations. (B) Follow-up tracing obtained the next day, showing diminution of the ST changes. (Reproduced from Goldberger AL. Myocardial infarction: Electrocardiographic differential diagnosis. 4th ed. St. Louis: Mosby; 1991.)

ST depressions). The ST elevations (current of injury pattern) usually persist for hours to days. During this same period, Q waves often begin to appear in the leads that show ST elevations. Once these changes have occurred, the ST segments start to return to the isoelectric baseline and the T waves become inverted during the evolving phase.

In the weeks or months after an infarct, what should you expect to happen to the Q waves and the ST-T changes just described? The answer is that you cannot make any certain predictions. In most cases the abnormal Q waves persist for months and even years after the acute infarction. Occasionally, however, the abnormal Q waves diminish in size

and even disappear entirely. In some cases, abnormal T wave inversions persist indefinitely. In others, improvement occurs, but minor nonspecific ST-T abnormalities such as slight T wave flattening may persist (see Figs. 9.4 and 9.5). Persistent ST segment elevations months to years after an MI (especially anterior) may represent a ventricular aneurysm.

## Normal and Abnormal Q Waves: A Brief Overview

A frequently encountered diagnostic problem is deciding whether Q waves are abnormal. Not all Q waves are indicators of MI. For example, a Q wave is normally seen in lead aVR. Furthermore, small "septal" q waves are normally seen in the left chest leads (I, aVL, and $V_4$ to $V_6$) and may be normal variants in one or more of leads II, III, and aVF. Recall from Chapter 4 the significance of these septal q waves. Recall that the ventricular septum depolarizes from left to right. Left chest leads record this spread of voltages toward the right as a small negative deflection (q wave) that is part of a qR complex in which the R wave represents the spread of left ventricular voltages toward the lead. When the electrical axis is horizontal, such qR complexes are seen in leads I and aVL. When the electrical axis is vertical, qR complexes appear in leads II, III, and aVF.

These normal septal q waves must be differentiated from the pathologic Q waves of infarction. Normal septal q waves are characteristically narrow and of low amplitude. As a rule, septal q waves are less than 0.04 sec in duration. A Q wave is generally abnormal if its duration is 0.04 sec or more in lead I, all three inferior leads (II, III, aVF), or leads $V_3$ to $V_6$.

What if Q waves with duration of 0.04 sec or more are seen in leads $V_1$ and $V_2$? A large QS complex can be a normal variant in lead $V_1$ and rarely in leads $V_1$ and $V_2$. However, QS waves in these leads may be the only evidence of an anterior septal MI. An abnormal QS complex resulting from infarction sometimes shows a notch as it descends, or it may be slurred instead of descending and rising abruptly (see Fig. 9.9). Further criteria for differentiating

normal from abnormal Q waves in these leads lie beyond the scope of this book, but the following can be taken as general guidelines/rules of thumb:

- An inferior wall MI should be diagnosed with certainty only when abnormal Q waves are seen in leads II, III, and aVF. If prominent Q waves appear only in leads III and aVF, the likelihood of MI is increased by the presence of abnormal ST-T changes in all three inferior extremity leads, or by abnormal Q waves in the lateral chest leads.
- An anterior wall MI should not be diagnosed from lead aVL alone. Look for abnormal Q waves and ST-T changes in the other anterior leads (I and $V_1$ to $V_6$).

Furthermore, *just as not all Q waves are abnormal, not all abnormal Q waves are the result of MI.* For example, slow R wave progression in the chest leads, sometimes with actual QS complexes in the right to middle chest leads (e.g., $V_1$ to $V_3$), may occur with left bundle branch block (LBBB), left ventricular hypertrophy, amyloidosis, and chronic lung disease in the absence of MI, in addition to multiple other factors. Prominent non-infarction Q waves are often a characteristic feature in the ECGs of patients with hypertrophic cardiomyopathy (Fig. 9.17). Non-infarction Q waves also occur with dilated cardiomyopathy (see Fig. 12.4). As mentioned previously, the ECGs of normal people sometimes have a QS wave in lead $V_1$ and rarely in leads $V_1$ and $V_2$. Prominent Q waves in the absence of MI are sometimes referred to as a *pseudoinfarct pattern* (see Chapter 25).

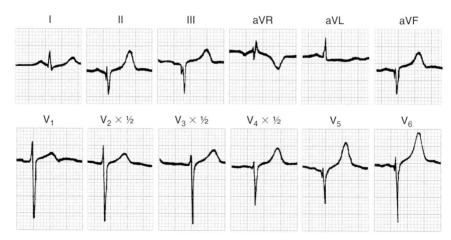

**Fig. 9.17** Hypertrophic obstructive cardiomyopathy (HOCM). Notice the prominent pseudoinfarction Q waves, which are the result of septal hypertrophy. (From Goldberger AL. Myocardial infarction: Electrocardiographic differential diagnosis. 4th ed. St. Louis: Mosby; 1991.)

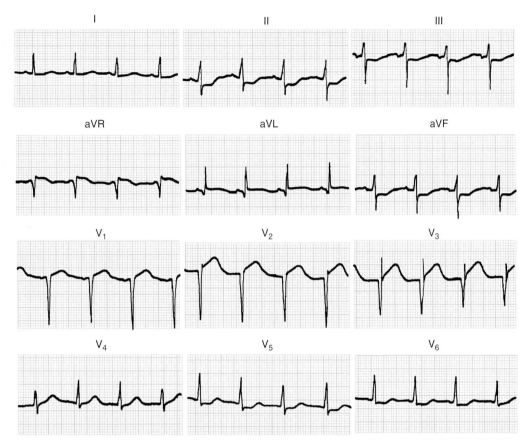

**Fig. 9.18** Anterior wall aneurysm. The patient had a myocardial infarction several months before this ECG was taken. Notice the prominent Q waves in leads $V_1$ to $V_3$ and aVL, the persistent ST elevations in these leads, and the reciprocal ST segment depressions in the inferior leads (II, III, and aVF). The persistence of ST elevations more than 2–3 weeks after an infarction suggests the presence of a ventricular aneurysm.

## VENTRICULAR ANEURYSM

A ventricular aneurysm may develop in some patients following a large MI (especially anterior). An aneurysm is a severely scarred portion of infarcted ventricular myocardium that does not contract normally. Instead, during ventricular systole the aneurysmal portion bulges outward while the rest of the ventricle is contracting. Ventricular aneurysms may occur on the anterior or inferior surface of the heart.

The ECG may be helpful in making the diagnosis of ventricular aneurysm subsequent to an MI. Patients with ventricular aneurysm frequently have persistent ST segment elevations after an infarct. As mentioned earlier, the ST segment elevations seen with acute infarction generally resolve within several days. The persistence of ST segment elevations for several weeks or more is suggestive of a ventricular aneurysm (Fig. 9.18). However, the absence of persisting ST segment elevations does not rule out the possibility of an aneurysm.

Ventricular aneurysms are of clinical importance for several major reasons. They may lead to chronic heart failure. They may be associated with serious ventricular arrhythmias. The aneurysmal LV may serve as a substrate for thrombus formation, which may result in a stroke or other embolic complications.

## MULTIPLE Q WAVE INFARCTIONS

Not infrequently, patients with advanced atherosclerotic heart disease may have two or more MIs

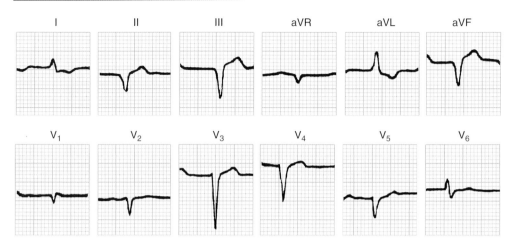

**Fig. 9.19** Multiple myocardial infarctions. This ECG shows evidence of previous anterior wall and inferior wall infarcts. Note the loss of normal R wave progression with QS complexes in chest leads $V_1$ to $V_5$, as well as the QS waves in leads II, III, and aVF.

at different times. For example, a new anterior wall infarct may develop in a patient with a previous inferior wall infarction. In such cases the ECG initially shows abnormal Q waves in leads II, III, and aVF. During the anterior infarct, new Q waves and ST-T changes appear in the anterior leads. (The ECG of a patient with anterior and inferior infarcts is presented in Fig. 9.19.)

## "SILENT" MYOCARDIAL INFARCTION

Most patients with an acute MI have symptoms. These include the classic complaint of crushing substernal chest pain. However, less "typical" presentations may occur as, or more, commonly (e.g., a sensation like indigestion, upper back pain, or jaw pain). Furthermore, clinicians must be aware that patients may experience few if any symptoms ("silent" MI). Therefore, it is not unusual for an ECG to show abnormal Q waves that indicate a previous infarction in a patient without a clinical history of definite MI. Clinicians should be aware that the absence of Q waves or prominent ST-T abnormalities does not exclude prior "silent" MI. (See Chapter 10 for discussion of silent ischemia.)

## DIAGNOSIS OF MYOCARDIAL INFARCTION IN THE PRESENCE OF BUNDLE BRANCH BLOCK

The diagnosis of infarction is more difficult when the patient's baseline ECG shows a bundle branch block pattern or a bundle branch block develops as a complication of the MI. The diagnosis of an MI

in the context of bundle branch blocks is challenging, and the ECG picture becomes more complex.

### Right Bundle Branch Block with Myocardial Infarction

The diagnosis of an MI can be made relatively easily in the presence of right bundle branch block (RBBB). Remember that RBBB affects primarily the terminal phase of ventricular depolarization, producing a wide R' wave in the right chest leads and a wide S wave in the left chest leads. MI affects the initial phase of ventricular depolarization, producing abnormal Q waves. When RBBB and an infarct occur together, a combination of these patterns is seen: The QRS complex is abnormally wide (0.12 sec or more) as a result of the bundle branch block, lead $V_1$ shows a terminal positive deflection, and lead $V_6$ shows a wide S wave. If the infarction is anterior, the ECG shows a loss of R wave progression with abnormal Q waves in the anterior leads and characteristic ST-T changes. If the infarction is inferior, pathologic Q waves and ST-T changes are seen in leads II, III, and aVF. (An anterior wall infarction with a RBBB pattern is shown in Fig. 9.20.)

### Left Bundle Branch Block with Myocardial Infarction

The diagnosis of LBBB in the presence of MI is considerably more complicated and confusing than that of RBBB. The reason is that LBBB disrupts both the early-mid and the later phases of ventricular stimulation (see Chapter 8). It also produces

## Acute Anterior STEMI and RBBB

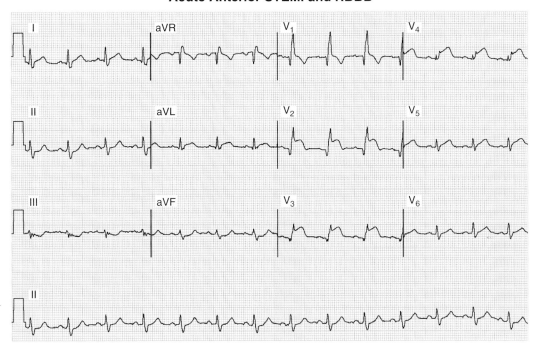

**Fig. 9.20** Acute anterior wall ST segment elevation myocardial infarction (STEMI) and right bundle branch block (RBBB). The wide QRS (about 120 msec) complexes with terminal R waves in leads V$_1$ and V$_2$ and a prominent S wave in lead V$_5$ indicate the presence of RBBB. The concomitant pattern of acute anterior MI is indicated by the ST segment elevations in leads V$_1$ to V$_4$ (also slightly in leads I and aVL) and Q waves in leads V$_1$ to V$_3$. Reciprocal ST depressions are seen in the inferior limb leads. Borderline left axis deviation is present. This combination points to a very proximal occlusion of the left anterior descending artery, with a large amount of ischemic/infarcting myocardium and increased risk of abrupt high-degree atrioventricular (AV) heart block with infranodal conduction block (see Chapter 18). (Reproduced with permission from Nathanson LA, McClennen S, Safran C, Goldberger AL. ECG wave-maven: Self-assessment program for students and clinicians. http://ecg.bidmc.harvard.edu.)

secondary ST-T changes. As a general rule, LBBB hides the diagnosis of an infarct. *Thus a patient with a chronic LBBB pattern who develops an acute MI may not show the characteristic changes of infarction described in this or the next chapter.*

Occasionally, the ECGs of patients with LBBB may show primary ST-T changes indicative of ischemia or actual infarction. Recall from Chapter 7, secondary T wave inversions of uncomplicated LBBB are usually best seen in leads with prominent R waves, e.g., leads V$_4$ to V$_6$. However, the appearance of T wave inversions in leads V$_1$ to V$_3$ (in leads with prominent S waves) is a primary abnormality that cannot be ascribed to the bundle branch block itself (Fig. 9.21).

The problem of diagnosing infarction with LBBB is further complicated by the fact that the LBBB pattern, itself, has features that closely resemble

those seen with infarction. Thus LBBB pattern can mimic an infarct pattern. As discussed in Chapter 8, LBBB typically causes slow R wave progression in the right-mid chest leads because of the reversed way the ventricular septum is activated (i.e., from right to left, the opposite of what happens normally). Consequently, with LBBB a loss of normal septal R waves is seen in the right chest leads. This loss of normal R wave progression may simulate the pattern seen with an anterior wall Q wave infarct.

Fig. 8.5 shows an example of LBBB with slow R wave progression. In this case, anterior wall infarction was not present. Notice also that the ST segment elevations in the right chest leads resemble the pattern seen during the hyperacute or acute phase of an infarction. ST segment elevation in the right chest leads is also commonly seen with LBBB in the absence of infarction.

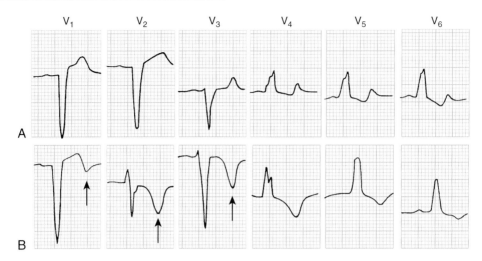

**Fig. 9.21** (A) Typical left bundle branch block pattern. Notice the slow R wave progression in the right precordial leads and the discordance of QRS and ST-T vectors reflected by the ST segment elevations in the right precordial leads and the ST depressions with T wave inversions in the left precordial leads. (B) Subsequently, the ECG from this patient showed the development of primary T wave inversions in leads $V_1$ to $V_3$ (*arrows*) caused by anterior ischemia and probable infarction. (Reproduced from Goldberger AL. Myocardial infarction: Electrocardiographic differential diagnosis. 4th ed. St. Louis: Mosby; 1991.)

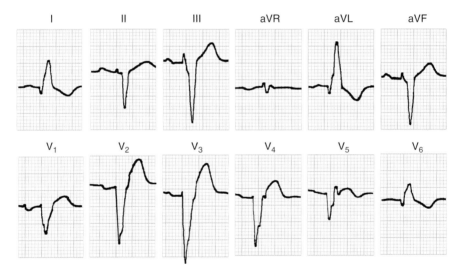

**Fig. 9.22** Chronic (prior) anterior wall infarction with left bundle branch block. Notice the prominent Q waves in the left chest leads as part of QR complexes (see text). (Reproduced from Goldberger AL. Myocardial infarction: Electrocardiographic differential diagnosis. 4th ed. St. Louis: Mosby; 1991.)

As a general rule, a patient with an LBBB pattern should not be diagnosed as having had an MI simply on the basis of slow ("poor") R wave progression in the right chest leads or ST elevations in those leads. However, the presence of Q waves as part of QR complexes in the left chest leads ($V_4$ to $V_6$) with LBBB generally indicates an underlying MI (Fig. 9.22). In addition, the appearance of ST segment *elevations* in the left chest leads or in other leads with prominent R waves suggests ischemia (see Fig. 9.22, lead $V_5$), as do ST segment *depressions* or *T wave inversions* in the right leads or other leads with an

| TABLE 9.1 | STEMI: Some Non-Atherosclerotic Causes |
|---|---|

1. Anomalous origin of a coronary artery
2. Carbon monoxide poisoning
3. Cardiac trauma: penetrating or non-penetrating; surgical
4. Coronary artery dissection, e.g., in context of late pregnancy or post-partum status, aortic dissection or connective tissue disease, or during percutaneous coronary interventions
5. Coronary artery embolism: infective or non-infective
6. Coronary artery spasm, e.g. due to drugs (e.g., ergot alkaloids or triptans; 5-fluorouracilcocaine; cocaine) or spontaneously occurring with or without underlying coronary disease
7. Kawasaki disease (and other causes of coronary vasculitis)
8. Myocarditis, acute (e.g., viral)
9. Pulmonary embolism, massive, with right-mid precordial ST elevations
10. Takotsubo syndrome

Note: The listed conditions may all be associated with actual myocardial infarction (necrosis), evidenced by ST elevations and increased serum cardiac enzyme biomarkers, identical to those typical of atherosclerotic STEMI.

rS or a QS morphology. The discussion of the ECG with ischemia and infarction continues in Chapter 10, which focuses on *subendocardial* ischemia and non-Q wave MI patterns.

## ST SEGMENT ELEVATION MI: NON-ATHEROSCLEROTIC CAUSES

We conclude this chapter by briefly calling attention to the clinically relevant fact that most, but not all ST segment elevation events are due to the classic mechanism of a ruptured or eroded atherosclerotic plaque leading to ischemia and infarction. A small but important subset of patients who present with ST elevations and serum enzyme biomarkers of infarction either do not have any coronary disease (e.g., those with traumatic injury to the myocardium or severe acute myocarditis) or who have non-atherosclerotic coronary disease (e.g., anomalous origin of a coronary artery, coronary arteritis, coronary vasospasm, takotsubo [stress] cardiomyopathy). Some of these entities, summarized in Table 9.1, are discussed in the next chapters.

# CHAPTER 10

# Myocardial Ischemia and Infarction, Part II: Non-ST Segment Elevation and Non-Q Wave Syndromes

Myocardial infarction (MI) may be associated with the appearance of classic ST segment elevations (STEMI), usually followed by T wave inversions as described in Chapter 9. Q waves may appear in one or more of these leads. However, in many cases, myocardial ischemia (with or without actual infarction) presents with ST segment depressions rather than primary ST elevations. Q waves are less likely to develop in these cases and the most affected areas are likely to be in the inner (subendocardial) layers of the left ventricle. In contrast, severe ischemia involving the full thickness of the wall, including the outer (epicardial) zones is likely to result in ST segment elevations. As discussed later, non-ST elevation MI may also present without characteristic ST-T changes (with normal ST segments, or nonspecific ST-T changes). In some cases, prominent T wave inversions without ST deviations are seen.

This chapter continues the discussion of acute coronary syndromes (ACS), as well as related conditions (e.g., takotsubo/stress cardiomyopathy syndrome; coronary vasospasm) that may be associated with ECG changes usually attributed to atherosclerosis-based coronary occlusion. The differential diagnosis of ST elevations, ST depressions and T wave inversions—the hallmark repolarization signatures of ischemia—is then described, along with an overview of the ECG in acute and chronic ischemic heart disease.

## SUBENDOCARDIAL ISCHEMIA

How can subendocardial ischemia occur without transmural ischemia? The subendocardium is particularly vulnerable to ischemia because it is most distant from the epicardial coronary blood supply and closest to the high pressure of the ventricular cavity. Therefore, the inner layers of the ventricle can become ischemic while the outer layer (subepicardium) remains normally perfused with blood.

The most common ECG change with predominant subendocardial ischemia is ST segment depression (Fig. 10.1). The ST depressions may be limited to the anterior leads (I, aVL, and $V_1$ to $V_6$) or to the inferior leads (II, III, and aVF), or they may be seen more diffusely in both lead groups. As shown in Fig. 10.1, the ST segment depressions most suggestive of subendocardial ischemia have a characteristic squared-off or downsloping shape.

Recall from Chapter 9 that acute transmural ischemia produces ST segment elevations, more technically referred to as a current of injury pattern. This characteristic finding results primarily from an injury current generated by the epicardial/subepicardial layers of the ventricle. With pure subendocardial ischemia, just the opposite occurs; that is, multiple ECG leads (sometimes, anterior and inferior) show ST segment depressions, except lead aVR, which often shows ST elevations.

To summarize: myocardial ischemia involving primarily the subendocardium usually produces ST segment depressions, whereas acute severe ischemia involving the epicardium/subepicardium and subendocardium produces ST elevations. This difference in the direction of the *injury current vector* is depicted in Fig. 10.2.

### ECG Changes with Angina Pectoris

The term *angina pectoris* (see Chapter 9) refers to episodes of chest discomfort caused by transient myocardial ischemia. Angina is a symptom of coronary artery disease. The "textbook" attack is reported

---

Please go to expertconsult.inkling.com for additional online material for this chapter.

as a dull, burning, or squeezing substernal pressure or heaviness, sometimes with radiation to the neck or jaw, or down one or both arms. This symptom is typically precipitated by exertion, emotional stressors, or exposure to cold and is relieved by rest and/or nitroglycerin.

Many (but not all) patients during episodes of classic angina have the ECG pattern attributable to subendocardial ischemia, with new or increased ST

segment depressions. When the pain disappears, the ST segments generally return to the baseline, although there may be a lag between symptom relief and remittance of ECG findings (Fig. 10.3 shows ST depressions during a spontaneous episode of angina.)

Clinicians should also be aware that some patients with angina do *not* show ST depressions during chest pain. Consequently, the presence of a normal ECG during an episode of angina-like chest discomfort does not rule out underlying coronary artery disease. However, the appearance of transient ST depressions in the ECG of a patient with characteristic anginal chest discomfort is a very strong indicator of myocardial ischemia.

### Exercise (Stress) Testing and Coronary Artery Disease

Many patients with coronary artery disease have a normal ECG while at rest. During exercise, however, ischemic changes may appear because of the extra

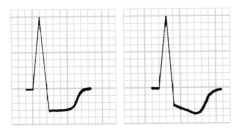

**Fig. 10.1** Predominantly subendocardial ischemia may produce ST segment depressions in multiple precordial and limb leads.

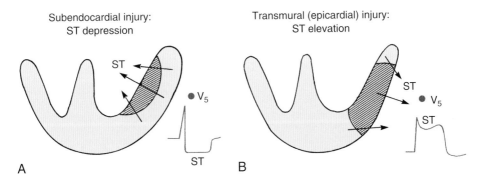

**Fig. 10.2** (A) With acute subendocardial ischemia the electrical forces (*arrows*) responsible for the ST segment are directed toward the inner layer of the heart, causing ST depressions in lead $V_5$, which faces the outer surface of the heart. (B) With acute transmural (epicardial) ischemia, electrical forces (*arrows*) responsible for the ST segment are directed toward the outer layer of the heart, causing ST elevations in overlying leads.

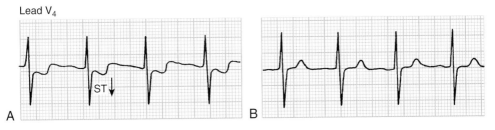

**Fig. 10.3** (A) Marked ST depressions are seen in lead $V_4$ of the ECG from a patient who complained of chest pain while being examined. (B) Five minutes later, after the patient was given sublingual nitroglycerin, the ST segments have reverted to normal, with relief of angina.

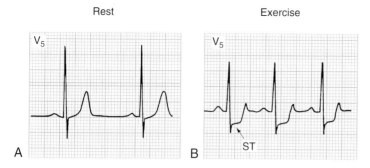

Rest                        Exercise

$V_5$                        $V_5$

A                        B          ST

**Fig. 10.4** (A) Baseline rhythm strip from the very positive (abnormal) exercise test of a patient with coronary artery disease. (B) Notice the marked ST depressions with only modest increased heart rate.

oxygen requirements imposed on the heart by exertion. To assist in diagnosing coronary artery disease, cardiologists often record the ECG while the patient exercises under controlled, closely monitored conditions. *Stress electrocardiography* is most often accomplished by having the patient walk on a treadmill or pedal a bicycle ergometer at increasing workloads. The test is stopped when the patient develops progressive angina, fatigue, dyspnea or diagnostic ST changes, or at patient request. When symptoms or ST changes do not occur with exertion, the test is considered negative, especially if the heart rate reaches 85% or more (or some other predetermined target) of a maximum estimated rate, usually predicted from the patient's age.

Fig. 10.4A shows the normal resting ECG of a patient, whereas Fig. 10.4B shows the marked ST depressions recorded while the same patient was exercising. The appearance of ST segment depressions constitutes a positive (abnormal) result. Most cardiologists accept horizontal or downward ST depressions of at least 1 mm or more, lasting at least 0.08 sec (two small boxes; 80 msec) as a positive (abnormal) test result (see Fig. 10.4B). ST depressions of less than 1 mm (or depressions of only the J point) with a rapid upward sloping of the ST segment are considered a negative (normal) or nondiagnostic ECG test response (Fig. 10.5).

The finding of prominent ischemic ST changes, with or without symptoms, occurring at a low level of activity is particularly ominous. Sometimes, these changes will be associated with a drop in blood pressure. *This combination of findings raises suspicion of severe three-vessel coronary disease and sometimes indicates high-grade obstruction of the left main coronary artery.*

Exercise (stress) electrocardiography is often helpful in diagnosing coronary artery disease in carefully selected patients. However, like virtually

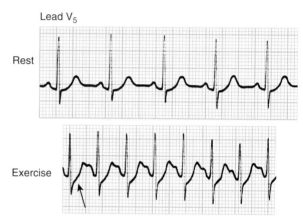

Lead $V_5$

Rest

Exercise

**Fig. 10.5** Lead $V_5$ shows physiologic ST segment depression that may occur with exercise. Notice the J junction depression (*arrow*) with sharply upsloping ST segments. (Reproduced from Goldberger AL. Myocardial infarction: Electrocardiographic differential diagnosis. 4th ed. St. Louis: Mosby; 1991.)

all medical tests, it yields both false-positive and false-negative results. For example, up to 10% of men without evidence of coronary obstructions and an even higher percentage of healthy women may have false-positive exercise tests. False-positive tests (defined here as ST depressions *without* obstructive coronary disease) can also be seen in patients who are taking digoxin and in patients who have hypokalemia, left ventricular hypertrophy (LVH), ventricular conduction disturbances (i.e., left bundle branch block, Wolff–Parkinson–White preexcitation pattern), or ventricular paced rhythms. (See also Chapter 24 on the Limitations and Uses of the ECG.)

False-negative tests can occur despite the presence of significant underlying coronary artery disease. *Therefore, a normal ("negative") exercise test does not exclude coronary artery disease.* The diagnostic accuracy of exercise tests may be increased in selected patients by simultaneous imaging studies, using echocardiography or nuclear medicine scans. *Pharmacologic stress testing*, an important and related topic, lies outside the scope of this text.

In summary, subendocardial ischemia, such as occurs with typical angina pectoris (or induced with stress testing) often produces ST segment depressions in multiple leads.

### "Silent" Myocardial Ischemia

A patient with coronary artery disease may have episodes of myocardial ischemia *without* angina, which is the basis of the term *"silent ischemia."* This important topic is discussed in Chapter 9.

### NON-Q WAVE INFARCTION

If ischemia to the subendocardial region is severe enough, actual infarction may occur. In such cases the ECG may show more persistent ST depressions instead of the transient depressions seen with reversible subendocardial ischemia, and will be associated with an abnormal increase in serum cardiac enzyme concentrations.

Fig. 10.6 shows an example of a non-Q wave infarction with persistent ST depressions. Is it possible for Q waves to appear with pure subendocardial infarction? The answer is that if only the inner half or so of the myocardium is infarcted, abnormal Q waves usually do not appear. Subendocardial infarction generally affects ventricular repolarization (ST-T complex) and not depolarization (QRS complex). However, as discussed at the end of this chapter, exceptions are not uncommon, and so-called *nontransmural* infarctions, particularly larger ones, may be associated with Q waves.

Another ECG pattern sometimes seen in non-Q wave infarction is T wave inversions with or without ST segment depressions. Fig. 10.7 shows an infarction pattern with deep T wave inversions. T wave inversions may also occur with non-infarctional ischemia.

To summarize: the major ECG changes with non-Q wave infarction are ST depressions and/or T wave inversions.

### Other ECG Changes Associated with Ischemia

In addition to the findings just described, myocardial ischemia may be associated with a number of other alterations in ventricular repolarization waveforms.

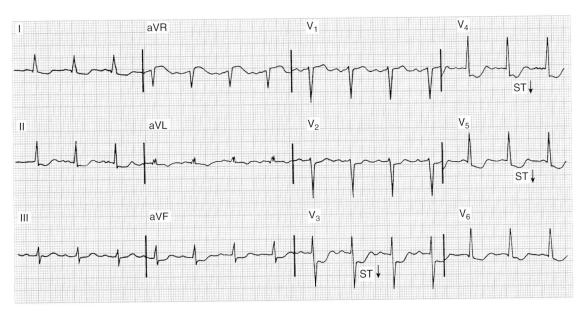

**Fig. 10.6** Non-Q wave infarction in a patient who complained of severe chest pain. Notice the marked, diffuse ST depressions in leads I, II, III, aVL, aVF, and V₂ to V₆, in conjunction with the ST elevation in lead aVR. These findings are consistent with severe ischemia, raising concern about multivessel disease and possibly left main obstruction. Other unrelated abnormalities include a prolonged PR interval (0.28 sec) and left atrial abnormality.

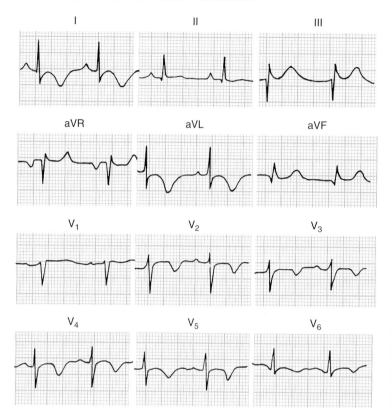

**Fig. 10.7** Evolving/acute non-Q wave infarction in a patient who complained of chest pain and also had elevated cardiac enzyme levels. Notice the deep T wave inversions in leads I, aVL, and $V_2$ to $V_6$. (Prominent Q waves in leads III and aVF represent an old inferior wall infarction.) Patients with acute myocardial infarction may have ST segment depressions or T wave inversions without Q waves.

Of note, in some patients the ECG may remain entirely normal during episodes of ischemia. In others, the ST-T complex may display only subtle changes. For example, you may see just slight T wave flattening or minimal T wave inversions. These findings are termed *nonspecific ST-T changes* (see Chapter 11).

Nonspecific ST-T changes may be abnormal, but they are never definite indicators of acute or chronic ischemic heart disease. They may also be caused by numerous other conditions, including physiologic alterations, drug effects, pulmonary disease, pericardial disease, cardiomyopathies, electrolyte, metabolic abnormalities (see Chapter 11), to name but some. Therefore, you should *not* make an ECG diagnosis of myocardial ischemia solely on the basis of nonspecific ST-T changes.

### Prinzmetal's (Variant or Vasospastic) Angina

*Prinzmetal's (variant) angina* is the symptom of another form of non-infarction ischemia. Recall that the ECG with classic angina shows the pattern

consistent with subendocardial ischemia, marked by ST segment depressions. A "variant" form of angina (first systematically reported by Dr. Myron Prinzmetal and colleagues in 1959) is seen in a small but important subset of patients. The term "variant" was adopted because during episodes of chest pain these patients have ST segment elevations, a pattern once thought diagnostic of acute MI. However, in Prinzmetal's angina the ST segment elevations are transient. After the episode of chest pain, the ST segments usually return to the baseline, without the characteristic evolving pattern of Q waves and T wave inversions that occur with actual infarction. Thus, Prinzmetal's variant angina is unusual from an ECG standpoint because it is associated with ST elevations rather than the ST depressions seen with classic angina.

Patients with Prinzmetal's (vasospastic) angina are also unusual from a clinical perspective because their chest pain often occurs at rest or at night, as opposed to with exertion or emotional stress. Prinzmetal's angina pattern is important because

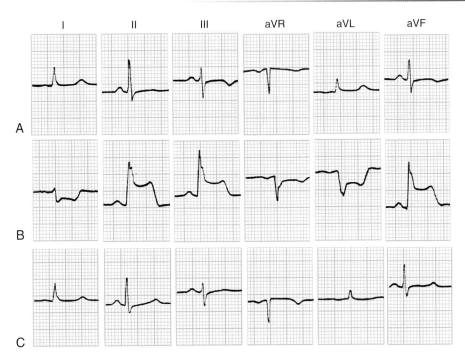

**Fig. 10.8** Prinzmetal's (variant) angina with transient ST elevations in a 30-year-old man with a history of angina with exertion and at rest. (A) The baseline resting ECG shows nonspecific inferior lead ST-T changes. (B) With chest pain, marked ST segment elevations occur in leads II, III, and aVF, and reciprocal ST depressions are seen in leads I and aVL. The rightward axis shift and slight widening of the QRS complex are most consistent with left posterior fascicular block (see Chapter 8). (C) The ST segments return to baseline after the patient is given nitroglycerin. Cardiac catheterization showed severe right coronary obstruction with intermittent spasm producing total occlusion and transient ST elevations. (Reproduced from Goldberger AL. Myocardial infarction: Electrocardiographic differential diagnosis. 4th ed. St. Louis: Mosby; 1991.)

it is a marker of coronary artery *spasm* sufficient to cause transient transmural ischemia. These episodes of spasm may occur in young adults with otherwise normal coronary arteries. In other cases, vasospasm is associated with high-grade coronary obstruction (Fig. 10.8). Ergonovine and related drugs may also cause coronary spasm in susceptible individuals. Increasing evidence implicates cocaine as another cause of coronary spasm, sometimes leading to MI.

Fig. 10.9 summarizes the diversity of ECG changes found in myocardial ischemia, with acute coronary syndromes.

## ACUTE STRESS/TAKOTSUBO CARDIOMYOPATHY

Trainees and practicing clinicians need to be aware of a distinct, non-atherosclerotic syndrome referred to by various terms including *acute stress* or *takotsubo cardiomyopathy*. Most, but not all patients with takotsubo cardiomyopathy are middle-aged to older

——————— Key Point ———————

The very diverse ECG changes seen with acute (and evolving) ischemic heart disease, also called acute coronary syndromes (ACS), include the following (see Fig. 10.9):

- Prominent ST segment deviations: elevations and/or ST segment depressions
- Prominent T wave alterations: inversions or increased positivity
- Nonspecific ST-T changes
- Pathologic Q waves
- Normal or nondiagnostic ECG findings

women who present with chest pain and ECG changes (ST elevations or depressions, or T wave inversions), and elevated serum cardiac enzyme levels mimicking the findings of a classic acute or evolving MI due to coronary occlusion (Fig. 10.10). Imaging studies

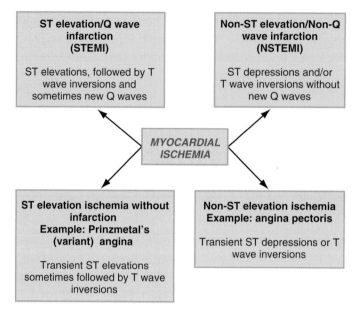

| **ST elevation/Q wave infarction (STEMI)**<br><br>ST elevations, followed by T wave inversions and sometimes new Q waves | **Non-ST elevation/Non-Q wave infarction (NSTEMI)**<br><br>ST depressions and/or T wave inversions without new Q waves |

*MYOCARDIAL ISCHEMIA*

| **ST elevation ischemia without infarction**<br>**Example: Prinzmetal's (variant) angina**<br><br>Transient ST elevations sometimes followed by T wave inversions | **Non-ST elevation ischemia**<br>**Example: angina pectoris**<br><br>Transient ST depressions or T wave inversions |

Note: Takotsubo and other stress cardiomyopathy syndromes may simulate any of the above.

**Fig. 10.9** Myocardial ischemia/myocardial infarction (MI) in acute coronary artery syndromes (ACS) may produces a diversity of ECG changes. T wave inversions may occur with or without infarction. Sometimes the ECG may show only nonspecific ST-T changes; rarely it may be normal.

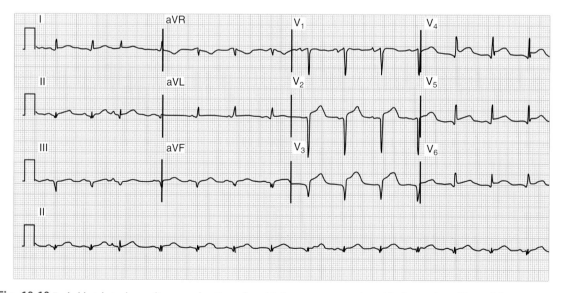

**Fig. 10.10** Probable takotsubo cardiomyopathy. Case of an elderly woman presenting with chest pain and heart failure symptoms whose ECG was consistent with anterior STEMI (along with inferior and anterior Q waves). Severe abnormal left ventricular wall motion was confirmed on echocardiography. Coronary angiography showed normal appearing coronary arteries. Serum cardiac enzyme biomarkers were elevated. Findings are most consistent with stress (takotsubo) cardiomyopathy. Third beat is a premature atrial complex.

## Early Repolarization

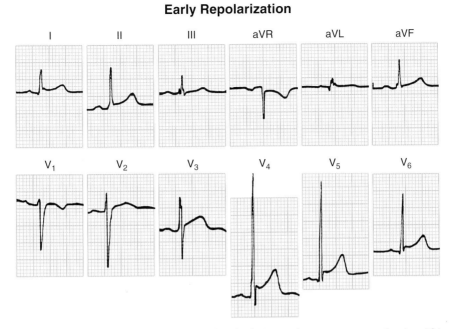

**Fig. 10.11** ST segment elevation, usually most marked in the chest leads, is sometimes seen as a normal variant. This early repolarization pattern may be confused with the ST segment elevations of acute myocardial infarction or pericarditis.

(echocardiographic and angiographic) may show left ventricular apical akinesis or dyskinesis (absence of contraction or outward "ballooning"). However, to qualify as a stress cardiomyopathy, epicardial coronary disease is not present. Instead, the pathophysiology may be related to coronary vasospasm and/or myocardial damage mediated by neurogenic and neurohumoral factors increasing myocardial oxygen demands in the context of emotional or physical stress. (In the popular press, this abnormality is sometimes called the "broken heart" syndrome.)[a]

## ECG DIFFERENTIAL DIAGNOSIS ISCHEMIA AND INFARCTION: ST-T CHANGES SIMULATING MI

### ST Elevations

Fig. 10.11 shows the ECG of a healthy young adult. Note the prominent elevation of the ST segments.

[a]Other forms of stress cardiomyopathy can occur with a variety of left ventricular wall motion abnormalities. For example, basilar or mid-cavity abnormalities of the left ventricular contraction may occur in certain forms of brain injury ("neurogenic stress cardiomyopathy"), also associated with a variety of ECG abnormalities. Prominent T wave inversions or tall positive T waves in concert with QT prolongation may occur, predisposing to torsades de pointes (see Chapters 16 and 21).

This finding, however, is not due to ischemia, but is a benign variant known as the *early repolarization pattern*. With benign early repolarization, the ST segments in the chest leads may rise to 2–3 mm above the (TQ) baseline. Although most common in young people, physiologic ST elevations can also occur in older persons, simulating the pattern of acute pericarditis or MI. However, the elevations of early repolarization are stable and do not undergo the evolutionary sequence seen with acute STEMI or *acute pericarditis* (Chapter 11). Furthermore, they are not associated with reciprocal ST depressions (except in lead aVR), contrary to what is often observed with acute MI.

ST segment elevations, resembling MI or pericarditis, may also occur with acute myocarditis (Chapter 12). Ventricular aneurysms may be associated with ST elevations that persist weeks to months or after an acute MI.

Chronic ST elevations are often seen in leads $V_1$ and $V_2$ in association with the patterns of *LVH* or *left bundle branch block (LBBB)* (Chapter 8).

Other causes of ST elevations include systemic hypothermia (J waves or Osborn waves, Chapter 11) in systemic hypothermia and the Brugada pattern (Chapter 21). A more comprehensive reprise of the differential diagnosis of ST segment elevations is given in Chapter 25.

## ST Segment Depressions: Differential Diagnosis

Subendocardial ischemia, as noted, is usually characterized by ST segment depression. However, not all ST depressions are indicative of subendocardial ischemia. For example, the ST-T changes associated with LVH (formerly referred to as the "strain" pattern) were discussed in Chapter 7. As shown in Fig. 7.12, the ST segment may be chronically depressed with LVH, simulating an acute coronary syndrome.

*Acute transmural ischemia* is another cause of ST segment depressions. Remember that acute anterior wall ischemia may be associated with reciprocal ST depressions in one or more of leads II, III, and aVF. Conversely, acute inferior wall ischemia may be associated with reciprocal ST depressions in one or more of the anterior leads (I, aVL, $V_1$ to $V_3$). Therefore, whenever you see ST depressions, you need to look at all the leads and evaluate these changes in context.

The ST segment may also be depressed by two important and common factors: *digitalis effect* and *hypokalemia* (see Chapter 11). Digitalis (most commonly prescribed as oral digoxin) may produce scooping of the ST-T complex with slight ST depressions, even the absence of elevated serum digoxin concentrations (see Fig. 20.1). The ST segment may also be moderately depressed in the ECGs of patients with a low serum potassium level (see Fig. 11.5). Prominent U waves may also appear. In some cases it may be difficult to sort out which factors are responsible for the ST depressions you are seeing. For example, a patient with left ventricular hypertrophy and systolic dysfunction may be taking digoxin and may also be having acute ischemia.

A comprehensive Instant Replay summary of the differential diagnosis of ST segment depressions is given in Chapter 25.

## Deep T Wave Inversions

Deep T wave inversions, as described previously, usually occur during the evolving phase of a Q wave MI (see Fig. 9.4B) and also sometimes with a non-Q wave MI (see Fig. 10.7). These deep inversions are the result of a delay in regional repolarization produced by the ischemic injury.

An important subset of patients with ischemic chest pain present with deep "coronary" T wave inversions in multiple precordial leads (e.g., $V_1$ or $V_2$ to $V_4$ or $V_5$) with or without cardiac enzyme elevations and with minimal or no ST elevations (Fig. 10.12). This pattern, called the *Wellens' syndrome* or the *LAD-T wave inversion pattern*, is typically caused by a tight stenosis (blockage) in the proximal left anterior descending (LAD) coronary artery system—these changes are often seen during a pain-free period in patients with intermittent chest pain.

## LAD-T Wave (Wellens') Pattern

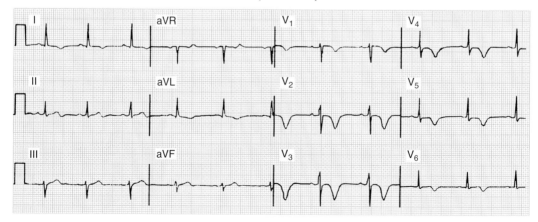

**Fig. 10.12** Patients with high-grade stenosis of the left anterior descending (LAD) coronary artery may present with chest discomfort and prominent anterior T wave inversions. Cardiac enzymes may be normal or minimally elevated. This finding is known as the LAD T-wave pattern or Wellens' pattern (named after the eminent Dutch cardiologist Dr. Hein J. J. Wellens).

However, just as not all ST segment elevations reflect ischemia, not all deep T wave inversions are abnormal. For example, T wave inversions are anticipated as a normal in leads with a *negative QRS complex* (e.g., in lead aVR). In adults the T wave may be normally negative in lead $V_1$ and sometimes also in lead $V_2$. Furthermore, as mentioned in Chapter 5, some adults, particular young to middle-aged women, have a persistent *juvenile T wave inversion pattern*, with negative T waves in the right and middle chest leads (typically $V_1$ to $V_3$).

In addition, not all abnormal T wave inversions are caused by MI. T wave inversions in the right chest leads may be caused by right ventricular overload (e.g., acute or chronic pulmonary embolism) and in the left chest leads by left ventricular overload (Chapter 7). Diffusely inverted T waves are seen during the evolving phase of pericarditis or myocarditis. Prominent T wave inversions may occur with the *takotsubo (stress) cardiomyopathy* (see earlier discussion).

Very deep, widely splayed T wave inversions (with a long QT interval and sometimes prominent U waves) have been described in some patients with cerebrovascular accident (CVA), particularly subarachnoid hemorrhage (*CVA T wave pattern*) (Fig. 10.13). The cause of these marked repolarization changes in some types of cerebrovascular injury (neurogenic T waves) is not certain, but they probably reflect marked changes in the autonomic nervous system function.

As described in Chapter 8, secondary T wave inversions (resulting from abnormal depolarization) are seen in the right chest leads with right bundle branch block (RBBB) and in the left chest leads with LBBB.

Deep T wave inversions ($V_1$ to $V_4$) may also occur after right ventricular pacing or with intermittent LBBB in normally conducted beats (*memory T wave pattern*; Chapter 21).

This brief discussion of non-infarctional factors that cause T wave inversions is by no means complete. However, the multiple examples should convey the point that *T wave inversions are not always indicative of myocardial ischemia*. Furthermore, in some cases, deep diffuse (*global*) T wave inversions may occur without any identifiable cause. A more comprehensive "instant review" summary of the differential diagnosis of T wave inversions is given in Chapter 25.

## ECG IN CONTEXT OF COMPLICATIONS OF MI

The major complications can be classified as mechanical/structural or electrical. *Mechanical* complications include heart failure, cardiogenic shock ("pump failure"), left ventricular aneurysm, rupture of the free wall of the heart or of a portion

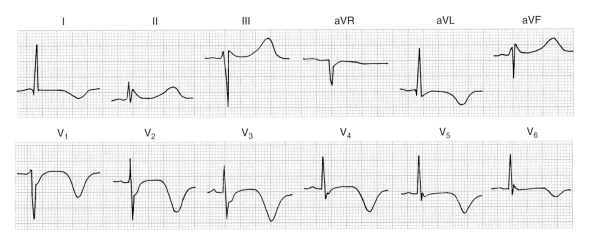

**Fig. 10.13** ECG of a patient with acute subarachnoid hemorrhage showing giant T wave inversions. Subarachnoid hemorrhage may cause deeply inverted T waves, usually with markedly prolonged QT intervals, simulating the pattern seen in myocardial infarction. (Reproduced from Goldberger AL. Myocardial infarction: Electrocardiographic differential diagnosis. 4th ed. St. Louis: Mosby; 1991.)

of the intraventricular septum, papillary muscle dysfunction, infarct extension and expansion, systemic or pulmonary embolism, and pericarditis. The *electrical* complications include the arrhythmias and atrioventricular (AV) or intraventricular conduction disturbances (bundle branch blocks) occurring as a consequence of ischemia or infarction. MI can cause virtually any arrhythmia, including sustained ventricular tachycardia (VT) or ventricular fibrillation leading to cardiac arrest. Acute MI is most likely to cause polymorphic VT, while sustained monomorphic VT in the clinical context of coronary disease usually indicates an underlying ventricular scar from prior MI. The topics of ventricular arrhythmias and sudden cardiac arrest are discussed in Part II of the book. Bundle branch blocks and AV heart blocks are discussed in Chapters 8 and 17. Both electrical and mechanical complications may occur together, particularly with more severe ischemia or extensive infarction.

## ECG AFTER CORONARY REPERFUSION

ECG recognition of acute MIs is important because such patients are generally candidates for emergency coronary reperfusion with catheterization/angioplasty-related procedures or with intravenous thrombolytic therapy. As noted in Chapter 9, systemic thrombolytic therapy has only proved helpful in cases of ST segment elevation MI (STEMI). Current evidence indicates that acute percutaneous coronary intervention (coronary angioplasty/coronary stenting) is even more efficacious than systemic thrombolysis in this setting and angioplasty-type procedures may also be useful in the emergency management of selected patients with non-ST segment elevation MI (non-STEMI).

Acute reperfusion therapies may alter the usual ECG evolution. Immediate reperfusion very early after the onset of an acute MI may be marked by the return of elevated ST segments toward the baseline, without development of new Q waves. Deep T wave inversions may evolve in leads that showed ST elevations. However, Q waves often appear even after successful reperfusion, although the intervention may lessen the amount of myocardium that is affected by the infarction. As a rule, the longer the time after the onset of ischemia or infarction, the less effect restoration of oxygenated blood flow has on acute or evolving ECG changes. Finally, the appearance of accelerated idioventricular rhythm

(AIVR) is most common in the context of coronary reperfusion (Chapter 16).

## THE ECG IN MI: CLINICAL OVERVIEW

Clinicians should recognize that the ECG is a reasonably sensitive but hardly perfect indicator of acute MI. Most patients with an acute MI or severe ischemia show the ECG changes described in Chapters 9 and 10. However, particularly during the early minutes or hours after an infarction, the ECG may be relatively nondiagnostic or even normal. Furthermore, an LBBB or ventricular pacemaker pattern may completely mask the changes of acute infarction. In the weeks to months following MI, the sensitivity of the ECG also decreases.

*Therefore, the ECG must always be considered in the clinical perspective of individual patient care, informed by experience and rigorous analysis.* Not all patients with acute MI will show diagnostic changes. Thus, the possibility of acute myocardial ischemia or infarction should not be dismissed simply because the ECG does not show the classic changes. Serial ECGs are usually more informative than a single one. On the other hand, ECG changes, exactly mimicking ischemia or infarction may be seen as normal variants or with other conditions not related to coronary artery disease.

In addition, as noted earlier, the traditional distinction between transmural and subendocardial (nontransmural) MIs on the basis of the ECG findings is an oversimplification and often invalid. In some patients, extensive infarction may occur without Q waves; in others, nontransmural injury may occur with Q waves. Furthermore, substantial evidence indicates that non-Q wave infarction may have as ominous a long-term prognosis as Q wave infarction.

For these reasons, cardiologists have largely abandoned the terms "transmural" and "subendocardial" when describing a clinically diagnosed infarction and instead use the descriptors STEMI, or non-STEMI, as appropriate. In addition, they encourage denoting the leads that show the changes and the magnitude of the changes. When Q waves are present from an acute infarct or previous one, these depolarization abnormalities should be noted and the leads specified.

Finally, clinicians involved in critical care should be aware that the classification of acute infarction based on ST elevations or ST depressions can be

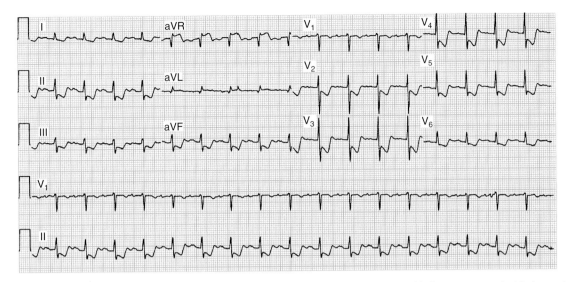

**Fig. 10.14** Left main coronary artery disease causing an acute coronary syndrome (ACS). An elderly man presented with chest pain and syncope. The ECG shows resting sinus tachycardia at a rate of about 110 with mild prolongation of the PR interval (approximately 200–210 msec), a leftward QRS axis (about −30°) and left atrial abnormality. The most striking findings are the widespread, very prominent downsloping ST depressions, seen in both limb (I, II, III, aVL, aVF) and precordial ($V_2$ to $V_6$) leads, with concomitant ST elevation in lead aVR (exceeding that in lead $V_1$). In concert, these findings are highly suggestive of severe three-vessel and/or left main coronary artery disease. The patient had elevated serum cardiac biomarkers and underwent cardiac catheterization with coronary angiography which revealed a critical distal left main stenosis, along with severe disease in the middle region of the left anterior descending coronary artery.

misleading. For example, acute ischemia due to left main obstruction (Fig. 10.14) or severe three-vessel disease may present with both changes: ST depressions in most of the anterior and inferior leads, with ST elevations in lead aVR and sometimes $V_1$. Posterolateral ST elevation MI may be associated with reciprocal ST depressions in $V_1$ to $V_3$. Failure to recognize this primary STEMI syndrome may result in delay in emergency reperfusion therapy.

# CHAPTER 11

# Drug Effects, Electrolyte Abnormalities, and Metabolic Disturbances

The ECG is importantly affected by a number of factors, including drug effects, electrolyte abnormalities, and a variety of other metabolic conditions. Indeed, the ECG may be the major, initial indicator of a life-threatening abnormality, such as hyperkalemia or tricyclic antidepressant toxicity. These topics are introduced in this chapter, along with a brief review of *nonspecific* versus more *specific ST-T changes.*

## DRUG EFFECTS

### Drugs Used to Treat Cardiac Arrhythmias

Numerous drugs, both "cardiac" and "non-cardiac," can affect the ECG. These changes may be mediated by direct effects on the electrical properties of a pacemaker, specialized conduction system, and atrial or ventricular cells. Drugs that alter autonomic nervous system activity (vagal and/or sympathetic) may also have important effects on pacemaker activity and conduction/recovery properties.

Cardiologists often use a shorthand classification system when referring to drugs primarily used to treat arrhythmias (Box 11.1). This system has a number of limitations, but is widely employed—so students and clinicians need to be aware of it.

*Class 1* drugs have a sodium channel blocking action, so they may prolong the QRS duration. The class I drugs are subdivided into A, B, and C groups. *Class 1A* drugs, such as quinidine, procainamide, and disopyramide, also prolong repolarization via potassium channel blocking effects. Therefore, they may prolong the QT(U) interval, leading to increased risk of *torsades de pointes* and *sudden cardiac arrest* (see Chapters 16 and 21). *Class 1B* drugs include lidocaine and mexiletine. *Class IC* drugs, such as flecainide and propafenone, used to treat atrial fibrillation and other supraventricular tachycardias,

are the most likely to produce clinically important widening of the QRS complex (intraventricular conduction delays) due to their prominent sodium channel blocking effects.

All "antiarrhythmic" class 1 (sodium channel blocking) drugs, along with many other pharmaceutical agents, may, paradoxically, induce or promote the occurrence of life-threatening ventricular arrhythmias by altering basic electrical properties of myocardial cells. These often unexpected *proarrhythmic drug effects*, which are of major clinical importance, are discussed further in Chapters 16 and 21.

Prolongation of the QT(U) interval with a life-threatening risk of torsades de pointes, a major type of ventricular *proarrhythmia*, can also occur with *class 3* drugs, notably ibutilide, dofetilide, sotalol (which also has beta-blocking effects), amiodarone (with beta-blocking, among multiple other effects), and dronedarone (Fig. 11.1). This QT(U) prolongation effect is also related to blocking of potassium channel function with prolongation of myocardial cellular repolarization.

Beta blockers (*class 2*) and certain calcium channel blockers (*class 4*) depress the sinus node and atrioventricular (AV) node, so that bradycardias may occur, ranging from mild to severe. Drug combinations (e.g., metoprolol and diltiazem) may produce marked sinus node slowing or AV nodal block, especially in the elderly. Carvedilol has both β-adrenergic and $α_1$-adrenergic (vasodilatory) effects, making hypotension a particular risk.

Limitations of this classification scheme include its failure to account for drugs with "mixed" effects (like amiodarone and sotalol) and the fact that important drugs, such as adenosine and digoxin, do not fit in. Instead, they are placed under the *class 5* or "other" category. Perhaps most important, as noted, is that the term "antiarrhythmic" agent does not take into account the potentially life-threatening *proarrhythmic* effects of many of these drugs (see Chapters 16 and 21). The major and large topic of the toxic effects of *digoxin* and related cardiac glycosides is discussed separately in Part III, Chapter 20.

---

**BOX 11.1** **Classification of Drugs Used to Treat Arrhythmias**

*Class 1:* Sodium channel blocking (conduction slowing) effects
  1A. Those also with potassium channel (repolarization) blocking effects (examples: quinidine; disopyramide; procainamide)
  1B. Those with mild to moderate sodium channel blocking effects (examples: lidocaine; mexiletine; phenytoin)
  1C. Those with most potent sodium channel blocking effects (examples: propafenone [also beta-blocking effects]; flecainide)
*Class 2:* Beta-blocking effects (examples: atenolol; carvedilol; metoprolol; nadolol; propranolol)
*Class 3:* Potassium channel (repolarization) blocking effects (examples: amiodarone; dofetilide; dronedarone; ibutilide; sotalol)
*Class 4:* Calcium channel blocking effects (examples: diltiazem; verapamil)
*Class 5:* Other (examples: glycosides, such as digoxin; adenosine)

---

## Psychotropic and Related Drugs

Psychotropic drugs (e.g., phenothiazines and tricyclic antidepressants) can markedly alter the ECG and in toxic doses can induce syncope or cardiac arrest due to a ventricular tachyarrhythmia or asystole. They may also prolong the QRS interval, causing a bundle branch block-like pattern, or they may lengthen repolarization (long QT(U) intervals), predisposing patients to develop torsades de pointes. Fig. 11.2 presents the classic ECG findings of tricyclic antidepressant overdose. Notice the triad of a prolonged QRS and QT interval, along with sinus tachycardia.

A variety of drugs used in psychiatric practice can prolong the QT interval, predisposing to torsades de pointes-type ventricular tachycardia. These drugs include methadone and the so-called "atypical" or "second generation" psychotropic agents (e.g., risperidone and quetiapine). This topic is discussed further in Chapter 16 as part of the very important clinical subject of *acquired long QT syndromes.*

Lithium carbonate, widely used in the treatment of bipolar disease, may cause sinus node pacemaker dysfunction or sinus exit block, resulting in severe bradycardia (Chapter 13).

Donezepil, used in the management of Alzheimer's disease, may induce or worsen bradyarrhythmias, due to its anticholinesterase effects that enhance the action of acetylcholine on the sinus and AV nodes.

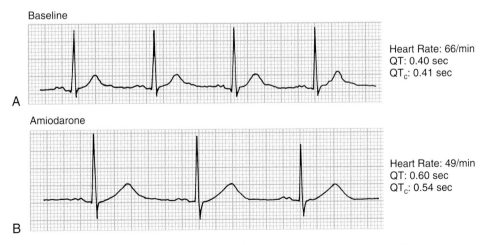

Baseline

Heart Rate: 66/min
QT: 0.40 sec
QT$_c$: 0.41 sec

A

Amiodarone

Heart Rate: 49/min
QT: 0.60 sec
QT$_c$: 0.54 sec

B

**Fig. 11.1** Effects of amiodarone. Note the very prominent prolongation of repolarization (long QT) produced by a therapeutic dose of amiodarone in this patient as therapy for atrial fibrillation. The heart rate also slows as a result of the beta-blocking effect of the drug. Note also the broad, notched P waves due to left atrial abnormality.

## Tricyclic Antidepressant Overdose

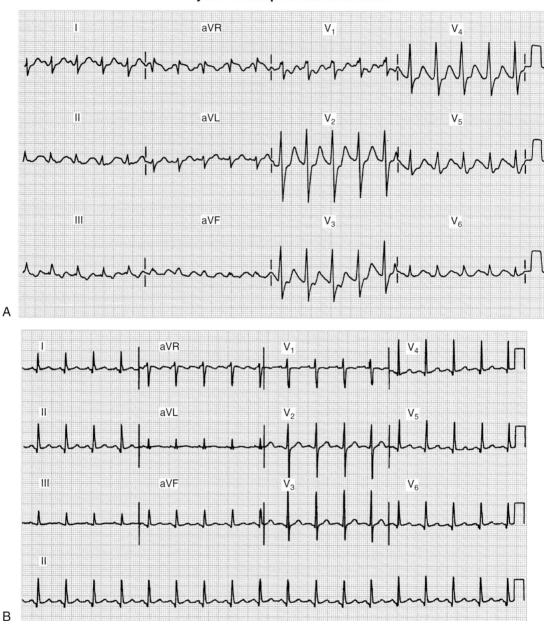

**Fig. 11.2** (A) This ECG from a patient with tricyclic antidepressant overdose shows three major findings: sinus tachycardia (from anticholinergic and adrenergic effects), prolongation of the QRS complex (from slowed ventricular conduction), and prolongation of the QT interval (from delayed repolarization). (B) Follow-up ECG obtained 4 days later shows persistent sinus tachycardia but normalization of the QRS complex and QT interval.

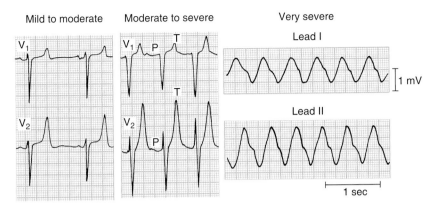

**Fig. 11.3** The earliest change with hyperkalemia is peaking ("tenting") of the T waves. With progressive increases in the serum potassium concentration, the QRS complexes widen, the P waves decrease in amplitude and may disappear, and finally a *sine wave* pattern leads to asystole unless emergency therapy is given.

## ELECTROLYTE DISTURBANCES

Abnormal serum concentrations of potassium and calcium can produce marked effects on the ECG. Hyperkalemia can, in fact, be lethal because of its cardiac toxicity.

### Hyperkalemia

As shown in Fig. 11.3, increasing degrees of hyperkalemia produce a distinctive sequence of ECG changes affecting both depolarization (QRS complex) and repolarization (ST-T segments). The normal serum potassium concentration is usually reported as between 3.5 and 5.5 mEq/L. The first change seen with abnormal elevation of the serum potassium concentration is narrowing and peaking of the T waves. As Fig. 11.4 demonstrates, the T waves with hyperkalemia have a characteristic "tented" or "pinched" shape, and they may become quite tall. With further elevation of the serum potassium concentration, the PR intervals become prolonged and the P waves are smaller and may disappear entirely. Continued elevations produce an intraventricular conduction delay, with widening of the QRS complexes (see Figs. 11.3 and 11.4). As the serum potassium concentration rises further, the QRS complexes continue to widen, leading eventually to a large undulating (sine wave) pattern and asystole, with cardiac arrest (Chapter 21).[a] The major cardiac electrophysiology changes of severe hyperkalemia are related at the cell membrane level to the depolarizing effects of excess potassium, resulting in reduced conduction velocity and automaticity.

Because hyperkalemia can be fatal, recognition of the earliest signs of T wave peaking may prove lifesaving. Hyperkalemia can occur in multiple clinical settings. The most common is kidney failure, in which the excretion of potassium is reduced. A number of drug classes may elevate serum potassium levels, including angiotensin-converting enzyme (ACE) inhibitors, angiotensin receptor blockers (ARBs), potassium-sparing diuretics (amiloride, eplerenone, spironolactone, triamterene), among others. Not uncommonly, hyperkalemia is multifactorial (e.g., intrinsic kidney disease, drug effects, dehydration).

### Hypokalemia

Hypokalemia may produce distinctive changes in the ST-T complex. The most common pattern comprises ST depressions with prominent U waves and overall prolonged repolarization (Figs. 11.5 and 11.6). The ECGs may show a characteristic "dip and rise pattern" reflecting these waveform perturbations. With hypokalemia the U waves typically become enlarged and may even exceed the height of the T waves. Technically the QT interval with hypokalemia may remain normal whereas repolarization is prolonged (as represented by the prominent U waves). Because the T wave and U wave often merge, the QT interval cannot always be accurately

[a]The major cardiac electrophysiology changes of severe hyperkalemia are related at the cell membrane level to the depolarizing effects of excess potassium, resulting in reduced conduction velocity and automaticity.

## Marked Hyperkalemia

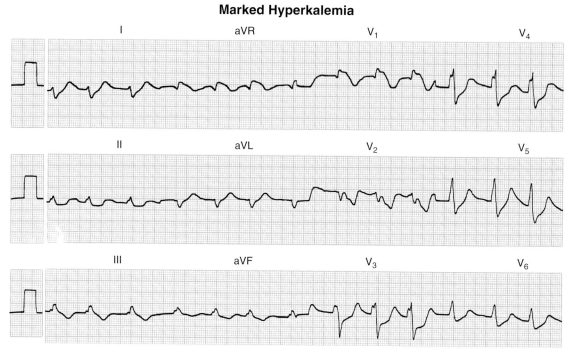

**Fig. 11.4** ECG of a patient with a serum potassium concentration of 8.5 mEq/L. Notice the absence of P waves and the presence of bizarre, wide QRS complexes.

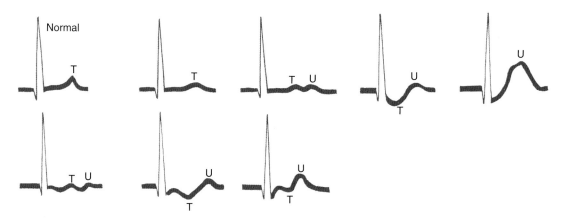

**Fig. 11.5** The ECG patterns that may be seen with hypokalemia range from slight T wave flattening to the appearance of prominent U waves, sometimes with ST segment depressions or T wave inversions. These patterns are not directly related to the specific level of serum potassium.

## Hypokalemia

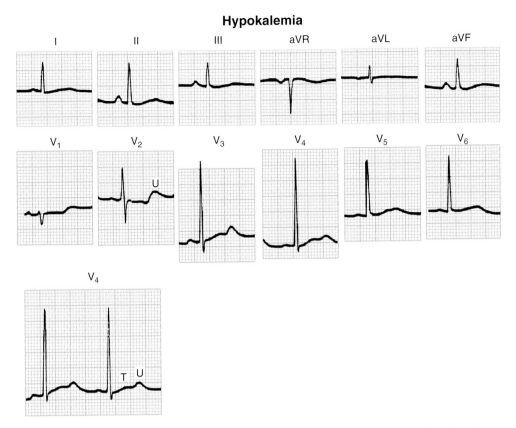

**Fig. 11.6** ECG leads from a patient with a markedly low serum potassium concentration of 2.2 mEq/L. Notice the prominent U waves, with flattened T waves.

measured. The term *T-U fusion wave* can be applied in such cases.[b]

### Hypercalcemia and Hypocalcemia

Ventricular repolarization (the plateau phase of the action potential) is shortened by hypercalcemia and lengthened by hypocalcemia (Fig. 11.7). In hypercalcemia, the shortening of the QT interval is due to shortening of the ST segment. With marked hypercalcemia the T wave appears to take off right from the end of the QRS complex. High serum calcium concentrations may lead to coma and death. A short QT interval in a patient with mental status changes is sometimes the first clue to the diagnosis of hypercalcemia. Hypocalcemia lengthens or prolongs the QT interval, usually by "stretching out" the ST segment. Of note, however, is that patients may have clinically significant hypocalcemia or hypercalcemia without diagnostic ECG changes (low sensitivity).

### Hypomagnesemia and Hypermagnesemia

Hypomagnesemia and hypermagnesemia are important because (1) they may be overlooked, and (2) they may play a role in the genesis of ventricular arrhythmias and contribute to other metabolic

---

[b]Hypokalemia causes membrane hyperpolarization (more negative resting potential) and also prolongs ventricular action potential (phase 3) duration. Via mechanisms that are insufficiently understood, the lowering of extracellular potassium reduces the outward repolarizing potassium current responsible for restoring the membrane potential to its resting (diastolic) negative value. This paradoxical effect (i.e., decreased extracellular potassium reducing the outward potassium current) appears to be mediated by a decrease in the effective number or responsiveness of certain types of potassium channels. The net effect of reducing the outward flow of positive (potassium) ions is to keep the membrane repolarized, prolonging action potential, and hence QT(U) duration.

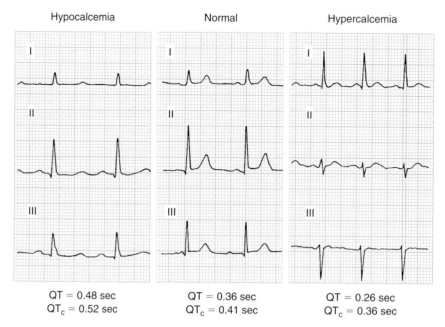

Hypocalcemia    Normal    Hypercalcemia

QT = 0.48 sec    QT = 0.36 sec    QT = 0.26 sec
$QT_c$ = 0.52 sec    $QT_c$ = 0.41 sec    $QT_c$ = 0.36 sec

**Fig. 11.7** Hypocalcemia prolongs the QT interval by stretching out the ST segment. Hypercalcemia decreases the QT interval by shortening the ST segment so that the T wave seems to take off directly from the end of the QRS complex.

disturbances. However, neither is associated with specific ECG alterations.

*Hypomagnesemia,* usually due to gastrointestinal or renal losses (e.g., with certain diuretics) may also play a pathogenetic role in causing or increasing the severity of hypokalemia. The ECG may be dominated by signs of the latter (see preceding discussion) in such cases. Hypomagnesemia has been implicated in ventricular arrhythmogenesis with acute myocardial infarction and also in torsades de pointes. Administration of intravenous magnesium is recommended empiric therapy in cases of torsades de pointes. Its infusion use may suppress the *early after-depolarizations* that initiate this type of polymorphic ventricular tachyarrhythmia (Chapter 16). Hypomagnesemia may also potentiate digitalis toxicity (Chapter 20). In addition, hypomagnesemia is important because it may foster hypocalcemia (see preceding discussion) by inhibiting release of parathyroid hormone.

*Hypermagnesemia* (usually due to renal failure or excessive intake) does not produce distinct ECG abnormalities, when only mildly or moderately elevated. Pronounced elevations may lead to a prolonged PR or QRS interval, as well as sinus

bradycardia. Extreme elevations, for example above 15–20 mEq/L, may contribute to cardiac arrest. Hypotension (due to vasodilation) and mental status changes may also occur with progressive increases in serum magnesium.

## OTHER METABOLIC FACTORS
### Hypothermia

Patients with systemic hypothermia may develop a distinctive ECG pattern in which a hump-like elevation is usually localized to the junction of the end of the QRS complex and the beginning of the ST segment (J point) (Fig. 11.8). These pathologic J waves, also called *Osborn waves,* are attributed to altered ventricular transmural action potential features with hypothermia. Patients with hypothermia are at increased risk of ventricular fibrillation, which may occur during rewarming.

### Endocrine Abnormalities

Most endocrine disorders do not produce specific changes on the ECG. In some instances, however, the ECG may play an important role in the diagnosis and management of hormonal abnormalities. For

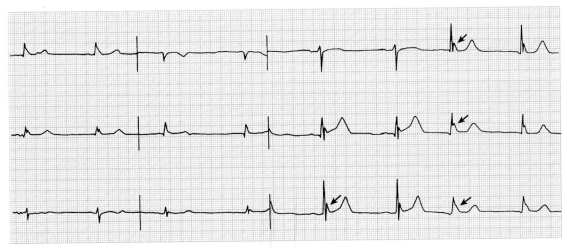

**Fig. 11.8** Systemic hypothermia is associated with a distinctive bulging of the J point (the very beginning of the ST segment). The prominent J waves (*arrows*) with hypothermia are referred to as Osborn waves.

example, hyperthyroidism (most commonly due to Graves' disease) is often associated with an inappropriately high resting sinus heart rate. The finding of an unexplained high sinus rate under basal conditions, therefore, should prompt consideration of hyperthyroidism, as should the sometimes unexpected finding of atrial fibrillation (see Chapter 15).

In contrast, hypothyroidism is typically associated with an excessively slow resting heart (sinus bradycardia). Severe hypothyroidism (myxedema) may lead to pericardial effusion, thereby causing *low voltage* QRS complexes. Low QRS voltage is strictly said to be present when the total amplitude of the QRS complexes in each of the six extremity leads is 5 mm or less, or 10 mm or less in the chest leads. Low (or relatively) QRS voltage is not a specific finding but can be related to a variety of mechanisms and causes, including increased insulation of the heart by air (chronic obstructive pulmonary disease) or adipose tissue (obesity); replacement of myocardium, for example, by fibrous tissue (in cardiomyopathy), amyloid, or tumor; or the accumulation of extracellular fluids (as with anasarca, or with pericardial or pleural effusions) (see Chapters 12 and 25).

### Metabolic Acidosis and Alkalosis

Acid–base abnormalities, by themselves, are not consistently associated with specific ECG findings. Metabolic acidosis is typically associated with

hyperkalemia and metabolic alkalosis with hypokalemia. The ECG morphologic appearance will be dominated by these electrolyte perturbations, both of which, when severe, may lead or contribute to cardiac arrest (see Chapter 21). Cardiac arrest, in turn, may quickly lead to respiratory and/or metabolic acidosis.

### ST-T CHANGES: SPECIFIC AND NONSPECIFIC

The concluding topic of this chapter is a brief review of the major factors that cause ST-T (repolarization) changes. The term *nonspecific ST-T change* (defined in Chapter 10) is commonly used in clinical electrocardiography. Many factors (e.g., drugs, ischemia, electrolyte imbalances, infections, and pulmonary disease) can affect the ECG. As already mentioned, the repolarization phase (ST-T complex) is particularly sensitive to such effects and can show a variety of nonspecific changes as a result of multiple factors (Figs. 11.9 and 11.10). These changes include slight ST segment depressions, T wave flattening, and slight T wave inversions (see Fig. 11.9).

In contrast to these nonspecific ST-T changes, certain fairly specific changes are associated with particular conditions (e.g., the tall, tented T waves of hyperkalemia). Some of these relatively specific ST-T changes are shown in Fig. 11.11. However, even such apparently specific changes can be misleading. For example, ST elevations are characteristic of acute

Normal T wave

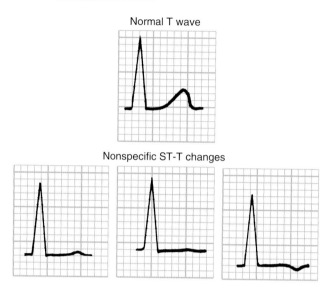

Nonspecific ST-T changes

**Fig. 11.9** Flattening of the T wave (bottom left and middle) and slight T wave inversion (bottom right) are abnormal but relatively nonspecific ECG changes that may be caused by numerous factors.

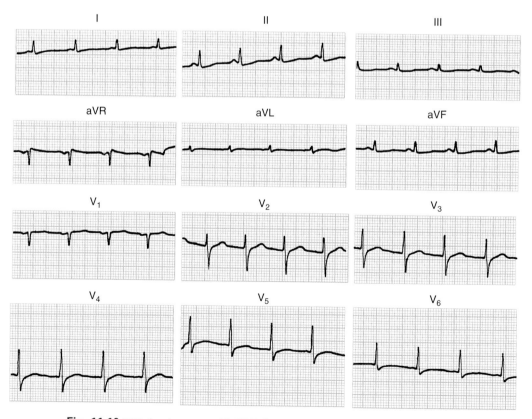

**Fig. 11.10** ECG showing nonspecific ST-T changes. Notice the diffuse T wave flattening.

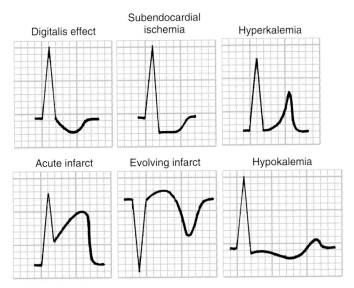

**Fig. 11.11** Examples of relatively specific ST-T changes. Note, however, that the changes are not absolutely specific for the abnormalities shown.

transmural ischemia, but they are also seen in ventricular aneurysms, pericarditis, and benign (normal) early repolarization. Similarly, deep T wave inversions are most characteristic of ischemia but may occur in other conditions as well (see Chapters 10 and 25).

In summary, repolarization abnormalities can be grouped into two general categories: (1) *Nonspecific* ST-T changes include slight ST segment deviation and flattening or inversion of the T wave. These changes are not diagnostic of any particular condition but must always be interpreted in clinical context. (2) Relatively *specific* ST-T changes are more strongly but not always definitively diagnostic of some particular underlying cause (e.g., hyperkalemia or myocardial ischemia).

# CHAPTER 12
# Pericardial, Myocardial, and Pulmonary Syndromes

A wide variety of major disease processes may alter the ECG. Particularly important are conditions affecting the pericardium (acute pericarditis, pericardial effusion, and constrictive pericarditis), the myocardium itself (not including ischemia and infarction, which are discussed separately in Chapters 9 and 10), and the pulmonary system, including pulmonary embolism (acute and chronic thromboembolic disease), chronic obstructive pulmonary disease, and pulmonary parenchymal disease.

## ACUTE PERICARDITIS, PERICARDIAL EFFUSION, AND CONSTRICTIVE PERICARDITIS

### Acute Pericarditis

Acute pericarditis (inflammation of the pericardium) may be caused by multiple factors, including viral or bacterial infection (e.g., tuberculosis), metastatic tumors, collagen vascular diseases (e.g. systemic lupus erythematosus), cardiac surgery, uremia, and myocardial infarction (MI). In clinical practice, the cause is often undetermined (idiopathic), and presumed viral.

As mentioned in Chapter 10, the ECG patterns of acute pericarditis resemble those seen with acute ST elevation MI. The early phase of acute pericarditis is also usually characterized by ST segment elevations. This type of *current of injury pattern* results from inflammation of the heart's surface (epicardial layer), which often accompanies inflammation of the overlying pericardium (Fig. 12.1).

One major difference between the ST elevations occurring with acute MI and acute pericarditis is their distribution. The ST segment elevations with acute MI are characteristically localized to the area of the infarct. The pericardium, in contrast, envelops the heart. Therefore, the ST-T changes occurring with pericarditis are usually more generalized and seen in both anterior and inferior lead distributions.

For example, in Fig. 12.1 note the elevations in leads I, II, aVL, aVF, and $V_2$ to $V_6$. Reciprocal ST depressions in pericarditis are usually limited to lead aVR, and sometimes $V_1$.

A second important difference is that the ST elevations seen with acute pericarditis tend to be less prominent than those with STEMI; however, multiple exceptions occur. The morphology of ST elevations with pericarditis also tends to maintain an upward concavity, whereas those with STEMI can be concave or convex. However, here again, multiple exceptions occur, precluding the application of "hard and fast" rules in differential diagnosis based primarily on ST-T morphology alone.

Third, acute pericarditis may not only affect ventricular repolarization (the ST segment), it also often affects repolarization of the atria, which starts during the PR segment (short period between the end of one P wave and the beginning of the next QRS complex) (Fig. 12.1). In particular, pericardial inflammation often causes an atrial current of injury, reflected by elevation of the PR segment in lead aVR and depression of the PR segment in other extremity leads and the left chest leads ($V_5$ and $V_6$).

---

## Key Point

With acute pericarditis the PR and ST segments typically point in opposite directions ("PR-ST segment discordance sign"), with the PR being elevated (often by only 1 mm, or so) in lead aVR and the ST usually being slightly depressed in that lead. Other leads may show combined PR depression and ST elevation. Because the elevation of the PR segment in lead aVR resembles a bent index finger, this pattern has been referred to informally as the "knuckle sign."

---

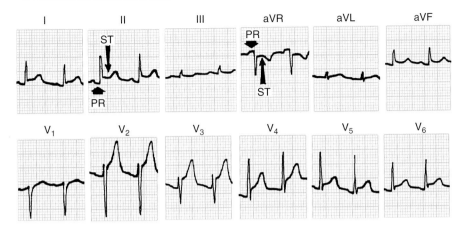

**Fig. 12.1** Acute pericarditis causing diffuse ST segment elevations in leads I, II, aVF, and V$_2$ to V$_6$, with reciprocal ST depressions in lead aVR. By contrast, a concomitant atrial current of injury causes PR segment elevations in lead aVR with reciprocal PR depressions in the left chest leads and lead II.

## Pericarditis: Evolving Pattern

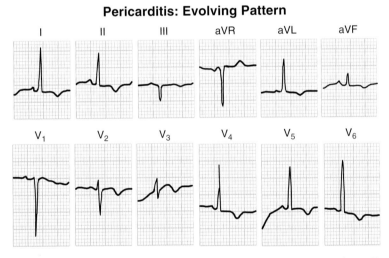

**Fig. 12.2** Note the diffuse T wave inversions in leads I, II, III, aVL, aVF, and V$_2$ to V$_6$.

PR segment deviations may also be useful in distinguishing the ECG of acute pericarditis from that of *benign early repolarization*. In younger adults the two patterns may coexist, causing further diagnostic confusion.

The ST segment elevations seen with acute pericarditis are sometimes followed (after a variable time) by T wave inversions (Fig. 12.2). The general sequence of ST elevations and T wave inversions is similar to that described for MI. In some cases the T wave inversions caused by pericarditis resolve completely with time and the ECG returns to normal.

In other cases the T wave inversions persist for long periods. Furthermore, very prominent T wave inversions (i.e., 5 mm or more in depth) are rare with pericarditis. Some patients with acute pericarditis never manifest evolving T wave inversions.

Another major difference between infarction and pericarditis is that pericarditis does not produce abnormal Q waves, such as those seen with certain infarcts. With MI, abnormal Q waves may occur because of the necrosis of heart muscle and the consequent loss of positive depolarization voltages (see Chapter 9). Pericarditis, on the other hand, generally causes only a superficial inflammation and does not produce actual myocardial necrosis.

Some patients have recurrent or relapsing episodes of pericarditis, which may occur intermittently or persist for sustained periods. The ECG findings are variable and may resemble those of acute or evolving pericarditis. Low voltage may occur if pericardial effusion is present or constrictive changes develop (see following discussion).

## Pericardial Effusion

*Pericardial effusion* refers to an abnormal accumulation of fluid in the pericardial sac. In most cases this fluid accumulates as the result of pericarditis. In some cases, however, such as myxedema (hypothyroidism) or rupture of the heart, pericardial effusion may occur in the absence of pericarditis. The major clinical significance of pericardial effusion is the danger of cardiac tamponade, in which the fluid actually "chokes off" the heart, leading to a drop in blood pressure and, in extreme cases, to cardiac arrest with *pulseless electrical activity* (PEA; see Chapter 21).

The most common ECG sign of pericardial effusion (with or without actual tamponade) is low voltage (or relatively low voltage) of the QRS complexes. The mechanism of the low voltage in this setting has not been established with certainty.

Different sets of criteria for high voltage were mentioned in the discussion of hypertrophy patterns (see Chapter 7). *Low voltage* (see Chapter 11) is strictly considered to be present when the total amplitude of the QRS complexes in each of the six extremity leads is 5 mm (0.5 mV) or less. Low voltage in the extremity leads may or may not be accompanied by low voltage in the chest leads, defined as a peak-to-trough QRS amplitude (total range) of 10 mm or less in each of leads $V_1$ to $V_6$. Clinicians should be aware that pericardial effusion may produce relatively low voltage (especially when compared to previous), without meeting absolute criteria just defined.

Fig. 12.2 shows an example of low voltage. A listing of other factors that can produce low QRS voltage is presented in one of the *Instant Replay* boxes in Chapter 25. One class of causes of low voltages includes myocardial deposition syndromes, in which the heart muscle gets infiltrated, and eventually replaced, with substances like amyloid or iron (hemochromatosis).

The mechanism of the low voltage QRS complexes differs based on the context. For example, obesity can cause low voltage because of the insulating effect of fat tissue that lies between the heart and the chest wall. Patients with emphysema have increased inflation of the lungs. This extra air also acts to insulate the heart. Replacement of, or damage to ventricular heart muscle tissue by fibrosis or amyloid can also cause low QRS voltages. Of the causes of low voltage, obesity, anasarca (generalized edema), pleural effusions, and emphysema are among the most common. However, when you see low voltage (particularly with unexplained sinus tachycardia), you need to consider the possibility of pericardial effusion because it can lead to fatal tamponade with pulseless electrical activity (see also Chapter 21).

*Electrical alternans* is a very distinctive finding that can occur with pericardial effusion especially when it is associated with tamponade or severe hemodynamic compromise (Fig. 12.3). This pattern is usually characterized by a periodic beat-to-beat shift in the QRS axis (ABABAB... type sequence) associated with mechanical swinging of the heart to-and-fro in a relatively large accumulation of fluid. The finding is usually most apparent in the mid-chest leads. *The triad of sinus tachycardia, electrical alternans, and low QRS voltage is virtually diagnostic of cardiac tamponade*, although *not* every patient with tamponade shows this pattern (i.e., it has high specificity, but only modest sensitivity).[a] Electrical alternans is most likely to occur with larger effusions, and therefore, has been associated with metastatic malignancy (e.g., breast or lung). However, alternans *per se* is not a unique marker for pericardial effusion due to any specific cause.

## Constrictive Pericarditis

Some conditions causing pericardial inflammation can lead to chronic fibrosis and calcification of the pericardial sac. Specific causes of pericardial constriction include cardiac surgery, trauma, infections such as tuberculosis (especially prevalent in

---

[a]Note that "electrical alternans" is a general term for alternation of one or more ECG waveforms on a beat-to-beat basis. The type of "total" electrical alternans (which usually affects the entire P-QRS-T) associated with pericardial effusion/tamponade is seen with sinus rhythm, and usually with sinus tachycardia. Practitioners should be aware that other forms of electrical alternans occur having nothing to do with pericardial disease. Probably the most common setting of QRS electrical alternans is (non-sinus) paroxysmal supraventricular tachycardia (PSVT). The ventricular rate is usually very fast (>200 beats/min) in such cases and the alternans is thought to be due to a subtle change in conduction patterns on a beat-to-beat basis. QRS alternans may also occur with monomorphic ventricular tachycardias (see Chapters 14 and 16).

## Electrical Alternans in Pericardial Tamponade

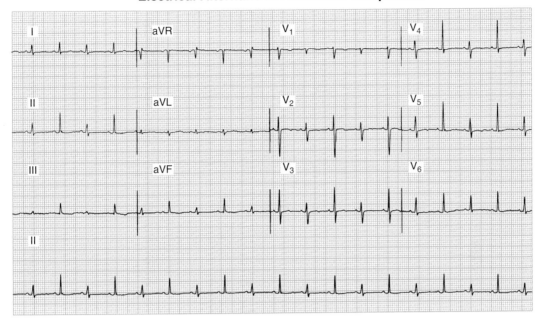

**Fig. 12.3** Electrical alternans may develop in patients with pericardial effusion and cardiac tamponade. Notice the beat-to-beat alternation in the P-QRS-T axis; this is caused by the periodic swinging motion of the heart in a large pericardial effusion. Relatively low QRS voltage and sinus tachycardia are also present.

developing nations), viral pericardial infections (which may have escaped notice in the acute phase), malignancy, connective tissue diseases, sarcoid, uremia (renal failure), and asbestosis. In some cases, no cause is evident and the term *idiopathic constrictive pericarditis* is applied.

Patients may present with evidence of heart failure (right-sided out of proportion to left) with elevated neck veins and even ascites. Usually, surgical treatment is required, with careful peeling ("stripping") of the pericardium (pericardiectomy) to allow the heart to fill normally and to decrease intracardiac pressures. *Constrictive pericarditis is important because it is one of the surgically curable forms of heart failure and may be mistaken for cirrhosis of the liver.*

Unfortunately, no single ECG pattern or constellation of findings is diagnostic of chronic constrictive pericarditis. Nonspecific ST-T wave changes and relatively low QRS voltages are most common. The PR/ST segment deviations may resemble those of acute pericarditis. However, atrial arrhythmias, especially atrial fibrillation, may preclude assessment of PR segment deviations.

Noninvasive diagnostic imaging tests, including chest radiography, echocardiogram with Doppler recordings, computed tomography, and magnetic resonance imaging studies, may be useful. But because imaging studies may be inconclusive, cardiac catheterization with careful hemodynamic measurements to test for elevation and equilibration of diastolic pressures, along with characteristic right heart pressure waveforms, is an essential part of the workup of patients prior to pericardiectomy.

## MYOCARDITIS

A variety of conditions (e.g., multiple viral infections, including HIV/AIDS, Lyme disease, autoimmune syndromes, etc.) may be associated with inflammation of the heart muscle (myocarditis). Individuals with myocarditis may have a wide range of symptoms and presentations, ranging from those who are asymptomatic to those who have severe heart failure and even sudden death. In some cases, pericarditis and myocarditis occur as part of the same inflammatory process (*myopericarditis* or *perimyocarditis*). In HIV/AIDS, myocarditis may be multifactorial—due to the

| BOX 12.1 | HIV/AIDS-Related ECG Changes: Selected List |
| --- | --- |

*Myocarditis/cardiomyopathy with reduced ejection fraction:* ST-T changes; intraventricular conduction abnormalities; left ventricular/left atrial overload/hypertrophy
*Pericardial effusion:* Low QRS voltage (may also be related to myocardial disease)
*Pulmonary hypertension:* Right atrial/right ventricular overload/hypertrophy
*Drug therapy for the disease and its complications:*
    Protease inhibitors: abnormalities due to ischemia/MI associated with premature or accelerated atherosclerosis
    Antibiotics: pentamidine, erythromycin-type; fluoroquinolones: QT prolongation with risk of torsades de pointes

primary infection, other viral, parasitic or bacterial infections, or therapeutic interventions (Box 12.1).

The ECG findings with myocarditis are also quite variable, ranging from nonspecific ST-T changes to the distinctive repolarization changes that occur with acute pericarditis. Occasionally, the ECG findings of severe myocarditis may exactly simulate those of acute MI, including ST elevations and even the development of pathologic Q waves. Atrial or ventricular arrhythmias can occur with myocarditis, as can atrioventricular (AV) or ventricular conduction disturbances. In rare cases, myocarditis can lead to sudden cardiac arrest/death.

## CHRONIC HEART FAILURE

Chronic heart failure (HF), often referred to as congestive heart failure or just heart failure, is a complex syndrome that may result from multiple causes, including extensive MI, systemic hypertension, myocarditis, valvular heart disease, and various cardiomyopathies. In some cases, more than one factor (e.g., hypertension and coronary disease) may play etiology roles. The ECG may provide helpful clues to a specific diagnosis in some patients:

- Prominent Q waves and typical ST-T changes, especially in middle-aged to older patients, suggest underlying ischemic heart disease with extensive underlying infarction.
- Left ventricular hypertrophy patterns (see Chapter 7) may occur with hypertensive heart disease, aortic valve disease (stenosis or regurgitation), or mitral regurgitation.

- Combination of prominent left atrial abnormality (or atrial fibrillation) and signs of right ventricular hypertrophy (RVH) should suggest mitral stenosis (see Fig. 24.1).
- Left bundle branch block (LBBB) (see Chapter 8) may occur with HF caused by ischemic heart disease, valvular abnormalities, hypertension, or cardiomyopathy.

In some patients, marked enlargement and decreased function of the left (and often the right) ventricle occur without coronary artery disease, hypertension, or significant valvular lesions. In such cases the term *dilated* (*"congestive"*) *cardiomyopathy* is applied. Dilated cardiomyopathy can be idiopathic, or it can be associated with chronic excessive alcohol ingestion (alcoholic cardiomyopathy), viral infection, hereditary factors, or multiple other etiologies. Dilated cardiomyopathy is a form of heart failure with very low left ventricular ejection fraction.

Patients with dilated cardiomyopathy from any cause may have a distinctive ECG pattern (the *ECG–HF* triad), characterized by the following findings:

1. Relatively low voltages in the extremity leads, such that the QRS in each of the six extremity leads is 8 mm or less in amplitude.
2. Relatively prominent QRS voltages in the chest leads, such that the sum of the S wave in either lead $V_1$ or lead $V_2$ plus the R wave in $V_5$ or $V_6$ is 35 mm or more.
3. Very slow R wave progression defined by a QS- or rS-type complex in leads $V_1$ to $V_4$.

When the ECG–HF triad is present (Fig. 12.4), it strongly suggests underlying cardiomyopathy but does not indicate a specific cause. The triad may occur not only with primary dilated cardiomyopathy but also with severe heart disease caused by previous infarction or significant valvular dysfunction. Furthermore, the ECG–HF triad has only modest sensitivity; that is, its absence does not exclude underlying cardiomyopathy.

## PULMONARY EMBOLISM (ACUTE AND CHRONIC)

The ECG is *not* a sensitive test for acute pulmonary embolism. In some cases the obstruction produced by an embolus in the pulmonary artery system can lead to ECG changes, but generally no single pattern is diagnostic. All of the following may be seen (Fig. 12.5):

## ECG-CHF Triad

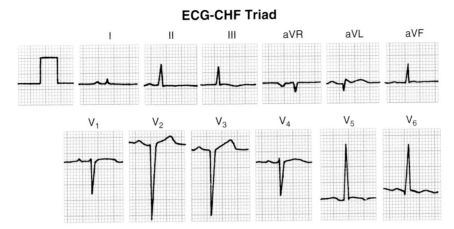

**Fig. 12.4** Severe idiopathic dilated cardiomyopathy in a young adult man with chronic heart failure. The triad of (1) relatively low QRS voltages in the limb leads, (2) prominent precordial QRS voltages, and (3) very slow R wave progression in the chest leads (rS in $V_4$) is highly suggestive of dilated cardiomyopathy. This finding is relatively specific, but not sensitive.

## Acute Pulmonary Embolism

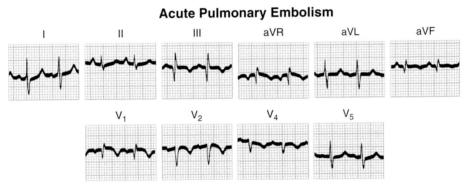

**Fig. 12.5** Features occasionally seen with pulmonary embolism include sinus tachycardia, S waves in lead I with Q waves and T wave inversions in lead III ($S_2Q_3T_3$ pattern), and slow R wave progression with T wave inversions in chest leads $V_1$ to $V_4$ resulting from acute right ventricular overload.

- Sinus tachycardia at rest. This finding is probably the most sensitive but least specific ECG finding with acute pulmonary embolism.
- Arrhythmias such as ventricular ectopy and atrial fibrillation or flutter may also occur. Massive pulmonary embolism may lead to ventricular fibrillation and sudden cardiac arrest (Chapter 21).
- A right ventricular overload (formerly called "strain") pattern, characterized by inverted T waves in leads $V_1$ to $V_3$ to $V_4$).
- The so-called "$S_1Q_3T_3$ pattern," with a new or increased S wave in lead I and a new Q wave in lead III with T wave inversion in that lead, as well as in lead aVF. This pattern, which may simulate

that produced by acute inferior wall MI, is probably due to acute right ventricular dilation.
- Shift of the mean QRS axis to the right, with or without frank right axis deviation.
- ST segment depressions consistent with diffuse subendocardial ischemia (Chapter 10).
- A new incomplete or complete right bundle branch block (RBBB) pattern: new rSR′ in lead $V_1$.
- A qR complex in $V_1$ of normal duration, especially with right axis deviation, is highly suggestive of acute or chronic right heart overload.
- Signs of right atrial overload: tall peaked P waves in the inferior leads, sometimes with a shift in P wave axis to the right.

## Chronic Lung Disease

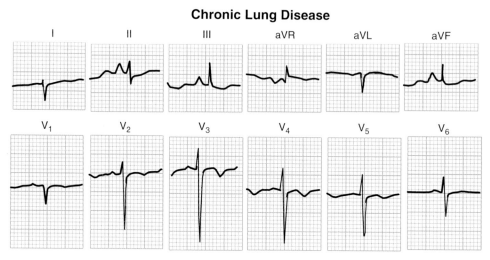

**Fig. 12.6** Note the characteristic constellation of relatively low voltages in the extremity leads, right axis deviation, right atrial overload pattern ("P pulmonale"), and slow R wave progression. The P wave axis is also more vertical than usual (almost +90°).

The appearance of these changes, particularly in combination, is suggestive but not diagnostic of pulmonary embolism. Even patients with large, acute pulmonary emboli may have only minor, nonspecific changes on their ECG. Thus, both the diagnostic sensitivity and the specificity of the ECG with pulmonary embolism are limited. Fig. 12.5 shows a classic example of the changes seen with pulmonary embolism. Note that these findings may also be due to other causes of acute (or subacute) right ventricular overload (*acute cor pulmonale*) due, for example, to severe pneumonitis, chronic obstructive airway disease, extensive pulmonary malignancy, pulmonary sarcoid or other causes of restrictive lung disease.

Patients with *chronic thromboembolic pulmonary hypertension (CTEPH)* due to recurrent pulmonary emboli may show signs of right ventricular overload or frank RVH (tall R in $V_1$, right axis deviation and right precordial T wave inversions), sometimes with peaked P waves due to right atrial overload. Identical findings may occur with primary pulmonary arterial hypertension (PAH).

## CHRONIC OBSTRUCTIVE LUNG DISEASE (EMPHYSEMA)

Patients with severe chronic obstructive lung disease with emphysema often have a relatively characteristic constellation of ECG findings (Fig. 12.6), including

(1) low QRS voltage, (2) slow R wave progression in the chest leads, (3) a vertical or rightward QRS axis in the frontal plane, and (4) right atrial overload. Excessive pulmonary air trapping causes the low voltage. The slow R wave progression results, in part, from the downward displacement of the diaphragm. Thus, with severe emphysema the chest leads, in their conventional locations, may actually be *relatively* higher than usual. In addition, right ventricular dilation may contribute to the delayed chest lead transition zone. Finally, the anatomically vertical position of the heart in the chest of a patient with emphysema (and sometimes right ventricular enlargement) causes the mean QRS axis to be vertical or even rightward (greater than +100°). Tall, relatively narrow (sinus-generated) P waves caused by right atrial overload (see Fig. 12.6) may be present, along with a vertical or rightward P wave axis (+90° or so).

### Pulmonary Parenchymal Disease

Other types of severe generalized pulmonary disease (e.g., due to idiopathic pulmonary fibrosis, sarcoidosis, metastatic tumor) may lead to ECG changes, including P pulmonale, RVH, right-mid precordial T wave inversions and QRS right axis shifts. However, these changes lack sensitivity, so that patients may have advanced pulmonary syndromes and few or no ECG findings of note.

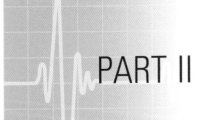

# PART II

# Cardiac Rhythm Disturbances

# CHAPTER 13
## Sinus and Escape Rhythms

Part II of this book deals with physiologic and abnormal cardiac rhythms. Systematically analyzing the cardiac rhythm from the ECG allows you to address two key sets of questions:

1. What pacemaker(s) is (are) controlling the heartbeat? There are three major possibilities:
   - Is the controller (driver) exclusively in the sinus node—the normal pacemaker?
   - Are sinus beats present, but interrupted by extra (ectopic) heartbeats? Ectopic beats, in turn, come in two general classes: (i) *premature*, occurring before the next sinus beat is due, or (ii) *escape*, occurring after a relatively short or long pause.
   - Is an entirely non-sinus (ectopic) mechanism controlling (driving) the heartbeat, as in the case of atrial fibrillation, atrial tachycardia, AV nodal reentrant tachycardia, ventricular tachycardia, or electronically paced rhythms (Chapter 22)?

2. Next you should ask: What, if any, is the signaling (communication link) between the sinus (or other supraventricular) pacemaker(s) and the ventricles? The physiologic situation ("normal sinus rhythm") occurs when every sinus depolarization results in a ventricular beat (at a HR of ~60-100 bpm), which requires timely conduction of the impulse through the atria, AV junction (AV node and His bundle) and the bundle branches, into the ventricular myocardium.

This chapter focuses on sinus rhythm and its variants, as well as on *escape* or *subsidiary* pacemakers, those that act as "backup electrical generators" when the sinus node fails to fire in a timely way or when the sinus impulse is blocked from stimulating the surrounding atrial tissue. Subsequent chapters deal with premature beats and the major

sustained ectopic rhythms, both supraventricular and ventricular, as well as with atrioventricular (AV) heart block and AV dissociation, and with preexcitation.

Projecting ahead, we discuss the most extreme form of disrupted AV signaling, called complete (third-degree) block (Chapter 17), in which sinus rhythm may still control the atria, but none of these sinus impulses traverse the AV junction to the ventricles. Instead the ventricles are electrically controlled by a lower (subsidiary) pacemaker, located in the AV junction or in the His–Purkinje–ventricular system.

Following that, we discuss another type of AV conduction anomaly, one associated not with delays, but with early or *preexcitation* of the ventricles, the substrate of the Wolff–Parkinson–White (WPW) patterns and syndromes (Chapter 18).

Keep in mind throughout the underlying principle: all normal and abnormal cardiac electrical function is based on two key properties of automaticity (impulse formation) and conductivity (impulse propagation and refractoriness).

## SINUS RHYTHMS
### "Normal" Sinus Rhythm

Sinus rhythm is the primary physiologic mechanism of the heartbeat. You diagnose it by finding P waves with a polarity predictable from simple vector principles (see Chapter 5). When the sinus (also called the sinoatrial or SA) node paces the heart, atrial depolarization spreads from right to left and downward toward the AV junction. An arrow (vector) representing the overall trajectory of this depolarization wavefront is directed downward and toward the (patient's) left. *Therefore, with normal sinus rhythm, the P wave is always positive in lead II and negative in lead aVR* (see Figs. 5.3 and 13.1), and the HR is between 60 and 100 bpm.

Please go to expertconsult.inkling.com for additional online material for this chapter.

========= Reminders =========

- If you state that the rhythm is "normal sinus" and do not mention any AV node conduction abnormalities, listeners will reasonably assume that each P wave is followed by a QRS complex and vice versa. A more technical, but physiologically unambiguous way of stating this finding is to say: "Sinus rhythm with 1:1 AV conduction."
- Strictly speaking, when you diagnose "sinus rhythm," you are only describing the physiologic situation in which the sinus node is generating P waves (upright in lead II, inverted in aVR). But this term, by itself, says nothing about AV conduction. *Sinus rhythm (i.e., activation of the atria from the SA node) can occur not only with normal (1:1) AV conduction but with any degree of AV heart block (including second- or third-degree), or even with ventricular tachycardia (a type of AV dissociation). In the most extreme case, a patient can have an intact sinus node consistently firing off impulses in the absence of any ventricular activation, leading to ventricular asystole and cardiac arrest (see Chapter 21).*

By convention, *normal sinus rhythm* in a resting subject is usually defined as sinus rhythm with normal (1:1) AV conduction and a normal PR interval at a heart rate between 60 and 100 beats/min. Sinus rhythm with a heart rate greater than 100 beats/min is termed *sinus tachycardia* (Fig. 13.2). Sinus rhythm with a heart rate of less than 60 beats/min is called *sinus bradycardia* (Fig. 13.3). However, be aware that the normal rate is context dependent. For an athlete at rest or during deep sleep, the

physiologic rate may be as slow as 30/min, transiently. In contrast, a young adult's heart rate during near maximal exercise may approach 200/min. Indeed, as discussed further below, if your spontaneous sinus rate during vigorous exertion were within the usually quoted "normal" range of 60–100/min, that finding would be distinctly abnormal. *For clarity, we follow those cardiologists who adopt the designation of "sinus rhythm" in preference to "normal sinus rhythm." Then you can add the rate, whether AV conduction is normal, what type of heart block is present, and whether there are ectopic beats. When useful, you can also designate when the ECG was recorded (e.g., rest, exercise, deep sleep).*

### Normal Sinus Rhythm
### (Sinus with 1:1 AV Conduction)

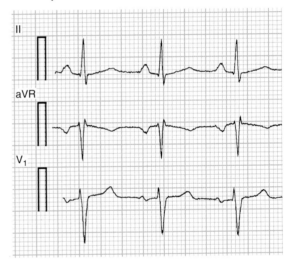

**Fig. 13.1** The heart rate is about 80 beats/min. Each QRS complex is preceded by a P wave that is negative in lead aVR and positive in lead II. The P wave in lead V₁ is usually biphasic with an initial positive component (right atrial activation) followed by a small negative component (left atrial activation).

### Sinus Tachycardia

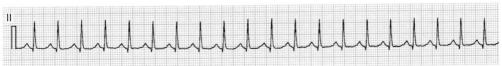

**Fig. 13.2** Sinus tachycardia. The heart rate is close to 150 beats/min. Note the positive (upright) P waves in lead II. There is nonspecific T wave flattening.

### Sinus Bradycardia

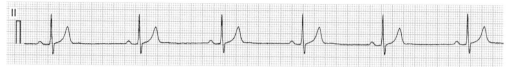

**Fig. 13.3** Sinus bradycardia. Sinus rhythm is present, but at a very slow rate of about 38 beats/min.

### Sinus Rhythm Shifting to Low Atrial Pacemaker

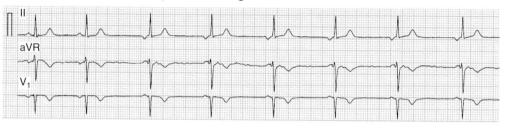

**Fig. 13.4** Note the change in P wave polarity from positive to negative in lead II. This shift from sinus bradycardia here to an ectopic (low) atrial escape rhythm may occur as a normal (physiologic) variant, especially with high vagal tone, or in a variety of other settings. When several different P waves occur, the term "wandering atrial pacemaker" is used (Chapter 21).

## REGULATION OF THE HEART RATE

The heart, like other organs, has a special nerve supply from the *autonomic nervous system*, which controls involuntary muscle cell activity and certain specialized pacemaker and conduction tissue. The autonomic nerve supply to the heart (in particular, the SA and AV nodes) consists of fibers with opposing effects: the *sympathetic nerves* and the *parasympathetic nerves*. Sympathetic stimulation increases the heart rate and the strength of myocardial contraction. Sympathetic stimulation is also mediated by secretion of circulating catecholamines (especially, norepinephrine and epinephrine), produced by the adrenal glands.

Parasympathetic stimulation (from the vagus system; 10th pair of cranial nerves) produces slowing of the sinus rate as well as increased conduction time through the AV nodal area. Parasympathetic stimulation can also cause a pacemaker "shift" from the SA node to the low right atrial area producing a so-called *low atrial rhythm*, with negative P waves in leads II, III, and aVF, and a positive P wave in lead aVR, with a short PR interval (Fig. 13.4).

In this way the autonomic nervous system provides a complex control system that automatically regulates the heart rate. Increased sympathetic nervous stimulation and/or decreased parasympa-

thetic (vagal) inactivation act as a cardiac accelerator, whereas increased parasympathetic and decreased sympathetic tone produce a braking effect. As a familiar example, when you are excited or anxious, or exercising, increased sympathetic stimuli (and diminished parasympathetic tone) result in an increased heart rate and increased contractility, producing the familiar sensation of a pounding or fluttering sensation in the chest (*palpitations*). Note that the sensation of "palpitations" (a frequent concern of patients leading to physician visits and referrals) may be associated with an entirely normal heartbeat, with isolated premature beats (atrial or ventricular), or, more seriously, with an actual run of ectopic (non-sinus) heartbeats (e.g., from atrial fibrillation or flutter, paroxysmal supraventricular tachycardia, or ventricular tachycardia).

## SINUS TACHYCARDIA

*Sinus tachycardia is sinus rhythm with a heart rate exceeding 100 beats/min.* In adults the heart rate with sinus tachycardia is generally between 100 and 180 beats/min. Even faster rates, transiently up to 200 beats/min or so, can be observed in healthy young adults during maximal exercise. (Of course, in newborns, heart rates of 145–150 are routine and not described as sinus tachycardia.)

Aging decreases the heart's capacity to generate very rapid sinus rates. This effect usually relates to decreased numbers of normally functioning sinus node cells and decreased autonomic system activity and responsivity. Elderly individuals (especially those older than 70 years) rarely show sinus tachycardia at rates above 140–150 beats/min even during maximal exertion. *Indeed, heart rates above this range in the elderly, especially at rest, usually indicate the presence of a non-sinus tachycardia (e.g., atrial fibrillation or flutter, or a paroxysmal supraventricular tachycardia).*

Fig. 13.2 shows an example of sinus tachycardia. Each sinus P wave is followed by a QRS complex, indicating sinus rhythm with 1:1 AV conduction. Sinus tachycardia (or bradycardia), however, as noted, can occur with any degree of AV block. Notice that the P waves are positive in lead II. With sinus tachycardia at very fast rates, the P wave may merge with the preceding T wave and become difficult to distinguish.

In general, sinus tachycardia occurs with any condition that produces an *increase* in sympathetic tone or a *decrease* in vagal tone (Box 13.1). Sinus tachycardia may occur with healthy or pathologic states, usually involving increased cardiac output needs or decreased vascular resistance. Recall that systemic cardiac output per minute is the product of stroke volume (how much blood the left ventricle pumps with each beat) multiplied by the heart rate (beats/min).

Treatment of sinus tachycardia associated with a pathologic condition must be directed at the *underlying* cause, e.g., infection, sepsis, internal bleeding, drugs (including certain "recreational" drugs like cocaine and herbal supplements with ephedra), pulmonary embolism hyperthyroidism, heart failure, acute anxiety, or alcohol withdrawal. Sometimes, more than one cause is present. In other cases, the cause may not be apparent. For example, *inappropriate sinus tachycardia* is a rare syndrome of unknown etiology, typically found in young females. The heart rate is more than 100 beats/min at rest (e.g., >90 beats/min averaged over a 24-hour period) without the expected decrease during sleep and with very rapid acceleration to 140–150 beats/min with minimal exercise. Prominent sinus tachycardia with standing, accompanied by symptoms of lightheadedness and palpitations, may also be due to the *postural tachycardia syndrome* (POTS). The etiologic basis of this condition, primarily seen in late adolescence and young adulthood, remains

---

| **BOX 13.1** | Sinus Tachycardia: Some Major Causes |
| --- | --- |

- *Physiologic*: Excitement; exertion; pregnancy
- *Pain*
- *Drugs*:
  - Cardiac vagal tone blockers (e.g., atropine and other anticholinergic agents)
  - Sympathetic tone stimulants (e.g., norepinephrine, epinephrine, dopamine, cocaine, amphetamines)
  - Alcohol (ethanol) intoxication or withdrawal. Unexplained increases in sinus rate may be an important clue to alcohol or other addictive drug withdrawal, especially in hospitalized patients
- *Fever*, many infections, and septic shock
- *Intravascular volume loss* due to bleeding, vomiting, diarrhea, acute pancreatitis, or dehydration. Unexplained increases in heart rate may be an early sign of internal bleeding or other volume loss
- *Chronic heart failure* (CHF): An increased resting heart rate in a patient with CHF may be the first sign of decompensation and is an adverse prognostic indicator
- *Pulmonary embolism*: As noted in Chapter 12, sinus tachycardia is the most common "arrhythmia" seen with acute pulmonary embolism
- *Acute myocardial infarction* (MI), which may produce virtually any arrhythmia. Sinus tachycardia persisting after an acute MI is generally a bad prognostic sign and implies extensive heart muscle damage
- *Seizures* (common with partial or generalized)
- *Endocrine dysfunction*:
  - Hyperthyroidism: sinus tachycardia occurring at rest may be an important clue to this diagnosis
  - Pheochromocytoma

---

uncertain. Ectopic atrial tachycardias originating in the high right atrium can simulate inappropriate sinus tachycardia (see Chapter 13).

## SINUS BRADYCARDIA

With sinus bradycardia, sinus rhythm is present and the heart rate is less than 60 beats/min (see Fig. 13.3). This arrhythmia commonly occurs in the conditions listed in Box 13.2.

Moderate sinus bradycardia usually produces no symptoms. If the heart rate is very slow (especially,

---

**BOX 13.2** Sinus Bradycardia: Some Major Causes

- *Physiologic variants*: Many, healthy people have a resting pulse rate of less than 60 beats/min, and trained athletes may have a resting or sleeping pulse rate as low as 35 beats/min. Sinus bradycardia is also routinely observed during sleep in healthy subjects
- *Obstructive sleep apnea* may be associated with marked sinus bradycardia and sinus pauses (up to 10 sec or more)
- *Drugs*:
  - Increasing cardiac vagal tone (e.g., digoxin, edrophonium, donezepil)
  - Decreasing sympathetic tone (e.g., metoprolol (and other primary beta blockers), sotalol, amiodarone, dronedarone)
  - Decreasing sinus node automaticity via calcium channel blockade channel mechanisms (e.g., verapamil, diltiazem)
  - Decreasing sinus node automaticity via reducing the inward (so-called "funny") sodium current regulating sinus node firing rate
  - Causing sinus node exit block (e.g., lithium carbonate)

- *Acute myocardial infarction* (MI): Sinus bradycardia with acute MI may be due to ischemia of the sinoatrial (SA) node itself, which is perfused from a branch of the right coronary or the left circumflex artery in most people. Also, inferoposterior infarcts may be associated with enhanced vagal tone, sometimes inducing profound sinus bradycardia
- *Endocrine*: Hypothyroidism
- *Metabolic*: Marked hyperkalemia or hypermagnesemia; anorexia nervosa
- *Seizure disorder*: Acute bradyarrhythmias may occur with complex partial seizures (ictal bradycardia); see below
- *Sick sinus syndrome* and related causes of sinus node dysfunction: Age-related degeneration of SA node; inflammatory processes; cardiac surgical and postsurgical causes
- *Hypervagotonia syndromes*:
  - Vasovagal reactions
  - Carotid sinus hypersensitivity
  - Certain forms of epileptic seizures (rare; usually temporal or frontal lobe origin)
- Intracranial hypertension

---

less than 30–40 beats/min in the elderly) lightheadedness and even syncope may occur. Treatment may require adjusting medications that slow the heart rate (e.g., beta blockers, calcium channel blockers, lithium carbonate, donezepil). If *inappropriate* sinus bradycardia causes symptoms of fatigue, lightheadedness, or syncope (sick sinus syndrome; see Chapter 18), or, if severe, symptomatic sinus bradycardia is due to doses of an essential medication that cannot be lowered, a permanent pacemaker is usually indicated (see Chapter 22).

When evaluating a patient with sinus bradycardia at rest it is also useful to assess the heart rate response to mild activity. Sometimes a formal exercise test is indicated. Some people are unable to appropriately increase the heart rate during exercise, which can cause symptoms of fatigue and shortness of breath. This condition, when not due to a drug or other reversible factor, is called *chronotropic incompetence*. In rare instances, when cardiac output is not sufficient to meet metabolic demands, a permanent electronic pacemaker might be indicated even when the resting heart rate is within the "normal" range (see Chapter 22).

## SINUS ARRHYTHMIA

In healthy people, especially younger subjects, the SA node does not pace the heart at a perfectly regular rate. Instead, a slight beat-to-beat variation is present (Fig. 13.5). When this variability is more accentuated, the term *sinus arrhythmia* is used.

The most common cause of short-term sinus arrhythmia is respiration. *Respiratory sinus arrhythmia* (RSA) is a normal finding and may be quite marked (up to 10–20 beats/min or more), particularly in children and young adults. The heart rate normally increases with inspiration and decreases with expiration because of changes in vagal tone that occur during the different phases of respiration. You can test this in yourself by measuring your heart rate during slow deep inspiration and fast, full expiration.

Respiration-related variations in heart rate are an important component of *heart rate variability*, often abbreviated HRV. Measurement of different parameters of HRV reflects the status of the autonomic nervous system and these measures are affected by cardiovascular status, age, medications, systemic diseases, and multiple other factors. In the

### Respiratory Sinus Arrhythmia

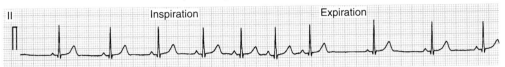

**Fig. 13.5** Respiratory sinus arrhythmia. Heart rate normally increases on inspiration and slows down with expiration as a result of changes in vagal tone modulation associated with or induced by the different phases of respiration (vagal tone decreases in inspiration and increases with expiration). This finding, a key aspect of *heart rate variability*, is physiologic and is especially noticeable in the resting ECGs of children, young adults, and athletes.

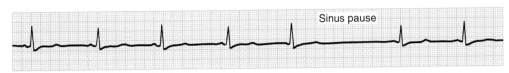

**Fig. 13.6** Sinus pause in a patient with sick sinus syndrome. The monitor lead shows sinus bradycardia with a long pause (about 2.4 sec).

### SA Exit Block

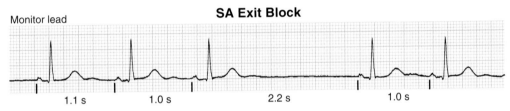

**Fig. 13.7** Pause due to 2:1 sinoatrial (SA) exit block. Note the sudden pause which is almost exactly twice the baseline PP interval. This distinctive finding is consistent with intermittent "exit block" of SA node depolarization, such that a P wave, which denotes atrial depolarization, does not occur even though the sinus pacemaker is firing appropriately. The reason for this "missing" P-QRS-T signal is that the sinus impulse is blocked intermittently from exiting the sinus node.

United States currently, HRV is primarily used as a research tool. (For more information on this important, but specialized topic, see the online supplement.)

## SINUS PAUSES, SINUS ARREST, AND SINOATRIAL BLOCK

In addition to sustained sinus bradycardia, sinus node dysfunction may occur intermittently, ranging from a mildly delayed beat (*sinus pause*; see Fig. 13.4) to long periods of asystole (*sinus arrest*). Two distinct mechanisms of sinus node dysfunction may be responsible for either sinus pauses or frank sinus arrest: sinus pacemaker failure and sinoatrial (SA) exit block. The former is due to an actual failure of the SA node to fire for one or more beats. The latter happens when the SA impulse is blocked from exiting the node and stimulating the atria (Fig. 13.6). SA

exit block may produce a pause that equals two or more PP intervals. From a clinical standpoint there is no significant difference between sinus node exit block or sinus pacemaker failure. Always look for reversible causes of SA node dysfunction, which may include drugs or electrolyte disturbances (see Box 13.2).

Sinus node dysfunction can happen spontaneously (sinus exit block; Fig. 13.7) or it can be induced by *overdrive suppression* of the sinus node by atrial fibrillation or atrial flutter resulting in a prolonged *post-conversion pause* when the atrial arrhythmia abruptly terminates or "breaks" (Fig. 13.8). Such pauses are an important cause of syncope in patients with paroxysmal atrial arrhythmias (and can be exacerbated by rate-controlling medications such as beta blockers or calcium channel blockers) resulting in a type of *tachy-brady syndrome* requiring a

## Sinus Arrest after Episode of Paroxysmal Atrial Fibrillation

Monitor lead

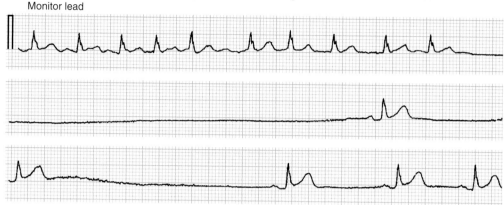

**Fig. 13.8** Sinus arrest following abrupt cessation of paroxysmal atrial fibrillation (AF). The mechanism is due to "overdrive suppression" of the sinoatrial node during the rapid stimulation of the atria during the AF. Such extended pauses may cause lightheadedness or syncope. This combination is an example of the tachy-brady syndrome. Resumption of sinus rhythm starts to occur after the prolonged sinus arrest. See also Chapters 15 and 19.

pacemaker as part of overall management (see Chapter 22).

### Secondary Pacemakers and Escape Rhythms

Why aren't sinus pauses or frank sinus arrest leading to syncope and sudden cardiac arrest even more prevalent? Recall that sinus node cells undergo spontaneous rhythmic depolarization (firing), making the SA node the primary physiologic pacemaker of the heart. However, almost any heart cell or cluster (e.g., atrial and ventricular myocytes, AV node cells, Purkinje fibers) is capable of generating spontaneous depolarizations and, therefore, initiating or maintaining the heartbeat.

The answer is that lower level (*secondary, escape*) pacemakers provide an essential backup mechanism when "higher level" pacemakers fail or conduction from them is blocked. The rate of spontaneous firing of the SA node is usually faster than that of secondary pacemakers. Thus, with every SA node firing, the wave of depolarization resets ("suppresses" or overdrives) these ectopic pacemakers. However, if the SA node fails to fire, the next in the hierarchy of ectopic pacemakers may "escape" or be uninhibited by this suppressive control and generate an *escape beat*.

The occasional failure of physiologic escape mechanisms to "rescue" the heart is noteworthy because it may precipitate syncope or even sudden

cardiac arrest. This finding suggests that the same factors suppressing the sinus node (e.g., drugs, ischemia, and exaggerated vagal tone) may also profoundly decrease the automaticity of these backup pacemakers.

Escape beats (or a sustained *escape rhythm* if sinus arrest persists) can appear from atrial cells (~60–80 beats/min), AV nodal cells (~35–60 beats/min), His–Purkinje cells (~25–35 beats/min), and ventricular myocytes, themselves (≤25–35 beats/min).

Atrial escape rhythms are characterized by regular P waves, slower than underlying sinus rhythm, with non-sinus P wave morphology (so-called "low atrial rhythm;" see Fig. 13.4).

In junctional escape rhythm (the terms *AV junctional, junctional, AV nodal,* and *nodal* are essentially synonymous), the atria are activated in a *retrograde* fashion, from bottom to top, producing negative P waves in leads II, III, and AVF, and a positive P wave in lead aVR (see Fig. 5.5).

With an AV junctional escape, the QRS complex will be normal (of "narrow" duration) because the ventricles are depolarized synchronously (unless a bundle branch block is also present). Furthermore, because the atria and ventricles are activated simultaneously during an AV junctional rhythm (not sequentially as with sinus rhythm), the QRS and P waves will occur at nearly the same time. As the result, an inverted P wave in lead II may appear: (1)

## Sinus Bradycardia and Junctional Escape Beats

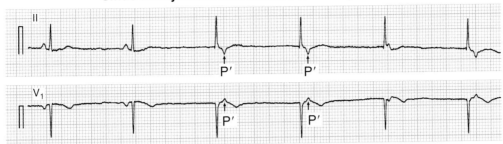

**Fig. 13.9** Atrioventricular (AV) junctional (nodal) escape rhythm. Simultaneous recording of lead II and lead $V_1$. The initial two beats show marked sinus bradycardia (at about 40 beats/min) followed by an even slower junctional escape rhythm (about 35 beats/min) with "retrograde" P waves (negative in lead II, just after the QRS complexes). These retrograde P waves may be confused with S waves in leads II, III, and aVF and with R waves in leads aVR and $V_1$. Therefore, they are sometimes called "pseudo S" and "pseudo R" waves, respectively. Always look for reversible causes of inappropriate sinus bradycardia and junctional escape rhythms, including certain drugs, hypothyroidism, and hyperkalemia.

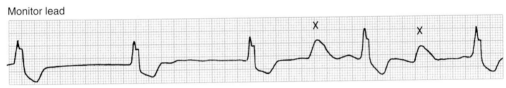

**Fig. 13.10** Idioventricular escape rhythm recorded during a cardiac arrest during attempted resuscitation. The waveforms marked "X" are chest compression artifacts. The underlying atrial mechanism, if any, cannot be determined (see also Chapter 21). Note also that the current recommended rate of chest compressions in adults is 100–120/min.

just before the QRS complex (with a very short PR interval), or more commonly (2) "buried" inside the QRS (where the P wave is invisible), or (3) just after the QRS (producing "pseudo-S waves" in leads II, III, and aVF and "pseudo-R'" waves in leads $V_1$ and aVR (Fig. 13.9).

Escape rhythms may also originate below the AV junction. Fascicular and idioventricular escape rhythms (Fig. 13.10) are slow, wide QRS rhythms that usually indicate a life-threatening situation. They are associated with low blood pressure, are unstable, and can transition abruptly into *pulseless electrical activity* or *asystole* with cardiac arrest (see Chapter 21). Emergency treatment of underlying reversible conditions (such as hyperkalemia, digitalis

toxicity, or other drug toxicity) is essential and temporary pacing is usually indicated.

It is important to understand that escape rhythms are not the primary arrhythmias but rather function as automatic backups or compensatory responses. The primary problem is failure of the higher order pacemakers or of AV conduction block. Therefore, diagnosis and treatment of these primary conditions are the goals (see Box 13.2).

In urgent conditions, intravenous atropine (a parasympathetic blocker) can be used to acutely increase the rate of atrial or junctional pacemakers. Sympathomimetic agents (e.g., dopamine or isoproterenol) increase both supraventricular and ventricular ectopic pacemaker rates.

# CHAPTER 14

# Supraventricular Arrhythmias, Part I: Premature Beats and Paroxysmal Supraventricular Tachycardias

## GENERAL PRINCIPLES

This chapter and the next two focus on rhythm disturbances with a rapid rate, namely: supraventricular (Fig. 14.1) and ventricular tachyarrhythmias.

====== Key Pathophysiologic Concept ======

For any rapid, abnormal heart rhythm to occur, two major factors have to be present:
- A *trigger* that initiates the arrhythmia.
- A *substrate* that allows the arrhythmia mechanism to continue (self-sustain).

Tachyarrhythmias, both supraventricular (Fig. 14.2) and ventricular (Chapter 16), usually start with premature beats that initiate arrhythmias by either *focal* or *reentrant* mechanisms (Fig. 14.2).

Focal tachycardias involve repetitive firing of an ectopic (non-sinus) pacemaker. In contrast, reentry involves the non-uniform spread of a depolarization wave through one pathway in the heart, with blockage along a second pathway. If block in the second pathway is *unidirectional*, the wave may be able to *reenter* it from the reverse direction and then loop around, traveling back down the first pathway, thereby creating an abnormal "revolving door" circuit.

Sometimes, an arrhythmia (e.g., atrioventricular nodal reentrant tachycardia; AVNRT) may be initiated by one mechanism (e.g., a premature beat from an ectopic atrial focus) and then sustained by another mechanism (e.g., reentry).

Please go to expertconsult.inkling.com for additional online material for this chapter.

The sinus or sinoatrial (SA) node (see Chapter 13) is the physiologic (natural or intrinsic) pacemaker of the heart. The SA node normally initiates each heartbeat, producing physiologic ("normal") sinus rhythm. However, pacemaker stimuli can arise from other parts of the heart, including the atrial muscle or pulmonary vein areas, the atrioventricular (AV) junction, or the ventricles.

Ectopic beats are most often premature; that is, they come before the next sinus beat is due. Examples include *premature atrial complexes* or *beats* (PACs or PABs/APBs, synonymously), *premature AV junctional complexes* (PJCs), and *premature ventricular complexes* (PVCs). Ectopic beats can also come after a pause (delay) in the normal rhythm, as in the case of AV junctional or ventricular *escape* beats (see Chapter 13). Ectopic beats originating in the AV junction (node) or atria are referred to as *supraventricular* (i.e., literally coming from *above* the ventricles).

This chapter and the next describe the major *non-sinus* supraventricular arrhythmias, and Chapter 16 deals with ventricular tachyarrhythmias.

## ATRIAL AND OTHER SUPRAVENTRICULAR PREMATURE BEATS

Premature atrial complexes (PACs)[a] result from ectopic stimuli arising from loci in either the left

[a]The terms premature atrial complexes or contractions, atrial premature beats, premature atrial depolarizations, and atrial extrasystoles are used synonymously. Most cardiologists prefer the designations premature atrial complex, beat, or depolarization because not every premature stimulus is associated with an actual mechanical contraction of the atria or ventricles. The same principle applies to the naming of ventricular premature complexes (Chapter 16).

**Major Narrow Complex
Tachycardias (NCTs)**

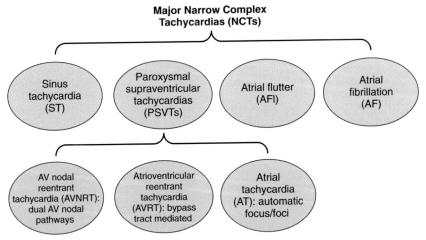

**Fig. 14.1** Classification of narrow complex tachycardias (NCTs). Rapid heart rhythms can be divided into *narrow (QRS) complex* and *wide (QRS) complex* tachycardias (WCTs); see Chapters 16 and 19. Wide complex tachycardias include ventricular tachycardia and any of the supraventricular tachycardias with aberrant ventricular conduction or conduction down a bypass tract (Chapter 19). Narrow complex tachycardias can also be classified based on regularity. Sinus tachycardia, atrial tachycardia or atrial flutter with pure 1:1 or 2:1 conduction, atrioventricular nodal reentrant tachycardia (AVNRT), and atrioventricular reentrant tachycardia (AVRT) are regular, but atrial fibrillation, multifocal atrial tachycardia, and atrial flutter or atrial tachycardia with variable degrees of atrioventricular (AV) block are irregular.

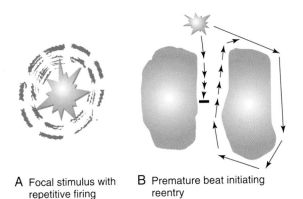

A Focal stimulus with repetitive firing

B Premature beat initiating reentry

**Fig. 14.2** Schematic showing basic mechanisms of tachy-arrhythmias: (A) *Focal arrhythmias*: repetitive firing of a group of cells. (B) *Reentrant arrhythmias*: repetitive motion of an electrical signal along a path around an "obstacle." The hallmark of reentry is that a premature ectopic beat (*star*) blocks in one conduction pathway due to its refractoriness. The signal then reaches the opposite side of this channel by the time it has recovered its conductivity. The signal then can conduct in the opposite way, completing a "reentrant loop" of excitation. Structures such as the AV node, accessory pathways, and viable tissue between the areas of scar (due to infarction or fibrosis) can provide the substrate for such abnormal circuits.

or right atrium, or interatrial septum, but not the SA node itself. After an atrial or junctional premature complex (JPC), the stimulus may spread normally through the His–Purkinje system into the ventricles. For this reason, the ventricular depolarization (QRS) is generally *not* affected by PACs or JPCs. The major features of PACs are listed in Box 14.1 and depicted in Figs. 14.3–14.6.

PACs may occur frequently or sporadically. Two PACs occurring consecutively are referred to as an *atrial couplet*. Sometimes, as shown in Fig. 14.4, each sinus beat is followed by a PAC. This pattern is referred to as *atrial bigeminy*.

## Clinical Significance

PACs, conducted and blocked, are very common. They may occur in people with normal hearts or with virtually any type of organic heart disease. Thus, the presence of PACs does not imply that an individual has cardiac disease. Supraventricular premature beats may be associated with emotional stress, excessive intake of caffeinated drinks, or the administration of sympathomimetic agents (epinephrine, albuterol, and other sympathomimetic agents). PACs may also occur with hyperthyroidism. PACs may produce *palpitations*; in this situation, patients may complain of feeling a "skipped beat"

| BOX 14.1 | Major Features of Premature Atrial Complexes |

- The atrial depolarization (P′ wave) is premature, occurring before the next sinus P wave is due.
- The QRS complex of the premature atrial complex (PAC) is usually preceded by a visible P wave that has a slightly different shape or different PR interval from the P wave seen with sinus beats. The PR interval of the PAC may be either longer or shorter than the PR interval of the normal beats. In some cases the P wave may be subtly hidden in the T wave of the preceding beat.
- After the PAC a slight pause generally occurs before the normal sinus beat resumes. This delay is due to "resetting" of the sinoatrial (SA) node pacemaker by the premature atrial stimulus. The slight delay contrasts with the longer, "fully compensatory" pause often (but not always) seen after premature ventricular complexes (PVCs) (see Fig. 16.9).
- The QRS complex of the PAC is usually identical or very similar to the QRS complex of the preceding beats. With PACs the atrial pacemaker is in an ectopic location but the ventricles are usually depolarized in a normal way. This sequence contrasts with the generation of PVCs, in which the QRS complex is abnormally wide because of

asynchronous ventricular depolarization (see Chapter 16).
- Occasionally, PACs result in *aberrant ventricular conduction*, so that the QRS complex is wider than normal. Figs. 14.5 and 14.6 show examples of such PACs causing delayed (aberrant) depolarization of the right and left ventricles, respectively.
- Sometimes, when a PAC is very premature, the stimulus reaches the atrioventricular (AV) junction just after it has been stimulated by the preceding beat. The AV junction, like other cardiac tissue, has an inherent refractory period. Therefore, it requires time to recover its capacity to conduct impulses. Thus a PAC may reach the junction when it is still *refractory*. In this situation the PAC may not be conducted to the ventricles and no QRS complex appears. The result is a so-called *blocked* PAC. The ECG shows a premature P wave *not* followed by a QRS complex (see Fig. 14.3B). After the blocked P wave, a brief pause occurs before the next normal beat resumes. The blocked PAC, therefore, produces a slight irregularity of the heartbeat. If you do not search carefully for blocked PACs, you may overlook them.

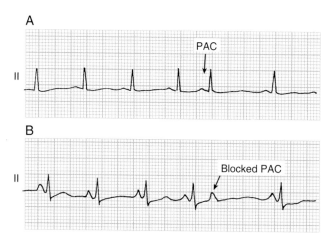

A

II

PAC

B

II

Blocked PAC

**Fig. 14.3** (A) Sinus rhythm with atrial ectopy. Note the premature atrial complex (*PAC*) after the fourth sinus beat (*arrow*). (B) Note also the blocked PAC, again after the fourth sinus beat (*arrow*). The premature P wave falls on the T wave of the preceding beat and is not followed by a QRS complex because the atrioventricular (AV) node is still in a refractory state.

or an irregular pulse (a type of palpitation). PACs may also be seen with various types of structural heart disease. Frequent PACs are sometimes the forerunner of atrial fibrillation or flutter (see Chapter 15) or other supraventricular tachyarrhythmias, as discussed in the next sections.

## PAROXYSMAL SUPRAVENTRICULAR TACHYCARDIAS (PSVTs)

Premature supraventricular beats (Box 14.2) may occur singly or repetitively. A sudden run of three or more such consecutive non-sinus beats constitutes an episode of paroxysmal supraventricular

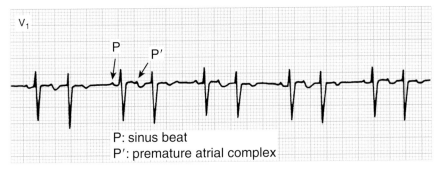

**Fig. 14.4** Sinus rhythm with atrial bigeminy. Each sinus beat is coupled to a premature atrial complex followed by a slight post-ectopic pause. This sequence is one of the causes of group beating pattern and must be distinguished from second-degree atrioventricular (AV) heart block in which the sinus P waves come "on time" and one is not conducted (see Chapter 17).

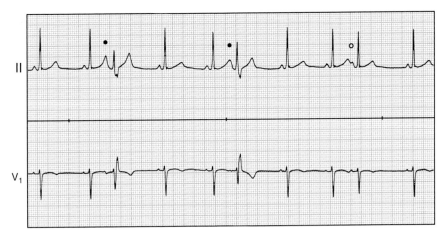

**Fig. 14.5** ECG shows sinus rhythm with three atrial premature beats. The first two (marked ·) are conducted with right bundle branch block aberrancy (rSR′ in lead $V_1$). The third premature atrial complex (○) is conducted with normal ventricular activation. Notice how the first two premature P waves come so early in the cardiac cycle that they fall on the T waves of the preceding sinus beats, making these T waves slightly taller or more positive.

## PACs with Intermittent LBBB

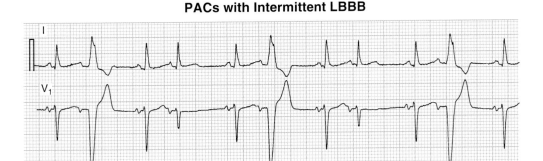

**Fig. 14.6** Sinus rhythm with premature atrial complexes (PACs) showing intermittent left bundle branch block (LBBB) aberration. Note that every second PAC conducts with an LBBB pattern of aberrancy.

tachycardia (PSVT). Episodes of PSVT may be nonsustained (i.e., lasting from a few beats up to 30 sec). Sustained episodes (greater than 30 sec) may last for minutes, hours, or longer. These episodes may stop spontaneously, after drug therapy, and

| BOX 14.2 | Classification of Major Types of Paroxysmal Supraventricular Tachycardia |
|---|---|

- Atrial tachycardia (AT) and related rhythms, including multifocal atrial tachycardia
- Atrioventricular nodal reentrant tachycardia (AVNRT)
- Atrioventricular reentrant tachycardia (AVRT) involving a bypass tract of the type seen in the Wolff-Parkinson-White (WPW) syndrome (see Chapter 18)

more rarely require emergency direct current (DC) cardioversion (Chapter 15) or, even more rarely, acute radiofrequency ablation therapy.

The detailed topic of PSVT is quite complicated. Furthermore, the term PSVT, itself, is somewhat misleading, because sometimes tachyarrhythmias in this class, as just noted, may be long-lasting or even incessant not just paroxysmal or intermittent. Therefore, the following brief discussion is intended to provide trainees and clinicians with an introduction and overview. Additional material is provided in the online supplement and in the bibliography.

The three major types of PSVT are shown in Fig. 14.7.

### Atrial Tachycardias

Classic ("monofocal") atrial tachycardia (AT) is defined as three or more consecutive PACs coming

Normal sinus rhythm

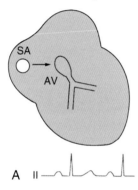

A

Atrial tachycardia (AT)

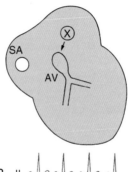

B

Atrioventricular nodal reentrant tachycardia (AVNRT)

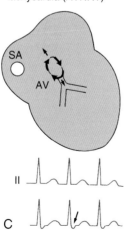

C

Atrioventricular reentrant tachycardia (AVRT)

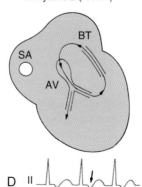

D

**Fig. 14.7** The three major types of paroxysmal supraventricular tachycardias (PSVTs). (A) The reference is normal sinus rhythm. (B) With (unifocal) atrial tachycardia (AT), a focus (*X*) outside the sinoatrial (SA) node fires off automatically at a rapid rate. (C) With atrioventricular (AV) nodal reentrant tachycardia (AVNRT) the cardiac stimulus originates as a wave of excitation that spins around the AV nodal (junctional) area. As a result, retrograde P waves may be buried in the QRS or appear just after the QRS complex (*arrow*) because of nearly simultaneous activation of the atria and ventricles. Rarely, they appear just before the QRS. (D) A similar type of reentrant (circus-movement) mechanism may occur with a manifest or concealed bypass tract (BT) of the type found in Wolff-Parkinson-White syndrome (see also Chapter 18). This mechanism is referred to as *atrioventricular reentrant tachycardia* (AVRT). Note the negative P wave (*arrow*) in lead II, somewhat after the QRS complex.

## Initiation of Atrial Tachycardia (AT)

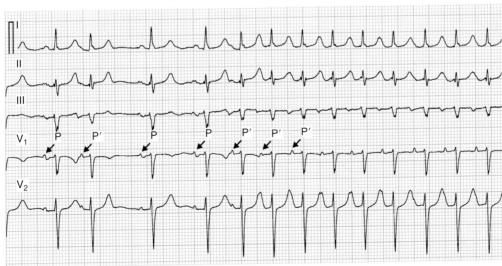

**Fig. 14.8** Atrial tachycardia (AT). P wave (*arrow*) indicates a sinus P wave; P′ (*with arrow*) indicates a premature atrial complex initiating and maintaining the AT. The P′ waves of the AT are best seen in lead $V_1$, and are more subtly detectable in lead III. They are difficult to see in leads I, II, and $V_2$ where they merge with the T waves, slightly distorting the T wave appearance. Note also that in this case the sinus P waves show left atrial abnormality (broad, biphasic P waves in lead $V_1$).

## Termination of Atrial Tachycardia

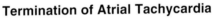

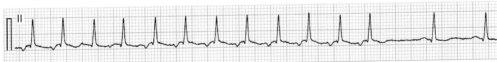

**Fig. 14.9** Cessation of atrial tachycardia (AT). After the AT focus stops firing, the last P′ wave conducts to the ventricles. Runs of AT almost always terminate with a QRS complex. Slight variation in the shape of the ectopic P waves during AT is related to slightly irregular heart rate and its superimposition on different portions of the preceding T wave. This is also typical for AT.

from a single atrial focus, with each having an identical, non-sinus P wave morphology (Fig. 14.8). The arrhythmic focus can be located in either the right or left atrium (sometimes in the proximal pulmonary vein areas), and fires off "automatically" in a rapid way. An important variant, discussed later, is *multifocal AT (MAT)*, in which the P waves vary because they represent ectopic foci originating from different sites (usually three or more) of abnormally increased automaticity.

### Initiation and Termination of Atrial Tachycardias

Atrial tachycardias are initiated by PACs, which may be conducted or blocked (i.e., not followed by a QRS).

Termination occurs when the ectopic atrial focus stops firing (either spontaneously or after administration of an antiarrhythmic drug). The last P wave of the tachycardia usually conducts to the ventricles producing a QRS complex at the end of the run. Therefore, *AT almost always terminates with a QRS complex* (Figs. 14.9 and 14.10). This is an important feature for differential diagnosis of other types of PSVTs (see later discussion).

### Conduction Patterns with Atrial Tachycardias and Other PSVTs

Conduction occurs over the AV node and His-Purkinje system with atrial tachycardias usually producing a *narrow QRS tachycardia*. However, if the

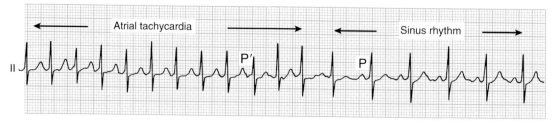

**Fig. 14.10** Atrial tachycardia terminating spontaneously with the abrupt resumption of sinus tachycardia. Note that the P′ waves of the tachycardia (rate: about 150 beats/min) are superimposed on the preceding T waves.

## Multifocal Atrial Tachycardia

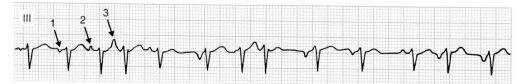

**Fig. 14.11** Multifocal atrial tachycardia. Note the rapidly occurring P waves showing variable shapes and PR intervals. This fast, irregular rhythm may be mistaken for atrial fibrillation. Arrows with numbers (1–3) above show a segment with multiple consecutive different P waves.

atrial rate is high, or the AV node is not normal, different degrees of delay and block can occur in any part of the conduction system (similar to that occurring with isolated PACs), producing not just PR prolongation, but QRS aberration (widening), and "dropped" (nonconducted) P waves, i.e., those that are not followed by QRS complexes. The latter produce a functional type of second-degree AV block, which may have a regular or irregular heart cadence, depending on the pattern of block.

Of note, if there is a preexisting bundle branch block or if a rate-related interventricular conduction delay (IVCD) occurs, the QRS during the AT or other PSVT will remain wide and can be confused with ventricular tachycardia (SVT with aberrancy) (see also Chapters 16 and 19).

### Multifocal Atrial Tachycardia: an Important Variant

Multifocal atrial tachycardia (MAT), as noted above, is a special variant of atrial tachycardia related to multiple sites of atrial stimulation (Fig. 14.11). The diagnosis of MAT requires the presence of three or more consecutive (non-sinus) P waves with different shapes at a rate of 100 or more per minute. MAT contrasts with classic (unifocal) AT, which involves only a single atrial focus and produces one repetitive,

non-sinus P wave. The PR intervals of P waves during MAT also vary. MAT is most often seen in patients with severe chronic lung disease. Because the ventricular rate is irregular and rapid, this arrhythmia may be mistaken for AF.

### Atrial Tachycardias: Clinical Considerations

Sustained AT can be observed in patients with apparently normal hearts, but often occurs in those with organic heart disease of varying types. The atrial rate can vary, usually between 100 and 250 beats/min. AT, particularly conducting at very rapid ventricular rates, may cause dizziness, lightheadedness, shortness of breath, but rarely syncope. Your patient may complain of palpitations. In susceptible individuals, AT can induce angina in patients with coronary disease or decompensation of chronic heart failure (CHF) in susceptible individuals. Short episodes may require no special therapy, but longer runs, or chronic episodes causing symptoms, are usually treated with antiarrhythmic drugs or radiofrequency (RF) catheter ablation (see later discussion), as well as reducing the dosage of, or eliminating, potentially provocative drugs. A careful history for "recreational drugs" or herbal and other over-the-counter medications is indicated. Sometimes AT can deteriorate into atrial fibrillation. As noted, MAT is usually seen in severe obstructive lung disease, but may also occur with heart failure syndromes.

## AV Nodal Reentrant Tachycardia

AV nodal reentrant tachycardia (AVNRT) is a supraventricular arrhythmia, usually paroxysmal, resulting from the reentry in the AV node area. Normally, the AV node behaves as a single electrical conduit connecting the atria with His–Purkinje-ventricular electrical network. However, in some people two functional conduction channels with different electrical properties (termed *dual pathways*) may be present. One AV nodal pathway has fast and the other has slow conduction speeds.

## Initiation and Maintenance of AVNRT

The mechanism of AVNRT initiation is presented in Fig. 14.12. During sinus rhythm the atrial signal engages both "fast" and "slow" pathways. It reaches the His bundle through the fast pathway first and

from there conducts to the ventricles. At the same time, it turns around and goes "up" the slow pathway, colliding with (and thereby extinguishing) the more slowly conducting downgoing signal. The surface ECG only registers sinus rhythm with a normal PR interval; there is no evidence of the "slow" pathway existence (beats 1 and 2 in Fig. 14.12).

If an early PAC arrives at the AV node, it blocks in both pathways (P′ wave after the second QRS) producing a blocked PAC. If the PAC arrives a little later, however, it blocks only in the "fast" pathway while conducting over the "slow" pathway (P′ after the fourth QRS) producing marked PR interval prolongation. The signal can then turn around (reenter) at the lower pathway junction and conduct up the fast pathway, which by this time has recovered its excitability (third beat from the right, indicated by upward arrow). Then the signal reenters the slow pathway at the top of the AV node and conducts down again starting a repetitive loop of reentry (indicated by the black arrows in the diagram of

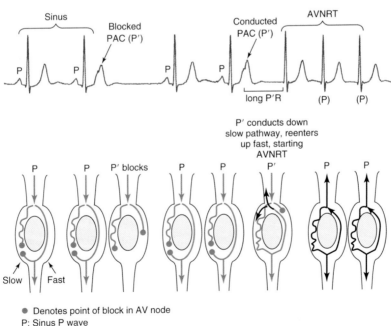

**DUAL AV Nodal Pathways: Substrate for AVNRT**

● Denotes point of block in AV node
P: Sinus P wave
P′: PAC
(P): Retrograde P wave due to reentry hidden in QRS

**Fig. 14.12** Mechanism of typical atrioventricular nodal reentrant tachycardia (AVNRT) initiation, involving *dual atrioventricular (AV) nodal pathways* and reentry. See text.

the last three beats). At every turn the signal activates the atria from the top and ventricles from the bottom of the circle.

Because the arrhythmia circuit operates within the AV node (between the atria and ventricles), the activation spreads nearly simultaneously up the atria and down the ventricles with every reentrant rotation of the signal. As a result, the P waves can be completely hidden ("buried") in the QRS complex (Fig. 14.13) or appear just after it. Very rarely they appear just before the QRS. Because of retrograde (bottom-to-top) activation of the atria, the retrograde P waves are negative in leads II, III, and aVF, sometimes producing subtle but distinctive "pseudo-S" waves and positive in leads $V_1$ and aVR where they are referred to as "pseudo-R'" waves that are absent during sinus rhythm (Fig. 14.14).

Besides this "typical" (slow–fast) AVNRT, there is a much rarer "atypical" form when the short circuit in the AV node moves in the opposite direction (down the fast and up the slow pathway, sometimes called "fast–slow" AVNRT). This sequence produces negative P waves in lead II, and positive P waves in aVR that come just in front of the QRS complexes.

### Termination of AVNRT

Unlike focal AT, which terminates when the ectopic focus stops firing, AVNRT is a self-perpetuating rhythm that will continue indefinitely unless a block develops in some part of the circuit. The block can occur in either fast (upgoing) or slow (downgoing) AV nodal pathway. The slow AV nodal pathway is more susceptible to vagal influences (see Fig. 14.15)

## Paroxysmal Supraventricular Tachycardia

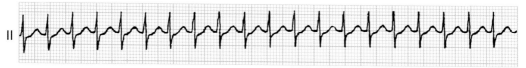

**Fig. 14.13** Atrioventricular nodal reentrant tachycardia (AVNRT). Notice the metronomic regularity with a rate of 170 beats/min. No P waves are visible because they are "buried" in the QRS due to simultaneous atrial and ventricular stimulation.

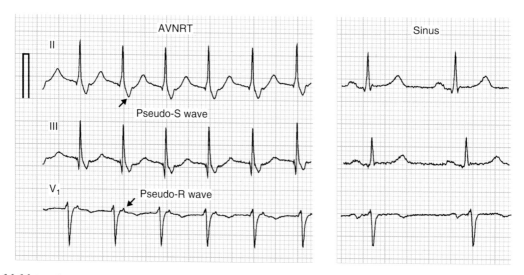

**Fig. 14.14** Pseudo-S waves (leads II, III) and pseudo-R' waves (lead $V_1$) caused by retrograde P waves during atrioventricular nodal reentrant tachycardia (AVNRT). Note that these waveforms disappear during sinus rhythm. Baseline artifact is present, along with LAA.

## Termination of AVNRT

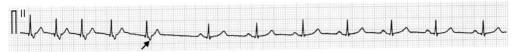

**Fig. 14.15** Atrioventricular nodal reentrant tachycardia (AVNRT) terminated with carotid sinus massage, a maneuver that increases vagal tone. The block of the reentrant conduction impulse occurs in the "slow" atrioventricular (AV) nodal pathway on its way down, before activation of the ventricles. Therefore, the QRS complex at the cessation of the arrhythmia is absent and the last ECG deflection is the retrograde P wave (negative in lead II, indicated by arrow). The P wave resembles an "S" wave and is sometimes called a "pseudo-S" wave with AVNRT. Note also the subtle progressive delay in the slow AV nodal pathway conduction seen prior to the arrhythmia termination, associated with longer RR intervals. Sinus rhythm then resumes abruptly.

or AV nodal blocking drugs (e.g., adenosine,[b] beta blockers, calcium channel blockers, or digoxin). The block in the slow pathway usually occurs just before the signal activates the ventricles from the bottom of the circuit; therefore, *the last arrhythmia deflection on the electrocardiogram is a retrograde P wave* (Fig. 14.15).

### AVNRT: Clinical Considerations

AVNRT produces a rapid and almost metronomically regular supraventricular rhythm with rates usually between 140 and 220 or so beats/min. Typically, AVNRT occurs in normal hearts and starts at a young age, particularly in young women. Until the arrhythmia is correctly identified, many of these patients are misdiagnosed as having "anxiety or panic attacks."

One of the most commonly reported symptoms at the onset of AVNRT is the sensation of palpitations characterized as a "flip-flop" sensation in the chest (resulting from the initiating PAC), followed by rapid, regular palpitations. The arrhythmia may start with the person suddenly changing position or may be associated with psychological or physiologic stress, pregnancy, or sympathomimetic drugs. Patients may complain of pulsations in the neck due to simultaneous atrial and ventricular contraction, producing "cannon A waves" on inspection of the jugular venous waves during the neck examination. AVNRT can also produce dizziness, lightheadedness, and rarely, syncope. In patients

with underlying coronary artery disease, PSVT may induce myocardial ischemia with angina.

### Atrioventricular Reentrant Tachycardia (AVRT)

Atrioventricular reentrant tachycardia (AVRT) involves an accessory atrioventricular bypass tract (see Chapter 18), which provides the substrate for reentry. Clinicians distinguish between two types of bypass tracts: *manifest* and *concealed*. Manifest bypass tracts can conduct the electrical signal in both directions: from the atria to the ventricles and in reverse. During sinus rhythm, this produces the classic triadic "signature" of Wolff–Parkinson–White syndrome (WPW): delta wave, short PR interval, and wide QRS (see Chapter 18).

Importantly, bypass tract conduction can produce wide or narrow complex reentrant tachycardias as part of the WPW syndrome depending on the direction of the reentrant loop. If the signal goes down the AV node and up the bypass tract, the ECG will have a narrow QRS (referred to as *orthodromic AVRT*). In contrast, if the signal goes down the bypass tract and up the AV node, a much less common finding, you will see a wide QRS; this reentrant variant is technically referred to as *antidromic AVRT*.

Importantly, clinicians should be aware that the majority of bypass tracts do *not* conduct the impulse from the atria to the ventricles and are therefore completely invisible (*concealed*) during sinus rhythm. Thus, you will *not* see the classic WPW signature. However, some concealed bypass tracts can conduct the impulse in the reverse direction (ventricles to atria), providing, in concert with the AV node and the infranodal conduction system, the second pathway necessary for reentry and the basis for a narrow complex tachycardia: namely, ortho-dromic AVRT (Chapter 18).

---

[b]Adenosine depresses the electrical activity in both the SA and AV nodes. Its very rapid action appears to be mediated by increasing an outward potassium current, hyperpolarizing the cells of both nodes. As a result, SA node automaticity is decreased, as are automaticity and conduction in the AV node area. Adenosine also is a vasodilator (accounting for its transient blood pressure lowering and facial flushing effects).

## AVRT: Initiation and Conduction

During sinus rhythm, retrograde conduction through the bypass tract usually does not occur because the signal gets to the ventricular end of the bypass tract through the normal conduction system while the atrium around it is still refractory from the preceding sinus beat (Fig. 14.16A).

A PVC that occurs close to the ventricular entrance of the concealed bypass tract can block the His-Purkinje system while conducting back to the atria through the bypass tract (Fig. 14.16B). *In fact, when a regular narrow complex tachycardia is initiated by a PVC, the mechanism is most likely AVRT* (see Figs. 14.16 and 14.17). Since the atria and ventricles activate one after another "in sequence" with AVRT as opposed to "in-parallel" as during AVNRT, the interval between the QRS and the P waves is longer in the former, and retrograde P waves are often visible superimposed on the ST-T wave.

Both the atrium and the ventricle are necessary to maintain the arrhythmia circuit, therefore AVRT always has a 1:1 AV relationship, as opposed to AT, which may be associated with 1:1 or variable conduction patterns. AVNRT almost always has a 1:1 AV relationship. *Thus, if you see more P waves than QRS complexes, AVRT and AVNRT can be effectively excluded.*

AVRT (as well as other PSVTs) also can produce *QRS alternans*—a periodic change in the QRS shape, occurring with every other beat (Fig. 14.18). This interesting pattern may be due to subtle conduction

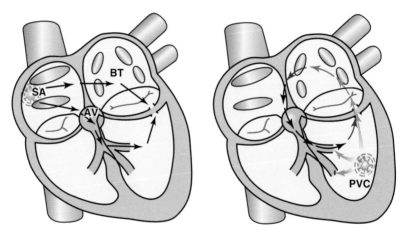

**Fig. 14.16** Atrioventricular reentrant tachycardia (AVRT) initiation by a premature ventricular complex (PVC). (A) During sinus (SA) rhythm there is no retrograde conduction across the bypass tract (BT) or atrioventricular (AV) node because of refractoriness from the previous SA beat. (B) A PVC (*star*) firing close to the bypass tract conducts to the atrium via the bypass tract, while simultaneously being blocked in the His-Purkinje system. This sequence initiates a narrow complex tachycardia in which the impulse travels down (antegrade conduction) the AV node–His-bundle branch system and reenters the atrium by going up (retrograde conduction) the bypass tract. AVRT may also be initiated by a premature atrial complex (PAC). See also Fig. 14.17 and Chapter 18.

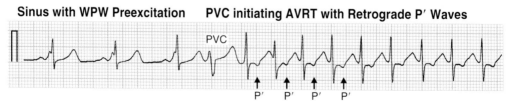

**Fig. 14.17** Atrioventricular reentrant tachycardia (AVRT) initiated by a premature ventricular complex (PVC). During sinus rhythm (first three beats) a short PR interval, wide QRS complex, and a delta wave are present, consistent with the classic Wolff-Parkinson-White (WPW) preexcitation pattern. A PVC (beat 4) initiates a narrow complex tachycardia. Retrograde P waves are visible as negative deflections in the middle of the T wave (*black arrows*). This finding corresponds to the mechanism depicted in Fig. 14.5.

## AVRT: QRS Alternans

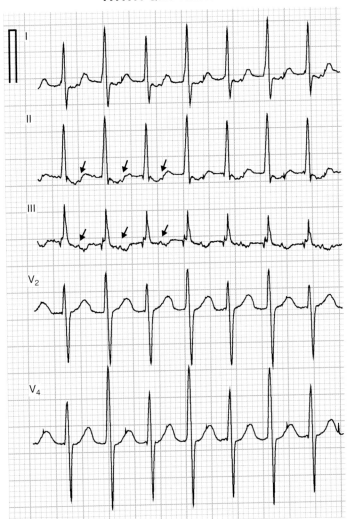

**Fig. 14.18** QRS alternans during atrioventricular reentrant tachycardia (AVRT). Note the periodically alternating pattern of QRS amplitudes ("ABABAB ...") best seen in leads $V_2$ and $V_4$. Retrograde P waves are seen in the middle of T wave in leads I and II (*arrows*). Alternans during paroxysmal supraventricular tachycardia (PSVT) should not be confused with alternans during sinus tachycardia (see Chapter 12), where it is an indicator of pericardial effusion, often cardiac tamponade (compare with Fig. 12.3). Also, alternans may occur with other types of PSVT (and, sometimes, ventricular tachycardia), so it is not specific for AVRT.

variations that occur at rapid rates. This type of alternans is different from the beat-to-beat alternans that may occur during sinus rhythm/tachycardia with pericardial effusion and tamponade, due to swinging of the heart to-and-fro in the pericardial effusion (Chapter 12).

### AVRT: Termination

Because AVRT uses the AV node to conduct electrical signals from the atria to the ventricles (during so-called *orthodromic AVRT*), this mechanism is susceptible to vagal influences and AV nodal

blocking agents, similar to the situation in AVNRT. With AVRT, the reentrant circuit often terminates in the AV node on *the way down before reaching the ventricles, producing a retrograde P wave at the end of arrhythmia run.*

### AVRT: Other Clinical Considerations

The first episode of AVRT usually presents in childhood or young adulthood in contrast to AVNRT, which is predominantly seen in young to middle-aged female subjects. AVRT occurs more frequently in men. The accessory bypass tracts, manifest or concealed, can be located on the left or right side of the heart (see Chapter 17). The symptoms, including palpitations and lightheadedness, as well as shortness of breath, are similar to AVNRT, discussed earlier.

## DIFFERENTIAL DIAGNOSIS AND TREATMENT OF PSVT

The differential diagnosis of PSVT can be difficult, even for seasoned cardiologists. P waves may not be clearly visible even if present because they are hidden in the T waves or ST segments, especially in a single monitor lead. Sometimes it is impossible to tell the exact mechanism of the arrhythmia (especially when initiation and termination of it are not recorded) unless an invasive electrophysiologic study is performed. A summary of major, differential diagnostic findings is presented in Table 14.1. More detailed diagnosis of this important topic is available in selected bibliographic references.

The most clinically useful diagnostic as well as therapeutic measures in terminating PSVT are aimed at achieving block in AV node conduction. These measures include vagal maneuvers, particularly the Valsalva maneuver and carotid sinus massage (CSM), and also pharmacologic interventions, especially intravenous adenosine.

*Clinical Note 1:* While performing CSM and adenosine injections, continuous ECG monitoring is critical to document response to the intervention. Resuscitation equipment, including an external defibrillator, should be available in case of unexpected reactions.

*Clinical Note 2:* Adenosine effect is blocked by methylxanthines (e.g., theophylline; caffeine) and potentiated by dipyridamole. An important electrophysiologic side effect of adenosine is induction of atrial fibrillation (which may or may not terminate spontaneously). Adenosine injection often creates an extremely uncomfortable feeling noted by patients (most frequent symptoms and signs are related to facial flushing, bronchospasm with dyspnea, and even transient asystole after arrhythmia termination). Patients should be warned that they may feel uncomfortable.

The response of PSVT to CSM (or other vagal maneuvers) or adenosine injection is summarized in Table 14.1.

### Management of Acute PSVT Episodes

The management of the first acute PSVT episode should start with vagal maneuvers (e.g., the Valsalva maneuver, CSM; see Fig. 14.15) followed by adenosine injection. Many patients who have had recurrent

| TABLE 14.1 | Differential Diagnosis of Supraventricular Tachycardias (SVT)* | | | |
|---|---|---|---|---|
| **Type** | **Sinus Tachycardia** | **Atrial Tachycardia (AT)** | **AVNRT** | **AVRT** |
| Onset/termination | Gradual | Abrupt | Abrupt | Abrupt |
| Heart (QRS) rate | Varies slightly with respiration and activity | Nearly constant rate between 100 and 250 | Nearly constant | Nearly constant |
| Typical initiation | Gradual, with acceleration of sinus P waves | PAC identical to subsequent P' waves of AT | Initiated by a PAC with a long PR interval | Initiated by a PVC or a PAC |
| P waves during the SVT | Sinus | Identical to each other (except with MAT) but different from sinus | Often pseudo-R' in $V_1$; pseudo-S in II, III, and aVF, or P waves invisible | Negative in II, III, and aVF, usually shortly after QRS complex |
| Vagal maneuvers or adenosine injection | Heart rate slows down, with possible transient AV block; (P waves continue) or SA block occurs | Rarely terminates; more commonly transient AV block may develop | Either no effect or PSVT terminates suddenly (usually ending with a P' wave) | Either no effect or PSVT terminates suddenly (usually ending with a P' wave) |
| SVT termination: last waveform seen | Gradual slowing of P-QRS rate; no abrupt termination | QRS complex | P' or QRS complex | P' or QRS complex |

*Note: This grouping does not include atrial fibrillation or flutter. The PSVT group includes only: AT, AVNRT, and AVRT.
AT, atrial tachycardia; AV, atrioventricular; AVNRT, atrioventricular nodal reentrant tachycardia; AVRT, atrioventricular reentrant ("reciprocating") tachycardia; MAT, multifocal atrial tachycardia; P', premature atrial P wave; PAC, premature atrial complex or beat; PSVT, paroxysmal supraventricular tachycardia; PVC, premature ventricular complex or beat.

episodes find ways to terminate the arrhythmias on their own (e.g., by coughing, deep breathing, using the Valsalva maneuver, squatting, facial immersion in cold water, or with CSM).

The success of vagal maneuvers for terminating PSVT is a highly specific, but only moderately sensitive, clue to a reentrant mechanism, namely either AVNRT or AVRT, not AT. Very rarely, ventricular tachycardias terminate during vagal stimulation. If adenosine is not available or is contraindicated, intravenous beta blockers or selected calcium channel blockers (diltiazem or verapamil) can be used, but may produce hypotension and depress myocardial function, particularly in subjects with heart failure. These longer-acting drugs can be beneficial in patients with extremely high sympathetic tone when the arrhythmia terminates with adenosine but immediately restarts. Digoxin can also be used (see Chapter 20). Rarely, synchronized external cardioversion is required to terminate PSVT (Chapter 15).

## Long-Term Management of PSVT

Long-term PSVT management depends on the episode frequency and degree of symptoms. If episodes are rare and mild, no specific treatment is necessary after termination. Avoidance of provocative agents may be helpful, e.g., excess caffeine or sympathomimetic drugs. In more severe cases prophylactic treatment with AV nodal blocking agents or antiarrhythmic drugs may be warranted. An early referral to an electrophysiology specialist is justified as the efficacy of ablation procedures is high (in AVNRT it is 97% or more), with very low major risks (e.g., complete heart block) when performed by experienced operators. Finally, clinicians should be aware that PSVT does not increase thromboembolic risk. Thus, anticoagulation is not indicated.

# CHAPTER 15

# Supraventricular Arrhythmias, Part II: Atrial Flutter and Atrial Fibrillation

This chapter discusses two of the most common and clinically important tachycardias: atrial flutter and atrial fibrillation (AF). Previous chapters have focused primarily on supraventricular tachycardias (SVTs) with organized atrial activity (manifest by discrete P waves, when not hidden in the QRS) and 1:1 atrioventricular (AV or VA) conduction.[a] In contrast, AF and atrial flutter are two related SVTs characterized by very rapid atrial rates that usually greatly exceed the ventricular rate (QRS response) (Fig. 15.1).[b] This finding indicates that some degree of physiologic (functional) AV block[c] is present. Furthermore, both arrhythmias involve *reentrant* mechanisms in which electrical impulses rapidly and continuously spin around "chasing their tails" in the atrial muscle (see Fig. 15.1). *The rapid atrial rate combined with reentrant activity generates continuous atrial activity, manifest as F (flutter) or f (fibrillatory) waves, rather than discrete P waves.*

However, clinicians should bear in mind that the classic "sawtooth" flutter waves or oscillatory waves of fibrillation are not always clearly apparent. Not surprisingly, both atrial flutter and AF are often mistaken for other supraventricular arrhythmias when these *F* and *f* waves, respectively, are confused with true P waves associated, for example, with sinus tachycardia with frequent atrial ectopy or with

(non-sinus) atrial tachycardias. These and other common mistakes in ECG reading are summarized in Chapter 24.

## ATRIAL FLUTTER: ECG CONSIDERATIONS

Atrial flutter is one of the major tachycardias because it: occurs commonly; usually indicates the presence of underlying structural/electrical atrial disease; is associated with increased risk of thromboembolism, and has specific therapeutic implications, as described below.

Atrial flutter most often involves a reentrant circuit located in the right atrium. The rhythm is sometimes termed *macroreentrant atrial tachycardia*. The reason is that, in contrast to reentry confined within the AV node (as with AVNRT), the reentrant circuit of atrial flutter is much larger (macroreentrant), with the impulse traversing the atrium from top to bottom. The lower part of the circuit passes through the narrow region between the inferior vena cava and the tricuspid valve annulus (cavo-tricuspid *isthmus*). As in the case of the paroxysmal supraventricular tachycardias (PSVTs), atrial flutter is most often initiated by a premature atrial complex (PAC).

Because the macro-reentrant circuit of atrial flutter has a stable rate (usually around 300 cycles/min; range 240–350 cycles/min) and follows a consistent path, the flutter (F) waves (i) occur at very regular intervals and (ii) are identical-in-appearance in any single lead recording.

Cardiologists further classify flutter as *typical vs. atypical* based upon the electroanatomy involved in the reentrant circuit. In typical (isthmus-dependent) atrial flutter, the most common variant, the reentrant circuit traverses the cavo-triscuspid isthmus in the lower right atrium. Typical atrial flutter can in turn be subclassified based on the direction

---

Please go to expertconsult.inkling.com for additional online material for this chapter.

[a] The term "1:1 AV or VA conduction" means that there is one atrial wave for every QRS complex, except in some cases of atrial tachycardia with AV block. Note also that in paroxysmal supraventricular tachycardia due to AV nodal reentry (AVNRT), retrograde P waves are present but often hidden in the QRS.

[b] Some authors do consider atrial fibrillation separately from the group of SVTs.

[c] Functional AV block (often 2:1) refers to physiologic limitations of the AV node in conducting excessively rapid stimuli due to its *inherent refractoriness*. In contrast, organic AV block (see Chapter 17) refers to impaired conduction in the AV node area associated with intrinsic (e.g., disease processes; excess vagal tone) or extrinsic (e.g., drugs) factors that impair conduction.

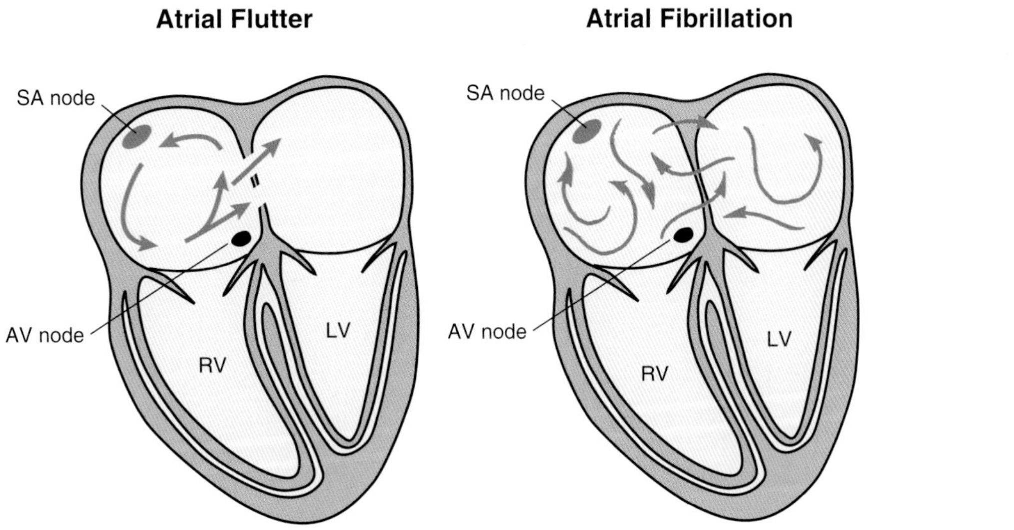

**Atrial Flutter**                    **Atrial Fibrillation**

**Fig. 15.1** Schematic comparing mechanisms of atrial flutter and atrial fibrillation (AF). Atrial flutter is typically due to a large reentrant wave, originating in the right atrium, initiated by a premature atrial complex. With the most common type of typical atrial flutter, the wave spreads in counterclockwise direction, involving the area near the tricuspid valve and inferior vena cava (cavo-tricuspid isthmus). In contrast, AF is sustained by multiple reentrant wavelets, not a single one, and often initiated by abnormal impulse formation in the area of the pulmonary veins in the left atrium. *AV*, atrioventricular; *LV*, left ventricle; *RV*, right ventricle, *SA*, sinoatrial.

(*counterclockwise* or *clockwise*) that the reentrant wave follows in going around the right atrium. The most common form of typical atrial flutter involves a counterclockwise loop, with the impulse going up the inter-atrial septum. Non-isthmus-dependent (so-called atypical) atrial flutter is much rarer, and the substrate for the circuit is often scar tissue within the left or right atrium, usually as a result of surgery, catheter ablation, or an idiopathic process.

Of interest, in atrial flutter the direction of the reentrant circuit can be predicted with reasonable accuracy from the ECG. With counterclockwise atrial flutter, the F waves are negative in the inferior leads, and positive in $V_1$. In most cases, the atrial depolarization rate is about 300 cycles per minute. The classic "sawtooth" pattern of F waves that are predominantly negative in leads II, III, and aVF and positive in $V_1$ with a very regular ventricular (QRS) rate of about 150/min (due to functional 2:1 AV block) is suggestive of counterclockwise type atrial flutter (Fig. 15.2A). Less often, a similar type of circuit gets initiated, but in the opposite direction, producing "clockwise" flutter. The polarity of the F waves will then be reversed: positive in leads II, III, and aVF, and negative in lead $V_1$ (Fig. 15.2B). Clockwise and

counterclockwise flutter can occur in the same patient and both are usually *isthmus-dependent*.[d]

The atrial rate during typical atrial flutter, as noted, is around 300 cycles/min (range about 240–330 cycles/min). Slower atrial rates can be due to drugs that decrease atrial conduction time. Fortunately, the AV node cannot usually conduct electrical signals at these rates to the ventricles—although a bypass tract in the Wolff-Parkinson–White (WPW) syndrome (see Chapter 18) may be able to conduct at rates of 300/min or so. Thus, with atrial flutter, *physiologic* AV block develops (commonly with a 2:1 A/V ratio) (Figs. 15.2 and 15.3). In the presence of high vagal tone, AV nodal disease, or AV nodal blocking drugs (e.g., beta blockers, digoxin, and certain calcium channel blockers) higher degrees of AV block can be seen, for example with a 4:1 conduction ratio (Figs. 15.3 and 15.4).

Often the AV nodal conduction shows more complex patterns and the degree of AV block varies

---

[d]The cavo-tricuspid isthmus is the most common area around which atrial flutter develops. However, it can develop around other atrial obstacles such as scars formed after cardiac surgery or areas of fibrosis following pericarditis, or even following ablation procedures in the left atrium used to treat atrial fibrillation.

## Typical Atrial Flutter Variants

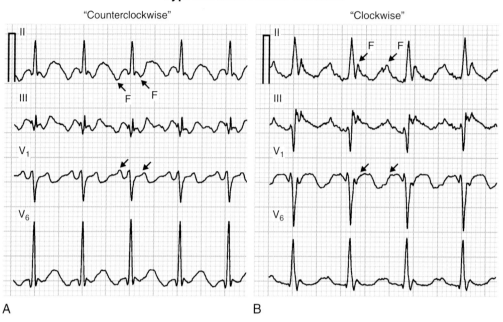

**Fig. 15.2** (A) Typical atrial flutter most commonly involves a reentrant ("merry-go-round"-like) circuit in the right atrium, proceeding in a highly consistent, counterclockwise pathway. The cycle length (rotation time) is about 200 msec, corresponding to an atrial rate of 300/min. Note that the "sawtooth" flutter (F) waves (*arrows*) are negative in the inferior leads (II, III, and aVF) and $V_6$, but positive in $V_1$. In the absence of drugs or atrioventricular node disease, the ventricular response is often exactly half the atrial rate (i.e.,150 beats/min). (B) With the "clockwise" variant, the flutter (F) waves are positive in the inferior leads and $V_6$, and negative in $V_1$. These variants have the same clinical implications.

in a periodic way, producing F wave/QRS ratios with repeating patterns (Fig. 15.4) of RR intervals (*group beating*). This phenomenon is attributed to multiple levels of block within the conduction system. Variable AV block may also be due to other mechanisms (e.g., AV Wenckebach), producing non-integer ratios of F waves to QRS complexes (Fig. 15.5).

Atrial flutter with 1:1 AV conduction (Fig. 15.6), although uncommon, constitutes a medical emergency and is most likely in three specific settings:
- In high catecholamine states (strenuous physical activity, infection, with high fever, shock, etc.).
- With certain antiarrhythmic medications, such as flecainide, which slow conduction through atrial tissue and therefore slow the flutter rate sufficiently (for example, from 300 to 220/min or less) such that the AV node is capable of conducting each of the F waves (1:1 conduction).
- In the presence of a bypass tract (WPW preexcitation syndrome) capable of rapid conduction (short refractory period).

*Because of the dangerously rapid ventricular rate, atrial flutter with sustained 1:1 AV conduction requires consideration of immediate synchronized electrical cardioversion.*

## ATRIAL FIBRILLATION (AF): ECG CONSIDERATIONS

Unlike atrial flutter, the reentrant waves of AF cannot be localized to any consistent, stable circuit in the atria. Most cases of AF are thought to originate in the area of pulmonary vein–left atrial junctions, involving the emergence of rapidly firing ectopic foci. With time, more and more of the atrial tissue becomes involved in the active maintenance of the arrhythmia, associated with the simultaneous formation of multiple unstable small (micro)-reentrant circuits (see Fig. 15.1). Therefore, atrial electrical activity on the ECG appears as irregular *f (fibrillatory) wavelets*, varying continuously in amplitude, polarity (reversing from positive or negative orientation in same lead), and frequency (changing cycle length,

## Atrial Flutter

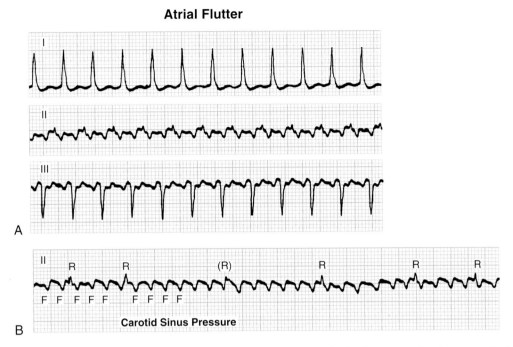

**Fig. 15.3** (A) Note the variable appearance of flutter waves in different leads. In lead I, the waves are barely apparent, leads II and III show the classic "sawtooth" appearance. The ventricular rate is about 160 beats/min, and the flutter rate is about 320 beats/min; thus 2 : 1 AV conduction is present. (B) Carotid sinus massage produces marked slowing of the ventricular rate by increasing vagal tone. *R*, R waves; (*R*), partially hidden R wave.

## Atrial Flutter with Variable AV Block

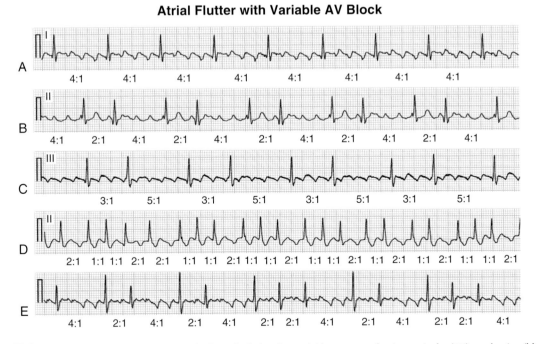

**Fig. 15.4** Atrial flutter from different patients (A through E) showing variable patterns of atrioventricular (AV) conduction (block). As shown, the block may alternate between two values. In other cases it is more variable.

### Atrial Flutter with Variable AV Block

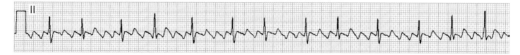

**Fig. 15.5** With atrial flutter, the ventricular response may be variable, but not always a simple ratio (½, ⅓, ¼) of the atrial rate. Even in these cases, the response usually shows some underlying patterns, in contrast to the random-appearing ventricular rate in atrial fibrillation.

### Atrial Flutter with 2:1 and 1:1 AV Conduction

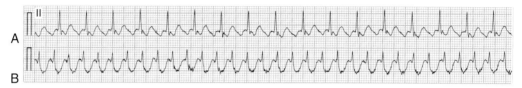

**Fig. 15.6** Atrial flutter with 2:1 atrioventricular (AV) conduction (A) compared with 1:1 (one-to-one) AV conduction (B) in the same patient. In the latter case, the flutter waves are hard to locate. Owing to the very rapid ventricular response (about 300 beats/min), atrial flutter with 1:1 conduction is a medical emergency, often necessitating direct current (DC) cardioversion.

### Atrial Flutter with Variable Block vs. Coarse Atrial Fibrillation

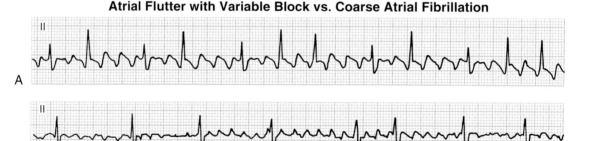

**Fig. 15.7** Atrial flutter with variable block (A) and coarse atrial fibrillation (B) are often confused. Notice that with atrial fibrillation the ventricular rate is completely erratic and the atrial waves are not identical from segment to segment, as they are with atrial flutter.

measured as the very brief interval from one f wave to the next).

Milder degrees of atrial activity "disorganization" or drugs that slow atrial activation may produce *coarse AF* with high amplitude f waves resembling atrial flutter (Fig. 15.7). Advanced rheumatic mitral stenosis may also be associated with coarse AF.

─────── Key Point ───────

Usually, the single best lead to identify the diagnostic irregular atrial activity of AF is lead V₁, where irregular f waves are likely to be most clearly seen (Fig. 15.8).

Severe atrial abnormalities (due to atrial dilation, fibrosis, or longstanding fibrillation, or drugs like digoxin) often result in *fine AF* with almost isoelectric (flat), very fast fibrillatory waves that can be confused with atrial asystole. Sometimes both fine and coarse f waves can appear in the same ECG.

### Atrial Fibrillation and AV Nodal Conduction

In AF, the AV node gets bombarded with highly disorganized impulses of different amplitude and frequency with atrial rates of up to 400–600/min. Most of the signals are blocked in the AV node and only a fraction conduct to the ventricles (see

## Atrial Fibrillation with a Slow Ventricular Response

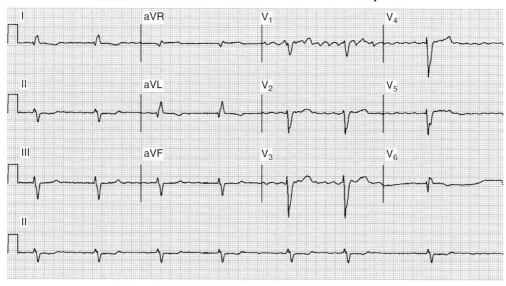

**Fig. 15.8** Atrial fibrillation (not flutter) is present with a very slow ventricular response. The fibrillatory waves are best seen in lead $V_1$. There is an atypical left bundle branch block pattern (see Chapter 8). The rsR′ in lateral leads (e.g., $V_6$ here) is highly suggestive of prior myocardial infarction (MI). A QR (or rsR′) complex is also present in leads I and aVL, also consistent with underlying MI. Left axis deviation and a long QT interval are noted as well. The patient had chronic heart failure due to severe coronary artery disease with prior "silent" MIs. The slow ventricular response raises the question of drug effect or excess (e.g., digoxin) or intrinsic atrioventricular (AV) node disease (see Chapters 17 and 20).

Figs. 15.7B and 15.8). Still, in the absence of AV nodal disease or certain drugs, the ventricular heart rate in AF is much higher than with sinus rhythm. Usually the mean QRS rate in untreated AF at rest is over 100 beats/min at rest, with often abrupt, inappropriate increases during exercise.

Due to random penetration of the impulses through the AV node, the RR intervals in AF are haphazardly irregular. However, when the ventricular rate gets very fast, this RR irregularity may become more difficult to appreciate; sometimes the rhythm appears regular (*pseudo-regularization*) and may be confused with other tachyarrhythmias such as PSVT (Figs. 15.9 and 15.10).

### Atrial Fibrillation with a Regularized Ventricular Response

There are three major settings where atrial fibrillation may occur with a regularized ventricular response, in contrast to the highly irregular cadence usually associated with this arrhythmia:
1. With *complete heart block*, in which case the ECG will usually show a regular, very slow ven-

tricular response, usually 40–50 beats/min or less (Fig. 15.11).
2. During sustained ventricular pacing (see Chapter 22).
3. With certain cases of digoxin toxicity (Chapter 20).

### ATRIAL FIBRILLATION VS. ATRIAL FLUTTER

Atrial flutter and AF are distinct but related arrhythmias. Although atrial flutter almost always occurs in the setting of structural heart disease, AF can develop in normal hearts. However, patients presenting with atrial flutter have an increased chance of manifesting AF on follow-up. Furthermore, AF and flutter can occur in the same patient, with the ECG showing transitions from one rhythm to the other. In such cases, the AF "organizes" into atrial flutter or atrial flutter "degenerates" into AF. However, at any given time there is usually one or the other (but not both) rhythms present. Although electrocardiographically these rhythms can appear quite similar, it is important to differentiate between them (Table 15.1) because of the differences in management. In

### Atrial Fibrillation with Rapid Ventricular Response

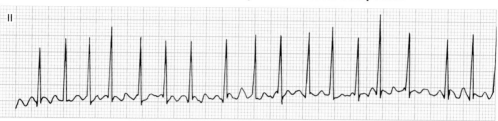

**Fig. 15.9** This patient with atrial fibrillation with a rapid ventricular response at rest had hyperthyroidism. (Note: the commonly used term rapid atrial fibrillation is actually a misnomer, because "rapid" is intended to refer to the ventricular rate rather than the atrial rate. The same is true for the term slow atrial fibrillation.) Note that the atrial fibrillation waves here have a "coarse" appearance which might lead to confusion with true (discrete) P waves or with atrial flutter.

### Atrial Fibrillation with Rapid Ventricular Response (Not PSVT)

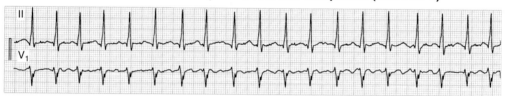

**Fig. 15.10** Atrial fibrillation with a rapid ventricular response. At rapid rates, the RR interval variability may be more subtle, leading to a mistaken diagnosis of paroxysmal supraventricular tachycardia (PSVT). See also Fig. 15.9.

### Atrial Fibrillation with Complete AV Heart Block

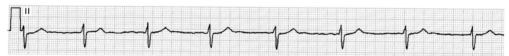

**Fig. 15.11** Complete atrioventricular (AV) heart block (see Chapter 16) can occur with underlying atrial fibrillation (or flutter); the ventricular response will be very slow, usually 50 beats/min or less, and regular. In this case, the narrow QRS complex indicates that the escape rhythm is in the nodal area. Such patients usually require both permanent pacing and anticoagulation.

particular, radiofrequency (RF) ablation is considered as first-line therapy in atrial flutter, but not in AF. The differences between the two arrhythmias, usually detectable by ECG, are based on the following:

- Atrial flutter has a single, stable reentrant pathway. Therefore, all flutter (F) waves look exactly the same in both shape and duration during any recording from the same patient. A simple, reliable way—the "calipers test"—to check for this finding is to measure the interval containing several consecutive clearly visible atrial waves and to move the calipers along the tracing. In case of atrial flutter, the subsequent F wave intervals will "map

out" perfectly. In AF, the shape and polarity of f waves often vary over the length of the tracing. Even if the shape of f waves appears similar, their timing will be "off" (Fig. 15.12).

- The propagation velocity of the signal through atrial tissue is limited and it takes a certain amount of time, termed the "cycle length" (usually at least 180 msec, equivalent to 4.5 small "boxes"), for the flutter signal to make a full rotation through the atrium. Therefore, atrial waves due to flutter generally cannot appear closer than 4 small boxes apart. An atrial cycle length shorter than 160 msec (4 small boxes or shorter) suggests AF. However,

| TABLE 15.1 | Differential Diagnosis of Atrial Fibrillation vs. Atrial Flutter | |
|---|---|---|
| **Feature** | **Atrial Flutter** | **Atrial Fibrillation** |
| Atrial wave morphology | Identical from one F wave to another | f waves vary continuously in shape and polarity |
| Atrial wave timing | Identical, i.e., F–F interval "map out" | Variable, i.e., f–f interval does not "map out" |
| Atrial wave cycle length | F–F intervals ≥180 msec (4.5 small boxes) | Variable f–f intervals can be <180 msec |
| Ventricular (QRS) response patterns | Constant (2:1, 4:1) F/QRS ratio, or group beating pattern(s) | Completely irregular (no pattern), unless complete heart block or ventricular pacing is present |

F, Flutter wave; f, fibrillatory wave.

you should be aware that so-called "coarse" AF can be present with cycle lengths of 180 msec or greater.

- In atrial flutter there is usually either a fixed ratio of F/QRS waves (2:1, 4:1) or a group beating due to a "patterned" ventricular response (e.g., 2:1-4:1). In cases of variable block, you are likely to see the exact RR interval of a given ratio repeat itself during the recording, generating a type of "group beating." In AF, the QRS interbeat intervals are completely erratic. *But be careful: as noted, when the ventricular rate is fast, this variability may be subtle, leading to the appearance of regularization (pseudo-regularization) and possible misdiagnosis.*

## Atrial Fibrillation: ECG Differential Diagnosis

Studies have repeatedly shown that atrial fibrillation is one of the most commonly misdiagnosed arrhythmias, both in terms of underdiagnosis and overdiagnosis, even by experienced observers. For instance, atrial fibrillation may be missed (false

### Atrial Fibrillation vs. Flutter: Calipers Test

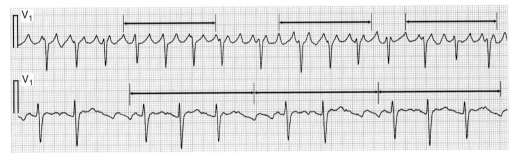

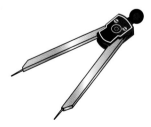

**Fig. 15.12** Coarse atrial fibrillation and atrial flutter may look very similar. A useful test (the "calipers test") is described in the text. It is based on the fact that in atrial fibrillation (top panel), the atrial (f) waves (remember these are not P waves) vary in timing and morphology, while in atrial flutter, the atrial (F) waves are identical. Thus, if you fix your calipers (or line up the distance with a 3 × 5 card) between two atrial waves and then "march" that interval forward or backward, the calipers will always hit the same point on F waves (bottom panel), but different ones on f waves (top panel).

negatives) especially when the ventricular rate is very fast (or very slow) and appears pseudo-regularized; when the ventricular rate is slow and regular (e.g., with ventricular pacing or complete AV heart block; see above); when intermittent higher amplitude or so-called "coarse" fibrillatory ( $f$ ) waves are mistaken for true P waves.

Specifically, there are four major fast, irregular patterns that may be mistaken for AF (i.e., false positives): (1) Artifact causing an irregular appearing baseline. This type of pseudo-AF may be due to poor electrode contact or to patient movement, including tremor from Parkinson's disease. (The RR intervals may be regular or irregular in such cases depending on the underlying mechanism.) (2) Sinus rhythm with frequent premature atrial complexes (PACs). (3) Multifocal atrial tachycardia (MAT). (4) Atrial flutter or atrial tachycardia with variable AV conduction. Sometimes the diagnosis is not clear from the available data. In such cases, obtaining longer rhythm strips may be helpful.

## ATRIAL FIBRILLATION AND FLUTTER: MAJOR CLINICAL CONSIDERATIONS

AF is the most common, major arrhythmia causing hospital admissions. Over 2 million Americans have intermittent or chronic AF, and the incidence rises with age. Nearly 10% of individuals 65 years or older develop AF. Over 20% of those over the age of 89 years will develop AF. In some patients, AF or atrial flutter occurs *paroxysmally* and may last only minutes or less, hours, or days. Some patients may experience only one episode or occasional episodes, whereas others have multiple recurrences. In some patients, AF is more persistent and may even become permanent (chronic), lasting indefinitely (Table 15.2).

### Symptoms and Settings

During the episodes, some patients are quite symptomatic (typically complaining of palpitations, fatigue, dyspnea, lightheadedness, or chest pain), whereas others have no specific complaints. Syncope can occur, usually as the result of the spontaneous post-conversion pauses upon arrhythmia termination (see "tachy-brady" syndrome, Chapter 13).

In the asymptomatic patient, AF may first be discovered during a routine examination or when the patient presents with heart failure or stroke. AF can occur in people with no detectable heart disease and in patients with a wide variety of cardiac diseases.

| TABLE 15.2 | Clinical Classification of Atrial Fibrillation (AF) Based on Duration |
|---|---|
| **Type** | **Description** |
| Paroxysmal | Recurrent AF (≥2 episodes) that terminates spontaneously in less than 7 days (usually less than 48 hours) |
| Persistent | AF that is sustained beyond 7 days, or lasting less than 7 days but necessitating pharmacologic or electrical cardioversion |
| Long-standing persistent | Continuous AF present for longer than 1 year |
| Permanent | AF lasting for more than 1 year in a patient in whom the decision has been made not to pursue restoration of sinus rhythm by any means |

The term *lone atrial fibrillation* is sometimes used to describe recurrent or chronic AF in patients without clinical evidence of heart disease. Paroxysmal AF may occur spontaneously, or it may be associated with excessive alcohol consumption in otherwise healthy individuals (*holiday heart syndrome*). In such cases, the arrhythmia often spontaneously reverts to normal sinus rhythm or is converted easily with pharmacologic therapy alone.

Changes in autonomic tone may provoke AF in susceptible individuals. Sometimes the arrhythmia is related to increased sympathetic tone (e.g., occurring during exercise or with emotional excitement). At other times, AF may occur in the context of abnormally high vagal tone (termed vagotonic atrial fibrillation). Of interest in this regard, evidence suggests that the risk of AF is higher in endurance athletes than non-athletes.

AF is also one of the most frequently observed arrhythmias in patients with organic (structural) heart disease. As noted, the frequency of occurrence of this arrhythmia rises with advancing age. Common pathologic substrates include coronary artery disease, hypertensive heart disease, and valvular heart disease. Patients with coronary artery disease may experience AF for the first time during an acute myocardial infarction (MI) or, more commonly, as a consequence of chronic ischemic myocardial disease, probably related to atrial dilation or fibrosis. Hypertensive heart disease is often associated with left atrial enlargement. AF is also commonly induced by chronic valvular heart disease, particularly when the mitral valve is involved. For example, severe rheumatic mitral stenosis or mitral regurgitation (of any cause) produces marked left atrial enlargement, a major predisposing factor for atrial tachyarrhythmias.

Numerous other conditions can also lead to AF. For example, patients with thyrotoxicosis (hyperthyroidism) may develop AF. The arrhythmia (or atrial flutter) is quite common after cardiac surgery. It may also occur with pericardial disease (especially recurrent or chronic), chronic lung disease, pulmonary emboli, cardiomyopathies of various types, certain forms of congenital heart disease (e.g., atrial septal defect), and other forms of heart disease. Severe obstructive sleep apnea (OSA) is associated with increased risk of AF (usually seen in the context of the patient's being overweight) and should always be suspected when the diagnosis of AF is first made. Not uncommonly, patients have more than one predisposing factor (e.g., hypertension, sleep apnea, mitral valve insufficiency and advanced age).

Chapter 25 includes a summary of important causes and contributors to AF (and flutter).

## Thromboembolic and Cardiac Function Complications

AF and flutter have two major clinical implications:

(1) First and foremost is the increase in thromboembolic risk (most importantly, stroke). Therefore, whenever AF or flutter is present on the ECG, the anticoagulation status of the patient should be reviewed and appropriate treatment promptly initiated. Anticoagulation should not be delayed pending rate control. Remember that recurrent paroxysmal arrhythmia does not markedly decrease thromboembolic risk compared to its persistent or chronic forms. The increase in stroke risk in AF/flutter is related to left atrial appendage thrombi formation caused by the loss of atrial contraction and stagnation of blood flow. It usually takes at least 48 hours of arrhythmia for the thrombi to start developing.

Among the highest risk groups for thromboembolism are patients with rheumatic heart disease or those with a mechanical prosthetic heart valve replacement (valvular atrial fibrillation). Several risk stratification schemes have been developed to predict the risk of stroke in patients with nonvalvular AF. The most common nonvalvular risk factors that increase thromboembolic risk include a history of hypertension, older age (≥65 years, with ≥75 years being higher risk), history of stroke or transient ischemic attack (TIA), history of diabetes mellitus,

and history of heart failure. Other factors, such as vascular disease (including myocardial infarction, carotid stenosis, peripheral arterial disease), and female gender have also been implicated in raising the risk of thromboembolism.

Current guidelines recommend warfarin in patients with AF related to valvular heart disease ("valvular" AF) and those with nonvalvular AF deemed at higher risk for thromboembolism. Several novel anticoagulants (NOACs) have been developed for prophylaxis in nonvalvular atrial fibrillation. These non-vitamin K antagonists include direct thrombin or Factor X inhibitors. Readers are referred to the Bibliography for additional clinical details and evolving guidelines.[e]

(2) The second important clinical implication is the risk of development or worsening of heart failure (HF). The exacerbation of HF can occur immediately due to decreased cardiac output from lack of atrial contraction, and the rapid rate that may be associated with ventricular ischemia and decreased time for ventricular filling. These pathophysiologic events, associated with increased filling pressures and lower cardiac output, can produce severe shortness of breath and even acute pulmonary edema. Furthermore, long-term (weeks to months) continuation of a rapid uncontrolled ventricular rate can, itself, lead to development of a *tachycardia-induced cardiomyopathy* with ventricular dilatation and decrease in the systolic function.

## TREATMENT OF ATRIAL FIBRILLATION/FLUTTER: ACUTE AND LONG-TERM CONSIDERATIONS

*The first two priorities in the acute treatment of AF and flutter are appropriate anticoagulation and rate control.* Potentially reversible causes and risk factors should be reviewed (e.g., hyperthyroidism disease and obstructive sleep apnea). For *long-term* management of AF and flutter, clinicians have two general treatment strategies: (1) *rate control* and (2) *rhythm control.*

### Rate Control

Rate control centers on limiting the ventricular response to AF, without attempts at restoring sinus

---

[e]Stroke prevention for patients with AF centers upon long-term oral anticoagulation. In patients who are intolerant of, or have a contraindication to, oral anticoagulants, a *left atrial appendage closure device* may be an alternative strategy. The device is inserted percutaneously, and is intended to prevent embolization of left atrial appendage clots to the systemic circulation.

rhythm. Rate control can be achieved by using AV nodal blocking agents (beta blockers, calcium channel blockers, and digoxin) or AV junctional (AVJ) ablation. The criteria of "optimal" rate control under chronic conditions are currently under investigation.

Rate control is usually the preferred treatment option in patients with the following:

- Permanent AF
- New-onset AF within the first 24 hours (which has approximately 50% chance of terminating spontaneously)
- Reversible acute illness when achievement and maintenance of sinus rhythm are unlikely until the cause is corrected (e.g., hyperthyroidism, metabolic abnormalities, especially hypokalemia, alcohol withdrawal, acute infection)
- Asymptomatic patients who can tolerate a lifetime of anticoagulation

Atrioventricular junction (AVJ) ablation (with pacemaker implantation) can be used in patients whose rate cannot be effectively controlled with medications. This procedure is a percutaneous one which electrically "disconnects" the atria from the ventricles and achieves excellent rate control without any further need for AV nodal blocking agents. The major downsides of AVJ ablation are that: (1) the patient becomes largely pacemaker-dependent, and (2) as with any of the other rate-controlling options, anticoagulation has to be continued indefinitely.

## Rhythm Control

Rhythm control strategy consists of two phases: (1) sinus rhythm restoration (by electrical or pharmacologic cardioversion) and (2) sinus rhythm maintenance.

Cardioversion can be achieved by using selected antiarrhythmic medications (chemical cardioversion), electrical cardioversion with direct current (DC) shock, or an intra-cardiac catheter ablation procedure. With any type of cardioversion, thromboembolic risk and anticoagulation history of the patient should be reviewed because of increase in risk of thromboembolism during and shortly after the transition to sinus rhythm.

Pharmacologic cardioversion in AF is of limited value. The rate of conversion to sinus rhythm with most antiarrhythmic medications is low. In selected patients, intravenous *ibutilide* may convert up to 50% of cases of recent onset AF and up to 70% of cases of atrial flutter. However, the drug can cause prominent QT prolongation and sometimes induce torsades de pointes. Therefore, very careful, continuous ECG monitoring is required during its administration. One advantage of chemical cardioversion is that there is no need for moderate or deep sedation, a requirement for electrical cardioversion.

Direct current (electrical) cardioversion (DCCV) is a safe and reliable method of restoring sinus rhythm in AF and flutter. A properly timed direct current shock administered through pads on the anterior and posterior chest (Fig. 15.13) depolarizes the whole heart, disrupting reentrant circuits and allowing the sinus node to "regain control" of the atria. It is essential to "synchronize" the shock with ventricular depolarization (R wave on the ECG). Unsynchronized shocks if delivered in the ventricular vulnerable period (around the peak of the T wave) can induce ventricular fibrillation, a variant of the "R on T phenomenon" (see Chapter 15).

Sinus rhythm maintenance can sometimes be achieved with antiarrhythmic drugs (see Chapter 11); drugs most often used are the class IC agents flecainide and propafenone, or class III agents sotalol, amiodarone, and dofetilide. Unfortunately, antiarrhythmic drugs are only modestly effective in maintaining sinus rhythm. Furthermore, most require monitoring for ECG changes that may forecast electrical instability: for example, QRS interval widening (flecainide, propafenone) and QT(U) interval prolongation with the serious, and potentially life-threatening proarrhythmic risk of torsades de pointes (Chapter 16). For instance, initiation of sotalol or dofetilide usually requires inpatient ECG monitoring. Another major limitation is that none of these antiarrhythmic agents maintains sinus rhythm reliably enough to discontinue anticoagulation.

Flecainide is not recommended for use in patients with coronary artery disease or with depressed left ventricular ejection fraction, and is not indicated in the treatment of chronic atrial fibrillation. Flecainide may increase AV conduction rates in atrial flutter and atrial fibrillation, and as such, concomitant use of an agent that slows AV conduction (e.g., a beta blocker) is usually recommended.

Ablation procedures using RF catheter-based technologies have become increasingly used both in sinus rhythm restoration and maintenance in AF and, especially, atrial flutter. *RF ablation is highly efficacious in treating typical atrial flutter, with close to a 90% long-term success rate in selected patients.* A linear

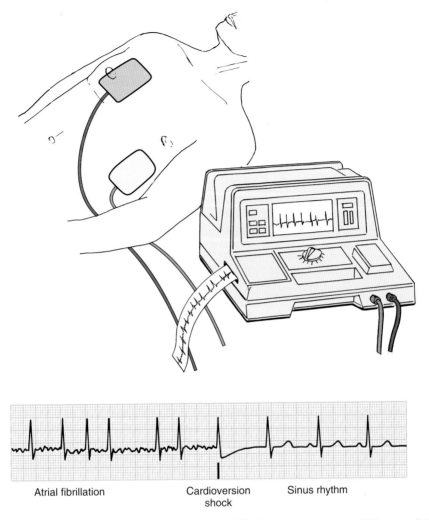

Atrial fibrillation          Cardioversion          Sinus rhythm
                                shock

**Fig. 15.13** Schematic of direct current cardioversion (DCCV) of atrial fibrillation to sinus rhythm. With external DCCV, an electric shock is administered to the heart via special electrode paddles placed on the chest wall. In the case depicted here, one electrode is placed on the anterior chest wall, to the left of the sternum; the other (indicated by dashed lines) is placed on the back, under the left scapula. The shock must be synchronized with the peak of the QRS complex to avoid inducing ventricular fibrillation, which may occur if the stimulus is delivered at the peak of the T wave.

lesion in the cavo-tricuspid isthmus using a percutaneously inserted ablation catheter is usually curative because it interrupts the underlying flutter pathway.

In contrast, ablation procedures for AF involve catheter access to the left atrium via a transseptal approach from the right atrium. The mainstay of current AF ablation is electrical disconnection of the pulmonary veins from the atrial tissue by RF energy or cryoablation using liquid-nitrogen-filled balloons. Choosing between rate and rhythm control and medication options, along with making decisions about the indications for and timing of ablation procedures, always need to be personalized.

Finally, lifestyle changes are increasingly recognized in reducing the burden of AF/flutter. These include weight loss, which may have multiple benefits, including improved control of hypertension and of obstructive sleep apnea. Stress management and avoidance of excess alcohol are also recommended.

# CHAPTER 16
# Ventricular Arrhythmias

The three preceding chapters have focused primarily on *supra*ventricular arrhythmias, especially those related to rapidly occurring electrical disturbances arising in the area of the sinus node, the atria, or the atrioventricular (AV) node (junction). Assuming normal ventricular conduction, these rapid rhythms all produce *narrow (normal QRS duration) complex tachycardias* (NCTs).

This chapter considers another essential ECG topic: ventricular arrhythmias—the major, but not the only cause of *wide complex tachycardias* (WCTs), those in which the QRS complex is prolonged in duration.

Ectopic (non-sinus) depolarizations frequently arise in the ventricles themselves, or in contiguous structures (e.g., valvular outflow tracts or the fascicular system), producing *premature ventricular complexes* (PVCs), *ventricular tachycardia* (VT), and in the most electrophysiologically unstable settings, *ventricular fibrillation* (VF) leading to immediate cardiac arrest (also see Chapter 21).

## VENTRICULAR PREMATURE COMPLEXES

Premature ventricular complexes[a] are premature depolarizations arising in the ventricles, analogous to atrial premature complexes (PACs) and premature junctional complexes (PJCs).

Not all premature atrial or ventricular premature depolarizations produce an effective mechanical response of the ventricles or atria, respectively. Therefore, we favor using the word "complex," not "contraction," as the "C" in PAC or PVC.

Recall that with PACs and PJCs, the early-occurring QRS complex is usually of normal ("narrow") width because the stimulus spreads synchronously through the bundle branches into the ventricles (unless a bundle branch block or some other cause of aberrancy is present).

With PVCs, however, the premature depolarizations typically arise in either the right or left ventricle. Therefore, the ventricles are not stimulated simultaneously, and the stimulus spreads through the ventricles in an aberrant and asynchronous manner. Thus, the QRS complexes are wide (0.12 sec or more) with PVCs, just as they are with the bundle branch block patterns.[b]

Examples of PVCs are shown in Figs. 16.1–16.12. Examples of ventricular tachyarrhythmias (VT and VF) are shown in Figs. 16.13–16.23.

---
### Key Point

The two major characteristics of PVCs are their:
1. *Premature timing*: they occur before the next normal beat is expected.
2. *Aberrant QRS-T appearance*: the QRS complex is abnormally wide (0.12 sec or more), and the T wave and QRS complex usually point in opposite (discordant) directions.

---

PVCs most often precede a sinus P wave. Occasionally they appear just after a sinus P wave but before the normal QRS complex. Sometimes, PVCs are followed by retrograde (non-sinus) P waves (negative in leads II, III, aVF) that arise because of a reversal in the stimulation direction (bottom to top, not top to bottom) of the atria. This sequence, called "VA" (ventriculo–atrial) conduction, may also occur in some cases of electronic ventricular pacing (see Chapter 22).

---

Please go to expertconsult.inkling.com for additional online material for this chapter.

[a]In the ECG literature and in clinical practice, the terms ventricular premature beat (VPB), ventricular premature depolarization, ventricular extrasystole, and premature ventricular complex or contraction (PVC) are used interchangeably.

[b]The basic electrophysiologic mechanisms responsible for PVCs are a subject of active investigation. PVCs may arise by at least three mechanisms: *reentrant waves*, increased *spontaneous depolarizations* of ventricular cells (enhanced automaticity), and *triggered activity* or *afterdepolarizations* (i.e., premature firing of ventricular cells triggered by the previous depolarization).

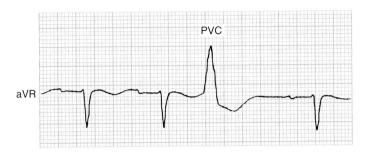

**Fig. 16.1** A premature ventricular beat or complex (PVC) is recognized because it comes before the next normal beat is expected and it has a wide, aberrant shape, very different from the QRS of supraventricular beats. (Notice also, as an unrelated finding in this example, the long PR interval in the normal sinus beats.)

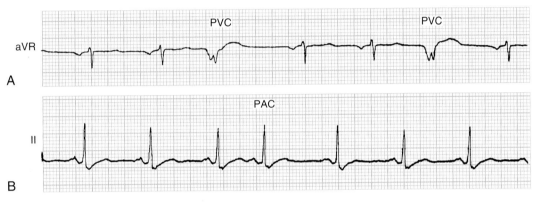

**Fig. 16.2** (A) Notice the wide, aberrant shape of a premature ventricular complex (PVC) compared to the QRS complexes of a premature atrial complex (PAC) (B), which generally resembles the other sinus-generated QRS complexes. (In this case the QRS of the sinus beats and the PAC all have right bundle branch block morphology.)

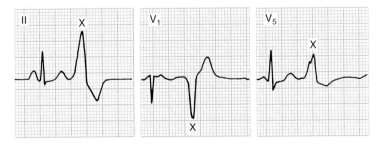

**Fig. 16.3** The same ventricular premature beat (X) recorded simultaneously in three different leads has different shapes. By comparison, notice that the multiform premature ventricular complexes shown in Fig. 16.11 have *different* shapes in the *same* lead.

## Features

A number of features of PVCs may have clinical relevance.

## Frequency

The frequency of PVCs refers to the number that is seen per minute or other unit of time. The PVC frequency may range from one or an occasional isolated premature depolarization to many.

Frequent PVCs may occur in various combinations. Two in a row (see Fig. 16.4) are referred to as a *pair* or *couplet*. Three or more in a row are, by definition, VT (see Fig. 16.5). Sometimes, as shown in Fig. 16.6A, isolated PVCs occur so frequently that each

Monitor lead

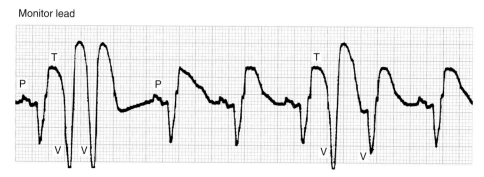

**Fig. 16.4** Two premature ventricular complexes are referred to as a *pair* or a *couplet*. They also show the "R on T" phenomenon.

## Nonsustained Ventricular Tachycardia

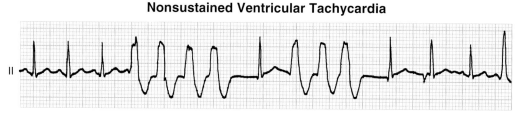

**Fig. 16.5** Two short bursts of nonsustained ventricular tachycardia.

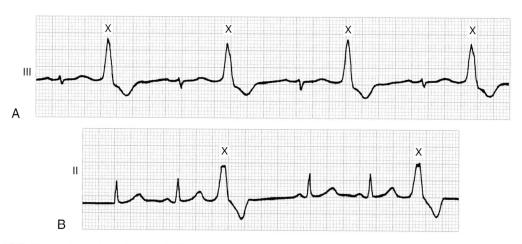

**Fig. 16.6** (A) Ventricular bigeminy, in which each normal sinus impulse is followed by a ventricular premature complex (*X*). (B) Ventricular trigeminy, in which a ventricular premature complex occurs after every two sinus beats.

normal beat is followed by a PVC. This produces a distinctive repetitive grouping of one normal beat and one PVC, which is called *ventricular bigeminy* (see Figs. 16.6 and 16.7). The repeating sequence of two normal beats followed by a PVC is *ventricular trigeminy*. Repeating sequences in which three normal

(or supraventricular) beats are followed by a PVC constitute *ventricular quadrigeminy*.

## Morphology and Axis
As you might predict from applying simple vector principles, the appearance of the PVCs will be

**Acute MI with PVCs**

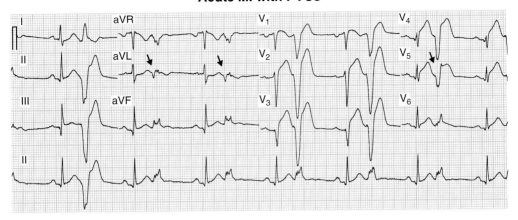

**Fig. 16.7** Frequent premature ventricular complexes (PVCs), with two morphologic patterns, with transient ventricular bigeminy, in a patient with an extensive acute ST segment elevation/Q wave myocardial infarction (MI). The coupling interval (between normal R waves and PVCs) is relatively short. Note the ST elevations in the precordial leads as well as in leads III and aVF, due to extensive ischemia. Q waves are present in leads $V_1$ to $V_4/V_5$. In addition, the Q waves in leads II, III, and aVF suggest prior MI. Note the PVCs with a QR configuration in leads aVL and $V_5$ (*arrows*) suggestive of myocardial infarction, even in the absence of pathologic Q waves in these leads in the normally conducted sinus beats.

different depending on the site(s) in the ventricles from which these beats originate.

- If the ectopic beat originates in the left ventricle, then right ventricular activation will be delayed and the QRS of the PVC will resemble a right bundle branch block (RBBB).
- If the ectopic beat comes from the right ventricle, then left ventricular activation is delayed, and the QRS resembles a left bundle branch block (LBBB).
- PVCs arising from the interventricular septum often show an intermediate (hybrid) pattern between that of RBBB and LBBB. These PVCs are usually relatively narrow as both ventricles get activated simultaneously from the middle of the ventricles. As a general principle, the further away from the middle region of the ventricles the ectopic beat's origin is, the wider will be its QRS duration.
- PVCs arising from the base (top) of the ventricles have an "inferior/rightward" QRS axis—pointing downward toward the positive poles of leads II, III, and aVF. In such cases cardiologists used the term "outflow tract" PVCs because the origin of the ectopic beats is inferred to be close to the pulmonary and aortic valves. Usually these PVCs have a LBBB-like shape. Outflow tract PVCs, those

originating in the right ventricular outflow tract (RVOT) or left ventricular outflow tract (LVOT), are among the most common variety of "benign" PVCs occurring in a structurally normal heart.
- In contrast, PVCs originating closer to the apex or the inferior wall activate the heart from the bottom up and have a "superior" axis, with a QRS complex that is predominantly negative in leads II, III, and aVF.
- PVCs originating in the area of a post-infarct myocardial scar often have a QR configuration. Finding this morphology in multiple leads should make you suspect an underlying infarct even when no Q waves are seen during sinus rhythm beats (see Fig. 16.7).

The sequence of ventricular *repolarization* after PVCs is such that ST-T waves are usually directed in the opposite direction to the main QRS deflection (QRS-T "discordance"), often with prominent ST segment elevations/depressions as expected (see Fig. 16.2). Clinicians need to recognize that these secondary ST-T changes are not indicative of ischemia and are similar to the QRS-T discordance findings in wide complex beats due to bundle branch block and ventricular pacing. In fact, concordance between QRS and ST-T directions during PVCs may be a sign of myocardial injury.

The same principles related to PVC morphology and axis apply to localization of the origin VT (a run of consecutive PVCs), which may be helpful in clinical management, as described later.

### Coupling Interval

The term *coupling interval* refers to the duration between the PVC and the QRS of the preceding normal beat. When multiple PVCs are present, *fixed coupling* often occurs, with the coupling interval approximately the same for each PVC (see Fig. 16.6). At other times, PVCs may show a *variable coupling interval*. Whether PVCs demonstrate fixed versus variable coupling does not usually have major clinical implications. (Interested readers can pursue this advanced topic, including *parasystolic rhythms*, in references given in the Bibliography.)

### Compensatory Pauses

As you may have noticed, PACs and PVCs are usually followed by a pause before the next normal sinus beat. The pause after a PVC is usually, but not always, longer than the pause after a PAC. A "fully compensatory" (or "complete") pause indicates that the interval between the normally sinus-generated QRS complexes immediately before and immediately after the PVC is twice the basic PP interval (Figs. 16.8 and 16.9). The basis of a compensatory pause is that

**Pauses After Premature Complexes**

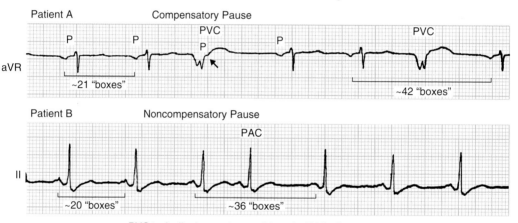

PVC typically does not reset SA node; PAC often does.

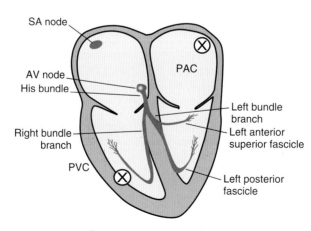

**Fig. 16.8** Difference between noncompensatory and compensatory pauses after premature atrial complexes (PACs) and premature ventricular complexes (PVCs), respectively. These are denoted by *Xs*. See text and Fig. 16.9.

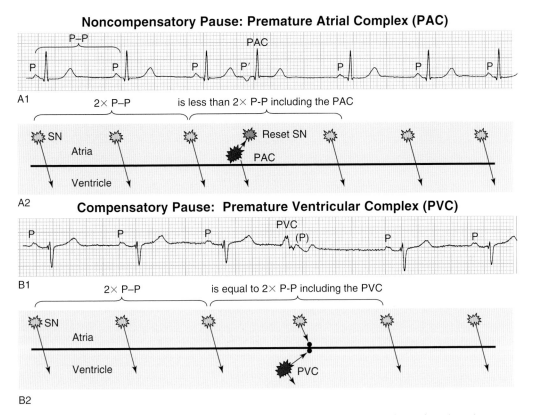

## Noncompensatory Pause: Premature Atrial Complex (PAC)

**Fig. 16.9** Mechanisms of noncompensatory pauses (panels A1 and A2) after premature atrial complexes (PACs) vs. compensatory pauses (panels B1 and B2) after ventricular premature complexes (PVCs), respectively. Schematics are shown below actual examples. The sinus node (*SN*) normally fires (*pink star*) at a relatively constant rate (P–P). In panel A2, a PAC (*red star*) depolarizes the sinus node and "resets" it (*grey star*). This resetting mechanism leads to a noncompensatory (incomplete) pause: the P–P interval surrounding the PAC is less than twice the usual sinus P–P interval. (Note also that the premature P wave in panel A1 is negative, indicating a low ectopic focus.) In contrast, a PVC (*red star* in panel B2) often conducts in a retrograde (backwards) way (i.e., from ventricles to atria), and is either blocked in the His-Purkinje system or collides with the native sinus beat (*P* in panel B1). In such cases, the native sinus pacemaker will continue to fire and not be "reset," leading to a fully compensatory (complete) pause after the PVC: the sinus P-QRS to sinus P-QRS interval surrounding the PVC will be = 2× the basic sinus P-P interval. See also Fig. 16.8.

the sinus node impulses are *not* affected (their timing is not reset) by PVCs,. Therefore, the sinus P waves coming after the PVC will occur "on time." A fully compensatory pause is more characteristic of PVCs than PACs because the latter often *reset* (delay) the timing of the sinus beats (see Fig. 16.9). However, clinicians should be aware that there are multiple exceptions to the "rule" that associates PACs with noncompensatory ("incomplete") pauses and PVCs with fully compensatory ones. For example, sometimes a PVC falls almost exactly between two normal beats; in such cases the PVC is said to be *interpolated* (Fig. 16.10).

## Uniform vs. Multiform PVCs

The terms *uniform* and *multiform* are used to describe the appearance of PVCs in any single lead. Uniform PVCs, i.e., those with identical appearance, arise from the same anatomic site (focus) (see Fig. 16.6). (Of course, uniform PVCs will have different shapes in different leads, just as normal beats do.) By contrast, multiform PVCs have different morphologies in the same lead (Fig. 16.11). Multiform PVCs often but not always arise from different foci. Thus, uniform PVCs are uni*focal*, but multi*form* PVCs are not necessarily multi*focal*. Uniform PVCs may occur in normal hearts and with underlying organic heart disease.

## Interpolated PVCs

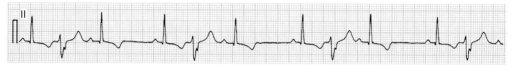

**Fig. 16.10** Sometimes premature ventricular complexes fall between two sinus beats, in which case they are described as *interpolated*. The underlying rhythm is sinus bradycardia at about 55 beats/min.

## Multiform PVCs

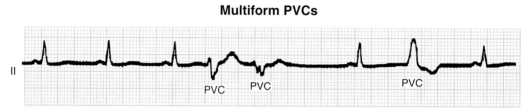

**Fig. 16.11** These multiform premature ventricular complexes have different shapes in the same lead. Compare this tracing with the one in Fig. 16.6.

Monitor lead

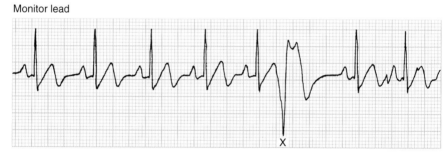

**Fig. 16.12** A ventricular premature beat (*X*) falling near the peak of the T wave of the preceding beat may be a predisposing factor for ventricular tachycardia or ventricular fibrillation, particularly when this "R on T" phenomenon occurs in the setting of acute myocardial ischemia or with long QT(U) syndrome.

Multiform PVCs usually indicate that organic heart disease is present, but are a nonspecific finding.

### "R on T" Phenomenon

The *R on T* (shorthand for *PVC on T*) *phenomenon* refers to PVCs that are timed so that they fall near the peak or trough (most positive or negative point) of the T wave of the preceding normal beat (Fig. 16.12). This short period of ventricular repolarization is associated with the greatest heterogeneity of refractoriness. An internal or external stimulus of sufficient magnitude and duration is most likely to induce VF during this so-called *vulnerable phase*.

There are four major settings where R on T beats (or their equivalent) may precipitate sustained VT or VF: (1) acute myocardial infarction (MI) or myocardial ischemia; (2) long QT(U) interval syndrome (discussed later in this chapter); (3) *commotio cordis* syndrome (Chapter 21); and (4) during direct current (DC) cardioversion, if the depolarizing stimulus is not synchronized with the QRS complex, and is instead inadvertently delivered near the peak of the T wave (Chapter 15). However, VT and VF most commonly occur without a preceding "R on T" beat, and most "R on T" beats do not precipitate a sustained ventricular tachyarrhythmia.

## PVCs: General Clinical Considerations

Occasional PVCs are very common in healthy people of all ages, as well as those with virtually any type of heart disease. These premature beats usually reflect increased automaticity of dormant ventricular pacemakers and may be provoked by adrenergic stimulation (stress, caffeine, sympathomimetic drugs, as well as by "recreational" drugs such as cocaine or other stimulants), electrolyte abnormalities (especially hypokalemia or hypomagnesemia), and certain types of drug toxicities (e.g., digoxin). Not infrequently, more than one factor may contribute to the occurrence of PVCs, such as hypokalemia and digoxin therapy.

As noted above, one of the most common locations for the origin of benign PVCs is the outflow tract; however, PVCs can arise from any area of the normal heart. In patients with organic heart disease, PVCs can result from acute ischemia, previous MI with fibrosis and scarring, abnormal stretch of muscle due to increased intra-cardiac pressure, increased sympathetic tone, and many other factors. Symptoms of PVCs can vary from none to bothersome palpitations.

Treatment approaches to a patient with PVCs depend on a number of factors. Asymptomatic PVCs, with or without heart disease, usually require no specific treatment. Very symptomatic PVCs sometimes respond to beta blockers. Efforts should be made to avoid antiarrhythmic medications in the suppression of PVCs because of serious, potentially lethal *proarrhythmic* side effects, including VT and VF (see Chapter 21).

Clinicians should be aware of a relatively uncommon but likely underappreciated syndrome referred to as *PVC-induced cardiomyopathy*. This term describes the occurrence of reversible left ventricular (LV) dysfunction that is solely or primarily attributable to very frequent PVCs (e.g., bigeminy and trigeminy). Patients with this syndrome may have 10,000–20,000 or more PVCs/day (close to 30% of the total beats/day) on Holter monitoring. The mechanism whereby frequent PVCs may actually induce LV dysfunction (not just be a marker of it) is not certain. Recurrent asynchronous activation of the ventricles may play a role in the pathogenesis of PVC-induced cardiomyopathy. The syndrome is important because it represents a potentially treatable form of cardiomyopathy. Therapeutic modalities include a trial of beta-blockade, careful consideration of antiarrhythmic therapy in selected patients, or catheter ablation

therapy, attractive because it may provide a definitive "cure." Suspicion of this syndrome is an indication for referral to a cardiac electrophysiologic (EP) specialist.

## VENTRICULAR TACHYCARDIAS: CLASSIFICATION SCHEMES

The usual (and arbitrary) definition of VT is three or more consecutive PVCs at a rate exceeding 100 or more beats/min (Figs. 16.13 and 16.14). As with narrow complex tachycardias, VTs can be due to focal (automatic or triggered) or reentrant mechanisms. Regardless of their electrophysiologic mechanism, runs of VT are usually initiated by PVCs.

From an initial diagnostic viewpoint, VT (Box 16.1) is classified along two "axes": the first based on its duration (Is the VT nonsustained or sustained?) and the second based on its appearance in any given lead (Is it monomorphic or polymorphic?).

## Monomorphic Ventricular Tachycardia: General Considerations

Similar to PVCs, the anatomic site of origin of monomorphic VT often can be determined by examining two features: QRS morphology and QRS axis. Arrhythmias coming from the left ventricle have a RBBB-like QRS shape (Fig. 16.15); the ones coming from the right ventricle have a LBBB-like shape, which are best seen in lead $V_1$ (Figs. 16.5 and 16.16). Those coming from the base (top) of the heart have QRS axes pointing in an inferior to rightward direction, toward leads II, III, and aVF;

---

**BOX 16.1**   Basic Classification of Ventricular Tachycardias

**Duration**
- *Nonsustained* ventricular tachycardia (VT): lasting 30 sec or less
- *Sustained* VT: longer than 30 sec in duration or requiring direct current (DC) shock due to hemodynamic instability

**Appearance (in any given lead)**
- *Monomorphic*: all QRS complexes look the same in a given lead
- *Polymorphic*: QRS shapes, directions, and sometimes rate vary from beat to beat

## Paroxysmal Nonsustained Ventricular Tachycardia

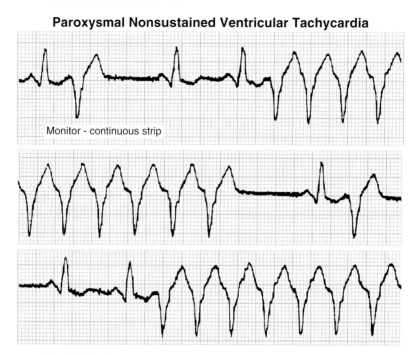

Monitor - continuous strip

**Fig. 16.13** The monitor lead shows short bursts of ventricular tachycardia.

## Sustained, Monomorphic VT Terminated by Direct Current Shock

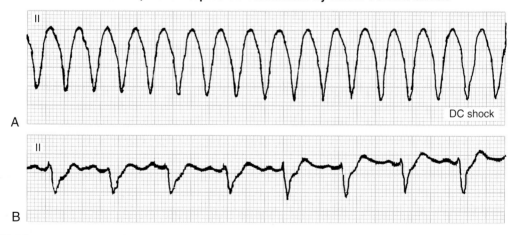

**Fig. 16.14** (A) Segment of a sustained run of monomorphic ventricular tachycardia. (B) Sinus rhythm restored after direct current (DC) cardioversion.

the ones coming from the inferior wall to the apex, in the opposite direction, have a superior axis (see Fig. 16.15).

VTs from the interventricular septum have a shape in between RBBB and LBBB and can have a relatively narrow QRS (about120 msec) when both ventricles are activated in parallel fashion from the middle (e.g., high interventricular septum) of the heart. Finally, the presence of QR configuration in more than one lead, with LBBB or RBBB configuration,

## Monomorphic VT: Prior MI

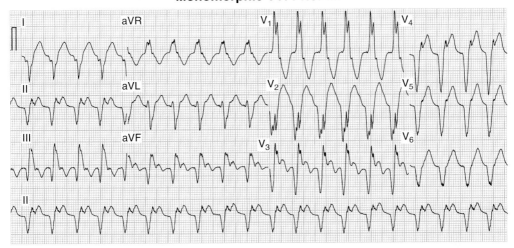

**Fig. 16.15** Monomorphic ventricular tachycardia (VT) originating in the left ventricle. Note the similarity of the QRS to that of a right bundle branch block in lead $V_1$, consistent with an impulse starting in the left ventricle and then depolarizing the right ventricle in a delayed manner. More subtly, the large Q waves (as part of QR complexes here) in leads II, III, and $V_2$ to $V_4$ suggest the presence of an underlying scar due to myocardial infarction (MI).

## VT: Right Ventricular Outflow Tract

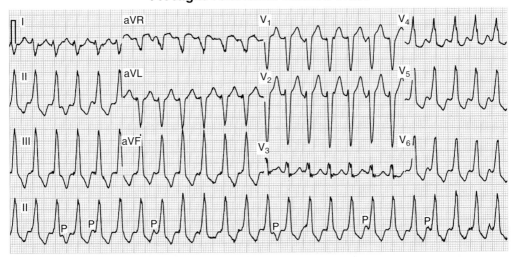

**Fig. 16.16** Monomorphic ventricular tachycardia (VT) originating in the right ventricular outflow tract. Note the QRS similarity to left bundle branch block in lead $V_1$, with an inferior-rightward QRS axis. A key finding indicating VT, as opposed to a supraventricular tachycardia with aberration, is the presence of underlying sinus P waves at a slower, independent rate, a sign of atrioventricular dissociation. See Chapter 19.

suggests that VT originates in the area of a myocardial scar due to a prior MI (see Fig. 16.15).

## Monomorphic Ventricular Tachycardia: Clinical Importance

Most middle-aged or older adults in the United States with monomorphic VT have underlying cardiac disease, most often a prior MI. Monomorphic VT can also occur in a structurally normal heart (such as with "outflow tract" VT; see Fig. 16.15) or with virtually any structural heart disease. Symptoms of VT depend on its rate and the systolic function of the heart. Common symptoms include a sensation of palpitations, shortness of breath, and lightheadedness. Patients with structurally normal hearts and preserved left ventricular function can maintain their cardiac output and tolerate very fast VT rates (over 200 beats/min) with relatively few symptoms, whereas in patients with depressed left ventricular ejection fractions this rate would most likely result in light-headedness, near-syncope, or frank syncope due to low cardiac output. Slow VTs, with rates between 100 and 130 beats/min are not unusual in patients receiving antiarrhythmic drugs and these episodes can be minimally symptomatic or completely asymptomatic.

Monomorphic VT in patients with a history of prior MI is usually caused by *reentry* around the areas of myocardial scar and not by acute ischemia. In the absence of other symptoms these patients do not need to be treated as having an "acute coronary syndrome." However, decreased cardiac output and increased oxygen demands during sustained VT can cause demand ischemia and degeneration of VT into VF; therefore DC cardioversion should be considered even if the patient appears stable.

## Polymorphic Ventricular Tachycardias

The term *polymorphic VT* describes a class of ventricular tachyarrhythmias characterized by a continuously varying pattern of QRS morphology in a given lead. The most useful clinical subclassification of polymorphic VT, based on the repolarization features of supraventricular beats, is between those (1) with underlying QT interval prolongation (long QT(U) syndrome) and (2) without QT interval prolongation (see also Chapter 21).

• The most important type of polymorphic VT with QT prolongation is torsades de pointes (TdP).
• Polymorphic VT without underlying repolarization prolongation can be further subdivided into *acute ischemic and nonischemic subsets*. Especially important in the latter category is a rare but important entity called *catecholaminergic polymorphic ventricular tachycardia* (CPVT).

### Torsades de Pointes (TdP)

As noted, the distinct and clinical major type of polymorphic VT that occurs in the setting of QT interval prolongation is called *torsades de pointes* (often abbreviated as TdP), from the French term meaning "twisting of the points" (Figs. 16.17 and 16.18). The hallmark of this tachycardia is the gradual variation in QRS direction (polarity) and amplitude in a given lead, such that each VT episode has a spindle-shaped "envelope" (see Fig. 16.18).

TdP is usually initiated by a PVC starting at the peak of a prolonged T-U wave, as a type of "R on T" beat (see Fig. 16.17). This sequence of events often starts with one or more PVCs followed by a post-ectopic pause and then second PVC on the T-U wave of the next supraventricular beat, which induces even more prolonged repolarization due to the pause.

---

Key Point

Sustained monomorphic VT in patients with structural heart disease is one of the major indications for implantable cardioverter-defibrillator (ICD) therapy (see Chapter 22). Sustained monomorphic VT in patients without known structural heart disease should include appropriate imaging (usually echocardiography and sometimes magnetic resonance) to rule out areas of myocardial scar that can serve as the substrate for reentry (e.g., subclinical myocarditis or cardiomyopathy). VT with LBBB morphology (i.e., originating in the right ventricle) can be the first sign of arrhythmogenic right ventricular cardiomyopathy/dysplasia (ARVC/D), a potential substrate for syncope or even sudden cardiac arrest. Importantly, therefore, the topic of sustained VT is closely related to that of sudden cardiac arrest/death, the subject of Chapter 21.

## Torsades de Pointes: Nonsustained

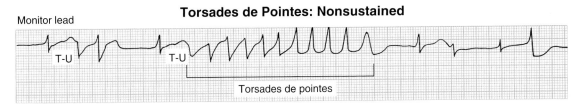

**Fig. 16.17** Notice the shifting polarity and amplitude of the QRS complexes during an episode of nonsustained torsades de pointes. QT(U) prolongation (0.52 sec) is present in the supraventricular beats (with possible underlying atrial fibrillation).

## Torsades de Pointes: Sustained

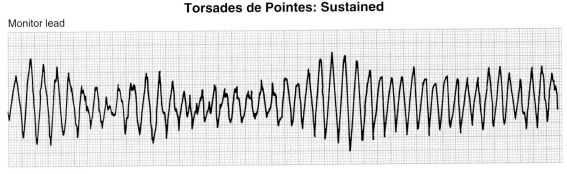

**Fig. 16.18** Classic example of the sustained torsades de pointes type of ventricular tachycardia. Notice the characteristic spindle-like pattern in which the QRS axis appears to rotate or turn in a systematic way. Fig. 16.17 shows a short, nonsustained run of the same arrhythmia, occurring in the setting of evident QT(U) prolongation.

TdP can occur with congenital (hereditary) or acquired QT interval prolongation, and can deteriorate into VF, causing sudden cardiac arrest (see Chapter 21).

QT prolongation syndromes that may give rise to TdP are usually classified as *acquired* or *congenital (hereditary)* (also see Chapter 25 for a more comprehensive list).

### Acquired Long QT Syndrome
Causes of acquired long QT syndrome include the following:
- Drugs, particularly quinidine (see Chapter 11 and Fig. 3.9) and related antiarrhythmic agents (disopyramide and procainamide), as well as ibutilide, dofetilide, sotalol, amiodarone, psychotropic agents (phenothiazines and tricyclic antidepressants), and many other non-cardiac drugs (e.g., methadone, pentamadine, haloperidol, erythromycin, and certain other antibiotics)
- Electrolyte imbalances, especially hypokalemia and hypomagnesemia, and, less commonly, hypocalcemia, which prolong repolarization

- Severe bradyarrhythmias (especially high-grade AV heart block syndromes)
- Miscellaneous factors, such as liquid protein diets.

### Hereditary Long QT Syndromes
Hereditary forms of long QT syndrome are related to abnormal ion channel function in the heart (especially involving transmembrane movement of potassium or sodium ions) resulting in prolonged repolarization. For a discussion of these so-called *channelopathies*, an important but more advanced concept, see the Bibliography.

Sometimes TdP is due to a combination of factors that "create a perfect storm" (e.g., hypokalemia, drug administration, and an unrecognized hereditary ion channel dysfunction that may become unmasked).

General principles of management of TdP include review and discontinuation of any possible QT-prolonging medications and correction of relevant electrolyte abnormalities (especially hypokalemia or hypomagnesemia). Intravenous magnesium may be helpful to shorten the QT even with normal serum magnesium levels and to suppress the PVCs that

## Polymorphic VT: Acute Ischemia

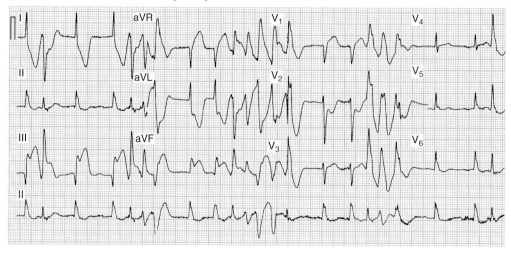

**Fig. 16.19** Polymorphic ventricular tachycardia (VT) in a setting of acute ST segment elevation inferior myocardial infarction. Note large ST with probable reciprocal anterolateral ST depressions. (However, this finding does exclude primary anterior wall subendocardial ischemia.)

trigger this arrhythmia. Increasing the heart rate by pacing, isoproterenol or dopamine infusion is sometimes employed to shorten the QT interval and make repolarization more homogeneous.

Polymorphic VT in the absence of QT interval prolongation *most often indicates ischemia*. It can be observed during acute MI (Fig. 16.19) but also with ischemia induced during exercise. The finding of polymorphic VT with no QT interval prolongation, especially during physical exertion, should prompt coronary artery evaluation. Much less frequent is CPVT (Chapter 20), which usually also presents during exertion and has been related to genetic defects in intracellular calcium handling. Most subjects are children or young adults. The Brugada syndrome (see Chapter 21) may also be associated with nonischemic polymorphic VT.

### The "Big Picture": Monomorphic vs. Polymorphic Ventricular Tachycardias

Clinicians should recognize that sustained ventricular tachycardia (VT) is an electrophysiologic syndrome and not a specific disease. As such, VT has multiple different basic mechanisms for its initiation and maintenance (e.g., reentry, different types of triggered activity, increased automaticity) as well as multiple different clinical substrates. The cardiologist's clinical overview of sustained ventricular

| **TABLE 16.1** | Sustained Monomorphic Ventricular Tachycardia: Major Clinical Substrates |
|---|---|

**I. No organic heart disease**
  A. Outflow tract: especially originating in the right and, more rarely, left ventricular outflow tract (RVOT or LVOT)
  B. Left ventricular: e.g., left bundle/posterior fascicular ventricular tachycardia

**II. Organic heart disease**
  A. Prior myocardial infarction (scar-related)
  B. Cardiomyopathies:
    1) Nonischemic dilated or nondilated
    2) Hypertrophic cardiomyopathy (HCM)
    3) Arrhythmogenic right ventricular dysplasia/cardiomyopathy (ARVD/C)
    4) Myocarditis: acute or chronic (e.g., viral, idiopathic, sarcoid, Chagas disease, etc.)
  C. Valvular heart disease
  D. Congenital heart disease (e.g., tetralogy of Fallot)
  E. Other (e.g., proarrhythmic effects of antiarrhythmic drugs without QT prolongation)

tachycardia (VT) is summarized in Tables 16.1 and 16.2. The first major division is into *monomorphic* vs. *polymorphic*. As described above, these two classes of VT are quite different in their clinical substrates and management. For monomorphic VT, the key follow-up question is whether the tachycardia is associated with underlying structural heart disease or not. Most patients with sustained monomorphic VT, especially middle-aged to older individuals, have organic heart disease. Occasionally, monomorphic VT is seen in the absence of organic heart disease.

| TABLE 16.2 | Sustained Polymorphic Ventricular Tachycardia: Major Clinical Substrates |
| --- | --- |

**I. With QT(U) prolongation (torsades de pointes)**
  A. Hereditary (congenital) long QT syndrome
  B. Acquired long QT syndrome
    1) Drug-induced:
      Cardiac agents (e.g., quinidine, sotalol, ibutilide, dofetilide)
      Non-cardiac agents (e.g., tricyclic antidepressants, methadone, haloperidol)
    2) Metabolic (e.g., hypokalemia, hypomagnesemia)
    3) Bradyarrhythmias (esp. high-degree atrioventricular block)
    4) Other (e.g., subarachnoid hemorrhage)
**II. Without QT(U) prolongation**
  A. Acute ischemia
  B. "Channelopathies"
    1) Catecholaminergic polymorphic ventricular tachycardia (CPVT)
    2) Brugada syndrome
    3) Short QT syndrome
**III. Bidirectional ventricular tachycardia**
  A. Digitalis toxicity
  B. CPVT

Polymorphic VT is usually divided in two groups: those associated with QT(U) prolongation in supraventricular beats and those without QT(U) prolongation. The former category is synonymous with torsades de pointes. The latter does not have a specific moniker and includes only a short list of clinical substrates. The most important one in adults is acute ischemia (with ST elevations and/or depressions). Polymorphic VT in the setting of acute ischemia may lead to ventricular fibrillation and sudden cardiac arrest (see Chapter 21). Other causes of polymorphic VT (e.g., catecholaminergic, Brugada syndrome) are described in this chapter and in Chapter 21. A rare subset of polymorphic category is bidirectional (bimorphic) VT in which the QRS complexes alternate in polarity from one beat to the next beat in a periodic fashion. Bidirectional VT is very rare and may occur with catecholaminergic polymorphic VT and with digitalis toxicity (see Chapter 20).

## ACCELERATED IDIOVENTRICULAR RHYTHM

Figs. 16.20 and 16.21 present examples of a distinctive arrhythmia called *accelerated idioventricular rhythm (AIVR)*, sometime referred to as *slow VT*. Recall that with typical VT the heart rate is more than 100 beats/min. With AIVR the heart rate is usually between 50 and 100 beats/min, and the ECG shows wide QRS complexes without associated sinus P waves.

### Accelerated Idioventricular Rhythm

aVF-Continuous strip

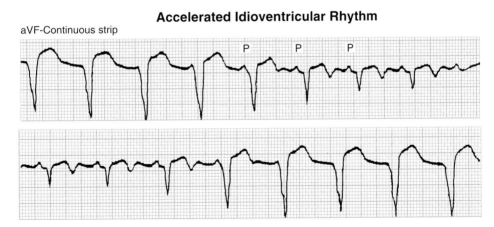

**Fig. 16.20** Accelerated idioventricular rhythm (AIVR) in a patient with an acute inferior wall infarction. The first four beats show the typical pattern of AIVR, followed by a return of sinus rhythm, then the reappearance of the AIVR. Notice that the fifth, sixth, twelfth, and thirteenth QRS complexes are "fusion beats" because of the nearly simultaneous occurrence of a sinus beat and a ventricular beat.

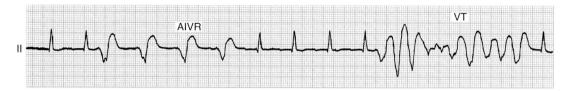

**Fig. 16.21** Accelerated idioventricular rhythm (AIVR) and nonsustained polymorphic ventricular tachycardia (VT) occurring together. Notice the "PVC on T" beats that initiate both the AIVR and the VT episodes.

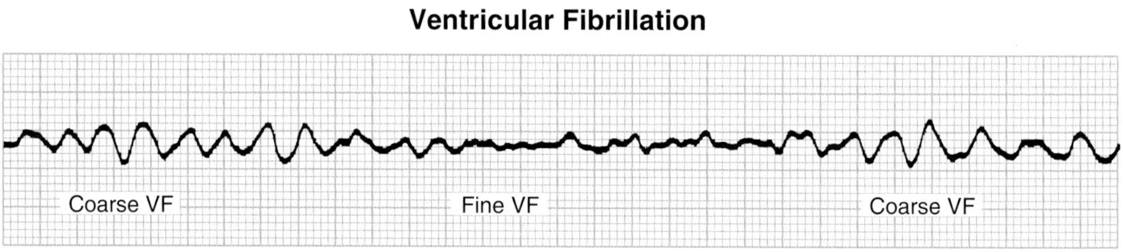

## Ventricular Fibrillation

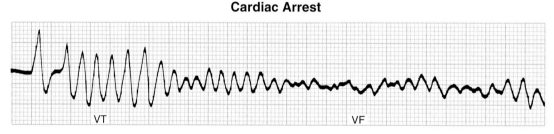

**Fig. 16.22** Ventricular fibrillation (VF) may produce both coarse and fine waves. Immediate defibrillation should be performed.

## Cardiac Arrest

**Fig. 16.23** Ventricular tachycardia (VT) and ventricular fibrillation (VF) recorded during the onset of cardiac arrest. The rapid "sine wave" type of VT seen here is sometimes referred to as *ventricular flutter*. The rapidity differentiates it from the sine-wave pattern of severe hyperkalemia (Chapter 11).

Underlying sinus rhythm with AV dissociation or retrograde ventriculo-atrial (VA) activation may be present.

AIVR is particularly common with acute MI, and may be a sign of *reperfusion* after the use of thrombolytic agents or after interventional coronary artery procedures, or it occur spontaneously. This arrhythmia is generally short-lived, lasting minutes or less, and usually requires no specific therapy. In most cases (see Fig. 16.15), AIVR appears to be a benign "escape" rhythm that competes with the underlying sinus mechanism. When the sinus rate slows, AIVR appears; when the sinus rate speeds

up, the arrhythmia disappears. More rarely (see Fig. 16.15), AIVR is initiated by premature beats rather than escape beats. This latter type is more likely to be associated with faster ventricular tachyarrhythmias.

## VENTRICULAR FIBRILLATION

Ventricular fibrillation (VF, Figs. 16.22 and 16.23) is a completely disorganized ventricular rhythm resulting in immediate cessation of cardiac output and cardiac arrest unless electrical defibrillation is performed in a timely way using unsynchronized DC shock. Based on the amplitude of fibrillatory waves, VF is sometimes arbitrarily classified as *coarse* or *fine*. VF can appear suddenly as a primary arrhythmia (from the baseline of normal sinus or another supraventricular rhythm) or, more commonly, as a "degeneration" of monomorphic or polymorphic VT. If left untreated, the typical progression is from coarse to fine VF, and then eventually to asystole (see Chapter 21).

## DIFFERENTIAL DIAGNOSIS OF WIDE COMPLEX TACHYCARDIAS

The differential diagnosis of wide complex tachycardias (WCTs), a major topic in clinical ECG interpretation, is discussed in Chapter 19. A boxed outline summary is presented in Chapter 25.

# CHAPTER 17

# Atrioventricular (AV) Conduction Abnormalities, Part I: Delays, Blocks, and Dissociation Syndromes

Normally, the only means of electrical communication (signaling) between the atria and ventricles is via the specialized conduction system of the heart. This relay network comprises the atrioventricular (AV) node, the bundle of His, and the bundle branch system (Fig. 17.1). The atria and ventricles are otherwise electrically isolated from each other by connective tissue in the indented rings (grooves) between the upper and lower chambers. The major exception occurs with Wolff–Parkinson–White (WPW) preexcitation, as described in Chapter 18.

The short (0.12–20 sec) physiologic delay between atrial and ventricular activation, represented by the PR interval, allows the ventricles near optimal time to fill with blood during and just after atrial contraction. Excessive slowing or actual interruption of electrical signal propagation across the heart's conduction system is termed *AV (atrioventricular) block* or *heart block*. The closely related topic of *AV dissociation* is discussed at the end of this chapter.

## Clinical Focal Points

Clinicians should try to answer two key questions when examining the ECG of a patient with apparent AV heart block:
1. *What is the degree of block:* first-, second-, or third-degree (complete)?
2. *What is the most likely level of the block:* in the AV node (nodal) or below the AV node (infranodal, i.e., in the His–bundle branch system)?

## WHAT IS THE DEGREE OF AV BLOCK?

Based on increasing severity of conduction impairment, three degrees of AV block/delay are described:
- *First-degree (PR interval prolongation)*: uniform slowing of conduction between the atria and ventricles (an increase in the normal AV delay described earlier), but without its interruption
- *Second-degree*: intermittent interruption of conduction, which may be further designated as Mobitz I (AV Wenckebach) or Mobitz II
- *Third-degree*: complete interruption of AV conduction, with a nodal or infranodal escape rhythm, or with asystole

In addition, two other important subtypes of second-degree AV block, namely *2 : 1 block* and *high-grade block* (also referred to as *"advanced second-degree AV block"*) will be discussed.

### First-Degree AV Block (PR Prolongation)

*First-degree AV block* (Fig. 17.2) is characterized by a P wave (usually sinus in origin) followed by a QRS complex with a uniformly prolonged PR interval greater than 200 msec. A more precise term is *PR interval prolongation* because the signal is not actually blocked, but rather is delayed. The PR interval can be slightly prolonged (e.g., 240 msec) or it can become markedly long (rarely up to 400 msec or longer).

### Second-Degree AV Block

*Second-degree AV block* is characterized by intermittently "dropped" QRS complexes. There are two major subtypes of second-degree AV block: Mobitz type I (AV Wenckebach) and Mobitz type II.

With *Mobitz type I, the classic AV Wenckebach pattern* (Figs. 17.3 and 17.4), each stimulus from the atria encounters progressively more "difficulty" in traversing the AV node en route to the ventricles (i.e., the node becomes increasingly refractory). Finally, an atrial stimulus is not conducted at all, such that the expected QRS complex is blocked ("dropped QRS"). This cycle is followed by recovery of the AV node, and then the whole cycle starts again.

The characteristic ECG signature of classic AV Wenckebach block, therefore, is of progressive lengthening of the PR interval from one beat to the next until a QRS complex is dropped. *Of note, the PR interval following the nonconducted P wave (the first PR interval of the new cycle) is always shorter than the PR interval of the beat just before the nonconducted P wave.* This can be a very useful (and clinically imperative)

means of differentiating Mobitz I block from Mobitz II, in which the PR interval is stable throughout the cycle.

The number of P waves occurring before a QRS complex is "dropped" may vary. The nomenclature is based on the *ratio* of the number of P waves to QRS complexes in a given cycle. The numerator is always one higher than the denominator. In many cases just two or three conducted P waves are seen before one is not conducted (e.g., 3:2, 4:3 AV block). In other cases, longer cycles are seen (e.g., 5:4, 10:9, etc.).[a]

As you see from the examples, the Wenckebach cycle also produces a distinct clustering of QRS complexes separated by a pause (the "dropped" QRS). Any time you encounter an ECG with this type of *group beating*, you should suspect AV Wenckebach block and look for the diagnostic pattern of lengthening PR intervals and the presence of a nonconducted P wave. As discussed in the following text, infranodal second-degree AV block (Mobitz type II) also demonstrates group beating with dropped QRS complexes, but without significant progressive PR interval prolongation (Fig. 17.5).

**Caution!** Be careful not to mistake group beating due to blocked premature atrial complexes (PACs) for second-degree AV block. In the former, the nonconducted P waves come "early;" in the latter the P waves come "on time" (see Chapter 14).

*Mobitz type II AV block* is a rarer and more serious form of second-degree heart block. Its characteristic feature is the sudden appearance of a single, nonconducted sinus P wave without two features seen in type I block: (1) progressive prolongation of PR

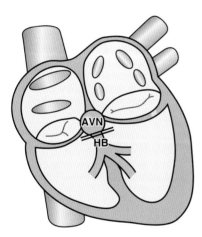

**Fig. 17.1** Nodal and infranodal blocks. Schematic depicts the two major locations (levels) of delay or actual block in the top of the atrioventricular (AV) conduction system. Block above the double line is AV nodal (*AVN*), whereas block below, involving the bundle of His (*HB*) and bundle branches, is infranodal.

[a]In some cases, however, the PR interval may not prolong noticeably, or it may even shorten. This atypical pattern is most common with very long cycles and long PR intervals. However, even in such atypical cases, the PR interval following the nonconducted beat will *always* be shorter than the PR interval before it.

## First-Degree AV Block

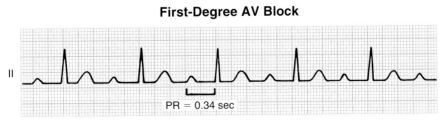

**Fig. 17.2** With first-degree atrioventricular (AV) "block," the PR interval is uniformly prolonged above 0.20 sec (200 msec) with each electrical cycle.

## Mobitz Type I (Wenckebach) Second-Degree AV Block

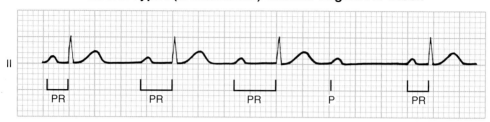

**Fig. 17.3** Sinus rhythm is present. The PR interval lengthens progressively with successive beats until one P wave is not conducted at all. Then the cycle repeats itself. Notice that the PR interval following the nonconducted P wave is shorter than the PR interval of the beat just before it.

## Mobitz Type I (Wenckebach) Second-Degree AV Block

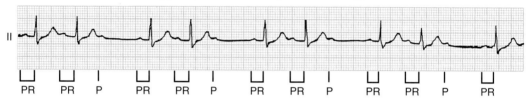

**Fig. 17.4** Sinus rhythm is present. The PR interval lengthens progressively with successive beats until one P wave is not conducted at all, as in Fig. 17.3. (The RR intervals may shorten, stay the same, or even prolong before the nonconducted P wave.) Mobitz type I (Wenckebach) block produces a characteristically syncopated rhythm with grouping of the QRS complexes ("group beating").

## Mobitz II AV Block with Sinus Rhythm

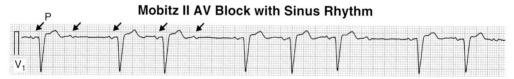

**Fig. 17.5** Mobitz type II atrioventricular (AV) second-degree heart block. Lead $V_1$ recording shows sinus rhythm (P wave; *arrows*) at a rate of about 75 beats/min (with left atrial abnormality). Most important, note the abrupt appearance of sinus P waves that are not followed by QRS complexes (nonconducted or "dropped" beats). Furthermore, the PR interval before the nonconducted P wave and the PR of the beat after (about 0.14 sec) are of equal duration. This finding contrasts with AV Wenckebach with 3:2 or higher ratios of conduction in which the PR interval after the nonconducted beat is noticeably shorter than the one before (see Figs. 17.3 and 17.4). The QRS of the conducted beats is also wide because of a left ventricular conduction delay. Mobitz II block is often associated with bundle branch abnormalities because the conduction delay is infranodal. Finally, note that the intermittent AV conduction pattern here gives rise to "group beating," also a feature of AV Wenckebach block.

intervals and (2) the noticeable shortening of the PR interval in the beat following the nonconducted P wave versus the PR before the nonconducted P wave.

A subset of second-degree heart block occurs when there are multiple consecutive nonconducted P waves present (e.g., P–QRS ratios of 3:1, 4:1, etc.). This finding is often referred to as *high-degree* (or *advanced*) AV block. It can occur at any level of the conduction system (Fig. 17.6). A common mistake is to call this pattern Mobitz II block or complete heart block.

### Third-Degree (Complete) AV Block

First- and second-degree AV heart blocks are examples of *incomplete* block because the AV junction conducts at least some stimuli to the ventricles. With *third-degree*, or *complete (third-degree) heart block*, no

## Advanced Second-Degree AV Block

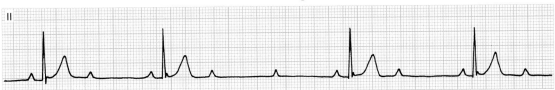

**Fig. 17.6** Modified lead II recorded during a Holter monitor ECG in a patient complaining of intermittent lightheadedness. The ECG shows sinus rhythm with 2:1 atrioventricular (AV) block alternating with 3:1 AV block (i.e., two consecutive nonconducted P waves followed by a conducted one). The term *high-grade* or *advanced second-degree AV block* is applied when the ECG shows two or more nonconducted P waves in a row.

## Third-Degree (Complete) AV Block

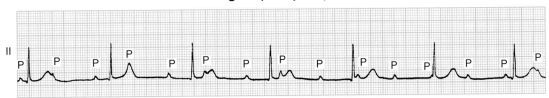

**Fig. 17.7** Complete heart block is characterized by independent atrial (P) and ventricular (QRS complex) activity. The atrial rate (sinus rate, here) is always faster than the ventricular rate. The PR intervals are completely variable. Some sinus P waves fall on the T wave, distorting its shape. Others may fall in the QRS complex and be "lost." Notice that the QRS complexes are of normal width, indicating that the ventricles are being paced from the atrioventricular junction. Compare this example with Fig. 17.8, which shows complete heart block with wide, very slow QRS complexes because the ventricles are most likely being paced from below the atrioventricular junction (idioventricular pacemaker).

stimuli are transmitted from the atria to the ventricles. Instead, the atria and ventricles are paced independently. The atria may continue to be paced by the sinoatrial (SA) node (or by an ectopic focus or by atrial fibrillatory activity). The ventricles, however, are paced by a nodal or infranodal escape pacemaker located below the point of block. The resting ventricular rate with complete heart block may be 30 beats/min or lower in some cases, or as high as 50–60 beats/min. This situation, when there is no "cross-talk" between the atria and ventricles and each of them is driven independently by a separate pacemaker at a different rate, is one generic example of *AV dissociation*. In the setting of complete heart block, AV dissociation almost always produces more P waves than QRS complexes (Box 17.1). However, as discussed later, AV dissociative rhythms is not unique to complete heart block. Examples of complete heart block are shown in Figs. 17.7 and 17.8.

Complete heart block may also occur in patients whose basic atrial rhythm is flutter or fibrillation.

> **BOX 17.1** **ECG With Sinus Rhythm and Complete Heart Block: Three Key Features**
>
> - P waves (upright in lead II) are present, with a relatively regular sinus rate that is typically much faster than the ventricular rate.
> - QRS complexes are present, with a slow (usually near-constant) ventricular rate.
> - The P waves bear no relation to the QRS complexes; thus, the PR intervals are variable.

In these cases, the ventricular rate is very slow and almost completely regular (see Fig. 15.11 and discussion below).

### WHAT IS THE LOCATION OF BLOCK? NODAL VS. INFRANODAL

Interruption of electrical conduction (see Fig. 17.1) can occur at any level starting from the AV node itself ("nodal block") down to the bundle of His

## Third-Degree (Complete) Heart Block

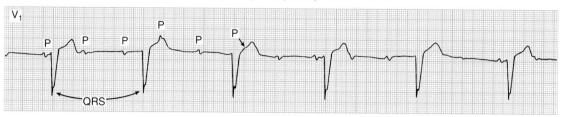

**Fig. 17.8** This example of sinus rhythm with complete heart block shows a very slow, idioventricular (note wide QRS) rhythm and a much faster independent atrial (sinus) rhythm. Left atrial abnormality (LAA) is also present.

| | |
|---|---|
| **BOX 17.2** | **Some Conditions that May Cause Temporary AV Conduction Impairment** |

- Autonomic factors (increased vagal tone with vasovagal syncope or obstructive sleep apnea). Trained athletes at rest may show a prolonged PR interval and even AV Wenckebach with sinus bradycardia that resolve with exercise
- Medications (especially beta blockers; digoxin, certain calcium channel blockers) and electrolyte abnormalities (especially hyperkalemia)
- Acute myocardial infarction, especially inferior (see text)
- Inflammatory processes (e.g., myocarditis, rheumatic fever, systemic lupus erythematosus)
- Certain infections (e.g., Lyme disease, toxoplasmosis)

| | |
|---|---|
| **BOX 17.3** | **Some Causes of Permanent AV Conduction System Damage** |

- Acute myocardial infarction, especially anterior wall
- Infiltrative diseases of the heart (e.g., amyloid, sarcoid, lymphomas)
- Degeneration of the conduction system, usually with advanced age (Lenègre's disease) or associated with cardiac calcification around the aortic and mitral valves (Lev's disease)
- Hereditary neuromuscular diseases (e.g., myotonic dystrophy, Kearns–Sayre syndrome, Erb's dystrophy)
- Iatrogenic damage to the conduction system as the result of valve surgery or arrhythmia ablations in the area of atrioventricular (AV) node and bundle of His; ethanol septal ablation for obstructive hypertrophic cardiomyopathy; transcatheter aortic valve implantation (TAVR)

and its branches (hence the term *infranodal block*). Although the AV node and infranodal structures represent a single, continuous "electrical wire," their physiology is quite different. *These differences often allow you to localize the level of block (nodal vs. infranodal) from the ECG, a distinction with important clinical implications.*

As general guidelines, clinicians should be aware that block at the level of the AV node (i.e., nodal):
- Is often caused by reversible factors (Box 17.2).
- Progresses slowly, if at all.
- In the case of complete heart block, is associated with a relatively stable escape rhythm.

In contrast, infranodal block:
- Is usually irreversible (Box 17.3).
- May progress rapidly and unexpectedly to complete heart block with a slow, unstable escape mechanism.

Therefore, infranodal block (even second-degree) generally requires pacemaker implantation.

Clues to nodal versus infranodal mechanisms of AV block include the following:
- Onset and progression
  - Nodal block usually occurs gradually. Conduction through the AV nodal cells is relatively sluggish (relying on slowly depolarizing calcium channels) and accounts for most of the PR interval duration. As the block progresses, a significant additional PR interval prolongation usually occurs before conduction fails leading to second- or third-degree block. (Analogy: consider the stretching of an elastic band before it snaps.)
  - In contrast, infranodal block usually happens abruptly. Conduction through the infranodal structures is relatively fast (relying on rapidly conducting sodium channels) and therefore accounts for only a very small portion of the PR

interval. As a consequence, when infranodal block develops there is minimal or no visible PR prolongation and the block (second- or third-degree) appears abruptly. (Analogy: consider the sudden snap of a metal chain under stress.)

- Escape rhythms
  - Because the AV node is located at the very top (proximal part) of the specialized conduction system, there are multiple potential escape or "backup" pacemakers located below the level of block, i.e., in the lower parts of the AV node as well as the bundle of His and its branches. Pure nodal and His bundle escape rhythms have narrow QRS complexes and a moderately low rate (e.g., 40–60 beats/min). However, the QRS complexes may be wide if there is an associated bundle branch block. As a result, complete block occurring at the nodal level is usually associated with an escape rhythm sufficient to maintain a hemodynamically adequate cardiac output (at least at rest).
  - In contrast, with infranodal block, there are fewer and less reliable potential escape pacemakers. Idioventricular escape mechanisms usually produce regular, wide QRS complexes with a very slow rate (i.e., 40 beats/min or less). In addition, the abrupt onset of the block can produce a life-threatening period of asystole.
- Autonomic and drug influences
  - The physiology of the AV node is similar to that of the sinus node and their functions tend to change in parallel. Both are sensitive to autonomic (sympathetic and parasympathetic) stimulation, as well as drugs affecting the autonomic nervous system (e.g., beta blockers, atropine, digoxin), as well as certain calcium channel blockers. For example, vagal stimulation can simultaneously produce both sinus bradycardia and AV block. This combination may be seen in vasovagal (neurocardiogenic) syncope, obstructive sleep apnea, or even during normal deep sleep.
  - Almost all medications causing sinus bradycardia (see Chapter 13) also decrease AV nodal conduction and can induce various degrees of heart block at the level of the AV node. Of note, adenosine has very potent suppressive activity on the AV (and SA) nodes and can induce transient complete heart block, an important effect to be aware of when it is used for differential diagnosis and termination of

supraventricular arrhythmias (see Chapter 13). Stimulation with sympathomimetic (e.g., dopamine, isoproterenol, and epinephrine) and anticholinergic drugs (atropine) increase the sinus rate and facilitate AV conduction.

- In contrast, infranodal conduction does not respond predictably to autonomic modulation or pharmacologic intervention. On occasion, antiarrhythmic sodium channel blockers such as quinidine, flecainide, or propafenone can produce infranodal block. They can also markedly worsen or unmask preexisting infranodal disease. Infranodal block often worsens with an increase in heart rate. Drugs causing tachycardia, such as atropine and sympathomimetics, may unexpectedly worsen conduction in infranodal block. However, beta agonists are useful in speeding up the rate of an idioventricular escape pacemaker in cases of complete infranodal block in emergency settings.
- QRS duration
  - The width of the QRS complexes depends in part on the location of the block. If the block is in the AV node proper, the ventricles are stimulated normally by a nodal pacemaker below the point of block and the QRS complexes are narrow (≤120 msec) (see Fig. 17.7), unless the patient has an underlying bundle branch block. If the block is within, or particularly below, the bundle of His, the ventricles are paced by an *infranodal pacemaker,* usually producing wide (>120 msec) QRS complexes (see Fig. 17.8). As a general clinical rule, complete heart block with wide QRS complexes tends to be less stable than complete heart block with narrow QRS complexes because the ventricular escape pacemaker is usually slower and less consistent. With infranodal disease there are often (but not always) other signs of conduction disease present (bundle branch blocks, hemiblocks, or nonspecific QRS widening).

## 2:1 AV BLOCK: A SPECIAL SUBTYPE OF SECOND-DEGREE HEART BLOCK

2:1 AV block occurs when every other QRS complex is "dropped" or, equivalently, every other P wave is not conducted. In such cases, it becomes difficult or impossible from the surface ECG to tell Mobitz I from Mobitz II type block simply because there are not two consecutive conducted PR intervals to compare with the subsequent nonconducted

### Sinus Rhythm with 2:1 AV Block

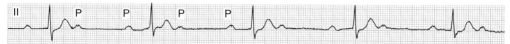

**Fig. 17.9** Sinus rhythm with 2:1 atrioventricular (AV) block. The very long and uniform PR intervals and narrow (normal) QRS complexes strongly suggest that the block here is in the AV node. Because the effective ventricular (QRS) rate is one half the sinus rate, the patient's pulse rate will be very slow (about 33 beats/min).

### Sinus Rhythm with 2:1 AV Block

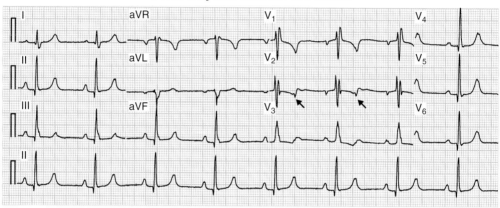

**Fig. 17.10** Sinus rhythm with 2:1 atrioventricular (AV) block. In this case, compared with Fig. 17.9, the QRS is wide due to a right bundle branch block. This finding increases the likelihood (but does not prove) that the block here is infranodal. This important pattern is easily missed because the nonconducted P waves (*arrows*) fall near the T wave of the preceding beats and therefore may be overlooked.

one. Here are two clues, which may be helpful in selected cases.

1. A very prolonged PR interval (>280 msec) in the conducted beats strongly suggests nodal (type I) block (Fig. 17.9).
2. A PR interval at the lower range of normal (120–150 msec), especially in association with QRS widening (bundle branch block pattern), strongly suggests infranodal (type II) block (Fig. 17.10). Unfortunately, intermediate values of PR intervals over a wide range (150–280 msec), are not diagnostic.[b]

---

[b]To help assess the need for a permanent pacemaker based on the level of block, an invasive electrophysiologic study can be done to record directly the signal transmission through the conduction system. In Mobitz I (nodal) block the signal blocks in the AV node without reaching the His bundle area. In Mobitz II (infranodal) block the signal reaches the bundle of His before being blocked, producing a characteristic deflection on the intracardiac recording.

**Cautions:**
- 2:1 AV block presents a very common pitfall in ECG analysis when the nonconducted P wave is hidden in the preceding T wave (see Chapter 24). In such cases, the rhythm may be misdiagnosed as "normal sinus" or "sinus bradycardia." If the PR interval of conducted beats is not prolonged (as often seen in infranodal block), the presence of AV block can be completely missed in a patient who urgently needs a permanent pacemaker.
- Also, care must be taken since blocked atrial bigeminy (see Chapter 14) can appear similar to 2:1 AV block, but PP interval differences usually allow you to distinguish between these two distinct diagnoses. In 2:1 AV block, the P waves come "on time," but with atrial bigeminy and blocked PACs, every other P′ wave is early (Fig. 19.3).

## ATRIAL FIBRILLATION OR FLUTTER WITH AV HEART BLOCK

With atrial fibrillation or flutter, the diagnosis of AV heart block is complicated. First- or second-degree AV block cannot be diagnosed in the presence of these conduction disturbances because of the lack of discrete P waves. However, with complete heart block, the two major clues are as follows (see Fig. 14.8):

1. Marked slowing (<50 beats/min) of the ventricular rate (sometimes with QRS widening and a change in morphology from baseline suggesting a fascicular/ventricular escape rather than conducted beats).
2. Regularization of the ventricular response (in contrast to the expected highly irregular QRS cadence in AF with intact AV conduction).

## GENERAL CLINICAL CONSIDERATIONS

### Symptoms

Symptoms of heart block vary depending on its degree as well as the time course of its development. PR interval prolongation (first-degree AV block) is usually asymptomatic (see Box 17.4). Occasionally, when the PR interval becomes so long that the P waves move close to the preceding QRS complexes, the patient may feel pulsations in the neck and even dizziness, due to near simultaneous atrial and ventricular contractions (see Chapter 22). This situation is similar to that seen in the pacemaker syndrome.

Second-degree block can produce sensations of skipped beats and exertional dyspnea due to inability to augment heart rate with exercise. Lightheadedness may occur if the heart rate is excessively slow. Mobitz

---

**BOX 17.4** | **Infections and Heart Block**

- Progressive PR prolongation in a patient with infective endocarditis is an ominous sign, suggesting the development of a perivalvular abscess.
- Lyme disease can produce any degree of heart block at the level of AV node, including complete heart block, often associated with severe symptoms. Occasionally syncope can be the first presentation of the disease. Almost always the block resolves with antibiotic therapy, but sometimes temporary pacing is required.

---

II (infranodal) block may result in syncope or even cardiac arrest.

Development of a complete heart block can be life-threatening, presenting with presyncope or syncope (Stokes–Adams attacks) due to a very slow escape rate or even to prolonged asystole. Severe bradycardia is more likely to occur with infranodal than nodal complete blocks due to the more abrupt onset and the slower rate of the escape rhythms in the former (see Chapter 13).

If the patient survives this initial episode of complete heart block, the primary complaints are usually severe exertional dyspnea and fatigue due to inability to augment heart rate and cardiac output with exercise, similar to that of second-degree AV block.[c] In addition, very slow rates due to AV heart block can induce severe QT(U) interval prolongation with torsades de pointes ventricular tachycardia (see Chapter 16), culminating in cardiac arrest (see Chapter 21).

### Treatment Approaches

The initial, emergency approach to a symptomatic patient with complete heart block should follow the current ACLS algorithms and appropriate measures, including preparation for transcutaneous/transvenous pacing if indicated. If the patient is hemodynamically stable, the level of block should be determined and potential causes reviewed (see Boxes 17.2 and 17.3). The important topic of AV block in acute infarction is considered next.

### AV HEART BLOCK IN ACUTE MYOCARDIAL INFARCTION

AV block of any degree can develop during acute myocardial infarction because of the interruption of blood supply to the conduction system and autonomic effects.

The AV node is usually supplied from the right coronary artery (and less frequently from the circumflex coronary artery). Occlusion of these vessels produces inferior myocardial infarction and block at the level of the AV node (Fig. 17.11). This block is usually transient and almost always resolves with time so that a permanent pacemaker is rarely needed, although temporary pacing might be necessary.

---

[c]Rarely, patients may have *congenital complete heart block* (which is usually at the AV nodal level, and associated with an escape rhythm with a narrow QRS and is not excessively slow). These individuals may be asymptomatic (other than noting a slow pulse) because of physiologic adaptations, including increased left ventricular dimension and stroke volume.

### Acute Inferior MI with Second-Degree AV Block

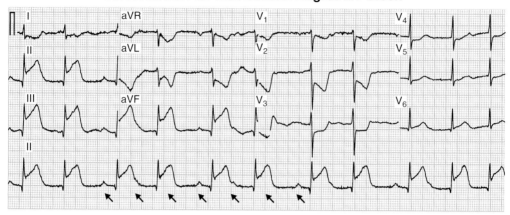

**Fig. 17.11** Sinus tachycardia with acute inferior (and probably posterolateral) ST segment elevation myocardial infarction (MI) with 3:2 atrioventricular (AV) Wenckebach block. Arrows point to the sinus P waves at a rate of about 100 beats/min. There is a 3:2 conduction pattern with AV Wenckebach block, indicating Mobitz I block. Note the subtle group beating pattern. The ST segment depressions in leads V₁ to V₃ are consistent with reciprocal change to the ST segment elevations laterally and probably posteriorly.

In contrast, the bundle of His, proximal portions of the right bundle branch, and left anterior fascicle of the left bundle branch are supplied by the septal branches of the left anterior descending (LAD) artery. Very proximal LAD artery occlusion producing anterior infarction may also cause infranodal heart block, often preceded by right bundle branch block (RBBB) or bifascicular blocks. This condition can progress abruptly to a complete heart block and often requires prophylactic pacemaker implantation (Fig. 17.12).

---

### Key Point

Prompt restoration of blood flow through the occluded coronary artery by angioplasty and stenting or thrombolysis may resolve infranodal block in anterior myocardial infarction.

---

## AV DISSOCIATION SYNDROMES

Cardiologists use the term *AV dissociation* in two related though not identical ways. This classification continues to cause considerable (and understandable) confusion among students and clinicians.

- AV dissociation is widely used as a *general* term for any arrhythmia in which the atria and ventricles are controlled by independent pacemakers. The

definition includes complete heart block, as described previously, as well as some instances of ventricular tachycardia or accelerated idioventricular rhythm in which the atria remain in sinus rhythm (see Chapters 16 and 19).

- AV dissociation is also used as a more *specific* term to describe a particular family of arrhythmias that are often mistaken for complete heart block. With this type of AV dissociation, very distinct from complete heart block, the SA node and AV junction appear to be "out of synch"; thus, the SA node loses its normal control of the ventricular rate. As a result the atria and ventricles are paced independently—the atria from the SA node, the ventricles from the AV junction. This situation is similar to what occurs with complete heart block. *However, in this type of AV dissociation, the ventricular rate is the same as or slightly faster than the atrial rate.* When the atrial and ventricular rates are almost the same, the term *isorhythmic AV dissociation* is used. (*Iso* is the Greek root for "same.")

  The critical difference between AV dissociation resulting from "desynchronization" of the SA and AV nodes from that of conduction failure and complete heart block is as follows: with AV dissociation (e.g., isorhythmic type) a properly timed P wave can be conducted through to the AV node, whereas with complete heart block, no P wave can stimulate the ventricles.

## Acute/Evolving Anterior MI and AV Heart Block

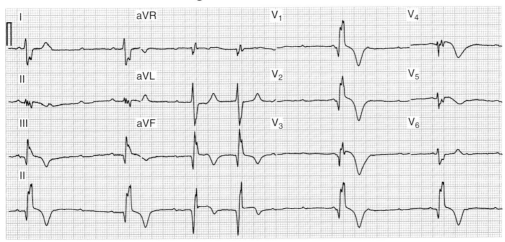

**Fig. 17.12** High-degree AV block (Mobitz II and complete) in recent anterior ST segment elevation myocardial infarction (STEMI). Multiple sinus nonconducted P waves are present. Third and fourth QRS complexes (narrow) appear relatively early and therefore are likely to be conducted. Wider QRS complexes (with right bundle branch block and right axis morphology) at a regular slow rate represent an idioventricular (fascicular) escape rhythm. The anterior and inferior ST segment elevations are present in both conducted and escape complexes. Q waves in anterior and inferior leads are consistent with evolving extensive anterior myocardial infarction, possibly due to a very proximal occlusion of a large "wrap-around" left anterior descending coronary artery. This situation requires emergency temporary pacing and reperfusion therapy.

## Sinus Bradycardia and AV Dissociation

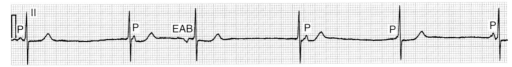

**Fig. 17.13** Sinus bradycardia and atrioventricular (AV) dissociation. The sinus rate is very slow at about 35 beats/min with a nodal escape rhythm at about the same rate. The third cycle is due to an ectopic atrial beat (*EAB*; note the negative P wave). This type of AV dissociation is not due to complete heart block, but a functional *desynchronization* of the sinus and nodal pacemakers. If the rate of the sinus node increases, 1:1 normal sinus rhythm should resume. Reversible factors, in general, include drugs (beta blockers, certain calcium channel blockers), enhanced vagal tone, and hyperkalemia.

## Isorhythmic AV Dissociation

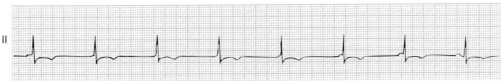

**Fig. 17.14** This common type of atrioventricular (AV) dissociation is characterized by transient *desynchronization* of the sinus and AV node pacemakers, such that they beat at nearly the same rate. Because they are "out of sync" with each other, the *P* waves (representing the sinus node pacemaker) appear to "slide" in and out of the QRS complexes (representing the AV node "escape" pacemaker). This type of AV dissociation, a minor arrhythmia, must be distinguished from actual complete AV block, a life-threatening conduction problem (compare with Figs. 17.7 and 17.8).

AV dissociation (Fig. 17.13) when used in the more specific context, therefore, can be regarded as a "competition" between the SA node and the AV node for control of the heartbeat. This situation may occur either when the SA node slows down (e.g., because of the effects of beta blockers or calcium channel blockers or with increased vagal tone) or when the AV node is accelerated (e.g., by ischemia or digitalis toxicity). Not uncommonly, isorhythmic AV dissociation is seen in healthy young individuals, particularly when they are sleeping.

Fig. 17.14 presents an example of *isorhythmic* AV dissociation, a common benign arrhythmia easily confused with complete heart block. Notice the P waves with a variable PR interval because the ventricular (QRS) rate is nearly the same as the atrial rate. At times the P waves may merge with the QRS complexes and become imperceptible for several beats. If the sinus rate speeds up sufficiently (or the AV junctional rate slows), the atrial stimulus may be able to penetrate the AV junction, reestablishing sinus rhythm.

# CHAPTER 18

# Atrioventricular (AV) Conduction Disorders, Part II: Preexcitation (Wolff–Parkinson–White) Patterns and Syndromes

The previous chapter focused primarily on disorders associated with *delays* in atrioventricular (AV) conduction, termed AV heart blocks. This chapter describes an entirely different class of AV conduction disorders, namely those related to abnormally early ventricular excitation (preexcitation). Our focus will be its most common presentations, namely Wolff–Parkinson–White (WPW) patterns and associated arrhythmia/conduction syndromes. This chapter also serves as an extension of the discussion of reentrant supraventricular tachycardias started in Chapter 14. A notable paradox is that both early ventricular excitation (preexcitation) and delayed ventricular excitation (as with bundle branch blocks and related intraventricular conduction disturbances described in Chapter 8) lead to a widened QRS complex. Another counterintuitive finding is that the classic ECGs of patients in sinus rhythm with a WPW pattern show a wide QRS, whereas when the characteristic reentrant type of paroxysmal tachycardia develops, the ECGs most often show a QRS of normal morphology and duration.

## PREEXCITATION VIA AV BYPASS TRACTS

The normal electrical stimulus (signal) generated by the SA node pacemaker travels to the ventricles via the atria and AV junction. The physiologic lag in conduction through the AV junction, which allows the ventricles time to fill, results in the normal PR interval (delay time) of 120–200 msec. Now consider the consequences of having an extra pathway between the atria and ventricles that provides an alternative means of activating the ventricles. This extra pathway (akin to a short-cut or short circuit) would literally *bypass* the AV junction, and in doing so, allow for early depolarization (preexcitation) of the ventricles. This situation is exactly what underlies the WPW pattern: a functional *atrioventricular (AV) bypass tract* connects the atria and ventricles, partly or fully circumventing conduction through the AV junction (Fig. 18.1).

Bypass tracts (also called *accessory or anomalous pathways*) represent persistent abnormal connections that form and fail to disappear during fetal development of the heart (but may stop conducting during later life). These abnormal conduction pathways, composed of short bands of heart muscle tissue, are usually located in the area around the mitral or tricuspid valves (AV rings) or interventricular septum. An AV bypass tract is sometimes referred to, historically, as a bundle of Kent.

## THE CLASSIC WPW TRIAD

Preexcitation of the ventricle during sinus rhythm with its classic triad signature produces the WPW signature (Figs. 18.2–18.4):
1. The PR interval is shortened (often but not always to less than 0.12 sec) because of the ventricular preexcitation.
2. The QRS complex is widened, giving the superficial appearance of a bundle branch block pattern. However, the wide QRS is caused *not* by a delay in ventricular depolarization but by early stimulation of the ventricles. The T wave is also usually opposite in polarity to the wide QRS in any lead,

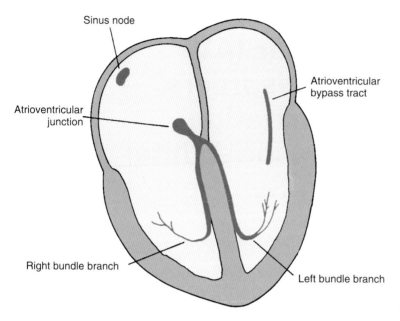

Sinus node

Atrioventricular bypass tract

Atrioventricular junction

Right bundle branch

Left bundle branch

**Fig. 18.1** Electroanatomy underlying the Wolff–Parkinson–White (WPW) preexcitation pattern. A small percentage of individuals are born with an accessory fiber (atrioventricular bypass tract) connecting the atria and ventricles.

## Wolff–Parkinson–White Preexcitation

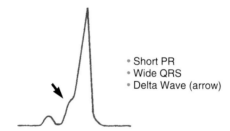

- Short PR
- Wide QRS
- Delta Wave (arrow)

**Fig. 18.2** Preexcitation via the bypass tract in the WPW pattern is associated with a triad of findings.

similar to what is seen with bundle branch blocks (another example of "secondary T wave inversions").

3. The upstroke of the QRS complex is slurred or notched. This notching, called a *delta* wave, is due to relatively slow conduction through the ventricular muscle from the bypass tract insertion site.

## The QRS Complex as a Fusion Beat in WPW

The QRS complex in sinus rhythm with WPW pattern, therefore, can be viewed as the result of a competition (race) involving two sets of signals, one going down the normal AV conduction system and the other down the (accessory) AV bypass tract. The signal going down the bypass tract usually reaches the ventricles first, while the signal going down the normal conduction system gets delayed in the AV node. Once the signal going down the normal conduction system passes the AV node, this activation wave "catches up" with the preexcitation wave by spreading quickly through the His-Purkinje system and activating the rest of the ventricles in the usual way. Thus the degree of preexcitation (amount of the ventricles activated through the bypass tract) is dependent on the relative speeds of AV nodal vs. bypass tract conduction—the greater the relative delay in the AV node, the larger portion of the ventricles that is activated through the bypass tract and the more apparent the delta wave will be. The QRS complex in WPW, therefore, can be viewed as a kind of fusion complex, resulting from the output of depolarization down the normal AV nodal pathway and down the accessory pathway.

Anomalous activation of the ventricles via a bypass tract can lead to QRS alterations mimicking bundle branch blocks, hypertrophy or infarction, as well as to secondary ST-T changes simulating ischemia. Figs. 18.2 and 18.3 show the WPW pattern,

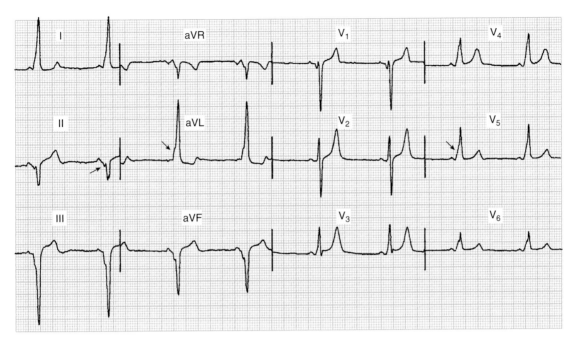

**Fig. 18.3** Notice the characteristic triad of the WPW pattern: short PR intervals, and delta waves (*arrows*) that are negative in some leads (e.g., II, III, and aVR) and positive in others (aVL and $V_2$ to $V_6$), and widened QRS complexes. The Q waves in leads II, III, and aVF are the result of abnormal ventricular conduction (negative delta waves) rather than an inferior myocardial infarction. This pattern is consistent with a bypass tract inserting into the posterior region of the ventricles (possibly posteroseptal in this case).

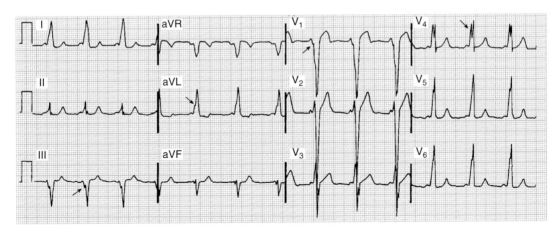

**Fig. 18.4** Another example of the WPW pattern with the triad of wide QRS complexes, short PR intervals, and delta waves (*arrows*). The finding of delta waves that are predominantly negative in lead $V_1$ and positive in the lateral leads is consistent with a bypass tract inserting into the free wall of the right ventricle. This pattern simulates a left bundle branch block pattern.

with its classic triad of a short PR interval, a widened QRS complex, and a delta wave.

## ECG Localization of Bypass Tracts

Atrioventricular bypass tracts can be located anywhere along the AV groove and interventricular septum. Some patients have more than one bypass tract. A useful exercise is to try to localize the area where the bypass tract inserts based on the pattern of preexcitation on the surface ECG. While many sophisticated algorithms have been developed to help facilitate this prediction, trainees and non-cardiologists may find a simple approach based on vector principles most useful and entirely sufficient for the non-expert.

Basically, if the bypass tract inserts into the lateral part of the left ventricle, the initial depolarization forces should be directed away from the left ventricle, and the QRS vector will point from left to right. In such cases, the delta waves will be negative in leftward leads I or aVL (and sometimes $V_6$) and positive in the right-sided leads $V_1$ to $V_2$. The resultant complex will resemble right ventricular hypertrophy, right bundle branch block (RBBB) or lateral wall myocardial infarction (MI) pattern.

---

=== Key Point ===

As a general rule: the initial QRS complex (delta wave) vector will point away from the area of the ventricles that is first to be stimulated by the bypass tract.

---

If the bypass tract inserts into the posterior region of the ventricles, the ECG usually shows positive delta waves in most of the precordial leads and negative delta waves in the inferior limb leads (resembling an inferoposterior infarct; see Fig. 18.3).

With right free wall preexcitation, the QRS complexes are predominantly negative in $V_1$ and $V_2$ (traveling away from right-sided leads), resembling a left bundle branch block (LBBB). The delta waves are typically biphasic or slightly negative in $V_1/V_2$ (together with a predominantly negative QRS complex) and positive in $V_6$ (Fig. 18.4). The QRS axis is horizontal or leftward.

Anteroseptal bypass tracts, the rarest WPW variant, may be associated with negative delta waves in leads $V_1$ and $V_2$ (resembling an anterior infarct). The frontal plane axis is more vertical.

## HIGHLIGHT: SOME POINTS OF CONFUSION

The terminology applied to preexcitation syndromes and accessory pathways is confusing to novices and clinicians. These bulleted notes are intended to help "disambiguate" selected terms and concepts.

- The terms "accessory pathway," "bypass tract," "anomalous pathway," and "bundle of Kent," are synonymous.
- There are two major classes of accessory pathways: *manifest* and *concealed*. Histologically they both represent atrial (not nodal) tissue.
- A *manifest* bypass tract is the key electrophysiologic finding in WPW and allows for antegrade (forward) conduction from atria to ventricles. Only a manifest bypass tract that conducts more rapidly than the AV junction will result in the classic WPW ECG triad: short PR, delta wave, and wide QRS.
- Not all bypass tracts (accessory pathways), however, are manifest. Some are never functional and are clinically irrelevant. Other bypass tracts may be capable of only retrograde conduction (i.e., from the ventricles to atria), but may or may not be capable of antegrade conduction due to functional or organic reasons. When bypass tracts conduct only in a retrograde direction they will be suspected on the surface ECG in sinus rhythm, although the patient may develop a classic narrow complex tachycardia that indirectly reveals their presence (see below). Therefore, such bypass tracts are termed *concealed*.
- The term "WPW pattern" applies only in cases when a bypass tract with antegrade conduction is manifest at least transiently during sinus or another supraventricular rhythm.

## BASIS OF NARROW COMPLEX TACHYCARDIA (NCT) WITH WPW

The presence of a bypass tract is a major substrate for the pathogenesis of paroxysmal supraventricular tachycardia (PSVT) due to reentry. The specific type of NCT typically seen with WPW (Figs. 18.5 and 18.6) involves a *reentrant loop* allowing impulse transmission down the AV junction, followed by retrograde conduction up the accessory pathway back into the atria, and then down the AV junction again and again. The QRS complex, therefore, will be normal in appearance given that the only antero-grade conduction from the atria to the ventricles is

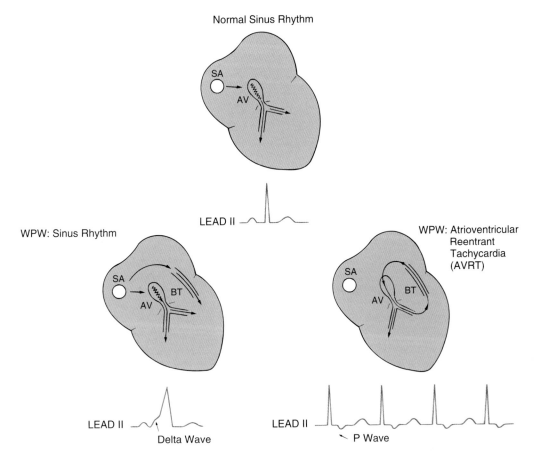

**Fig. 18.5** Conduction during sinus rhythm in the normal heart (*top*) spreads from the sinoatrial (SA) node to the atrioventricular (AV) node and then down the bundle branches. The jagged line indicates physiologic slowing of conduction in the AV node. With the Wolff–Parkinson–White (WPW) syndrome (*bottom left*), an abnormal accessory conduction pathway called a bypass tract (*BT*) connects the atria and ventricles. With WPW preexcitation, during sinus rhythm the electrical impulse is conducted quickly down the bypass tract, preexciting the ventricles before the impulse arrives via the AV node. Consequently, the PR interval is short and the QRS complex is wide, with slurring at its onset (delta wave). WPW predisposes patients to develop an atrioventricular reentrant tachycardia (AVRT) (*bottom right*), in which a premature atrial beat may spread down the normal pathway to the ventricles, travel back up the bypass tract, and recirculate down the AV node again. This reentrant loop can repeat itself over and over, resulting in a tachycardia. Notice the normal QRS complex and often negative P wave in lead II during this type of bypass-tract tachycardia.

down the AV node (and not involving the bypass tract). This type of highly regular NCT is called *atrioventricular (AV) reentrant tachycardia* (AVRT). As noted, when patients with WPW are in sinus rhythm, they may show a wide QRS due to antegrade conduction down the bypass tract. If they develop PSVT due to AVRT (using the bypass tract for retrograde conduction), their QRS waveform will "paradoxically" change from a wide complex morphology during the slower sinus rate to a narrow complex

one during the AVRT episode.[a] The WPW abnormality predisposes patients to AVRT because of the presence of the accessory conduction pathway. These tachycardias are usually initiated when a precisely

---

[a]Patients with PSVT due to antegrade conduction down the AV node/ His–Purkinje system and retrograde conduction up the bypass tract (AVRT) usually show a narrow complex tachycardia (NCT; see also Chapter 19). However, if a bundle branch block is already present or develops due to the increased rate, this variant of PSVT will appear as a wide complex tachycardia (WCT), simulating ventricular tachycardia.

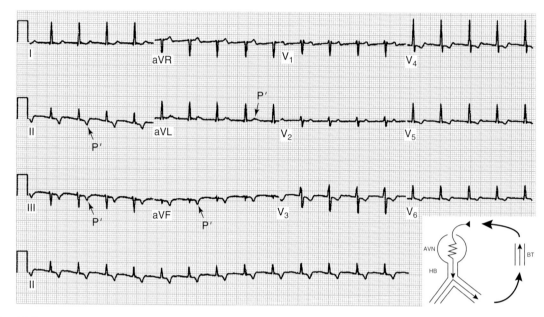

**Fig. 18.6** Example of a classic bypass-tract-mediated narrow complex tachycardia. This type of PSVT is referred to as atrioventricular reentrant tachycardia (AVRT). Technically, it is called orthodromic AVRT since the reentrant loop goes down the normal conduction system—AV node and His bundle–Purkinje network—and back up the concealed bypass tract (see inset). This mechanism is similar to AV nodal reentrant tachycardia (AVNRT), discussed in Chapter 14. Indeed, the two may be indistinguishable from the surface ECG. In general, with AVRT, the P′ wave, if seen, is usually retrograde (negative in lead II) and located in the ST segment or T wave, further away from the preceding QRS than in typical AVNRT, because of the additional time for the signal to conduct through the ventricular myocardium before reaching the bypass tract and conducting up to the atria. With AVNRT, the retrograde P wave is usually hidden within the QRS, or comes just after it, producing a pseudo-S and pseudo-R waves (typically in leads II and aVR, respectively). *AVN,* atrioventricular node; *HB,* His bundle; *BT,* bypass tract.

timed premature atrial complex travels down the AV junction and then back up the bypass tract, or premature ventricular premature complex travels up the accessory pathway and then back down the AV junction. The resulting reentrant circuit is termed *orthodromic* AVRT (Fig. 18.6). This type of reentry is closely related to that seen with the other major type of paroxysmal supraventricular tachycardia described in Chapter 14, namely that associated with dual pathways in the AV node (termed *AV nodal reentrant tachycardia,* or AVNRT).[b]

A paroxysmal supraventricular tachycardia based on a reentrant loop that conducts in the opposite direction, namely, down the bypass tract and up the AV node, is termed *antidromic* AVRT. This bypass tract variant is much less common than the orthodromic type of AVRT. With antidromic AVRT,

because of antegrade conduction down the bypass tract (as opposed to the AV node with orthodromic AVRT), the QRS complex will show a wide complex tachycardia (WCT) (see Chapter 19).

## Key Point: WPW Pattern vs. WPW Syndrome

Use the term "WPW syndrome" to apply to patients with the "WPW pattern" who also have arrhythmias related to the bypass tract. The WPW pattern does not mean that the patient also has arrhythmias; just that the characteristic ECG triad is present. Conversely, a narrow complex tachycardia (AVRT) may be due to a concealed bypass tract without evidence of the full WPW triad in sinus rhythm. Thus, all patients with the WPW pattern have a bypass tract, but not all patients with bypass-tract-mediated tachycardias will show evidence of preexcitation when they are in sinus rhythm.

[b]Clinicians should be aware that a confusing taxonomy has been used to label bypass-tract-mediated tachycardias. Synonymous terms include: atrioventricular reentrant (reentry) tachycardia (AVRT), which is the currently preferred usage; circus movement tachycardia (CMT), and AV reciprocating tachycardia (also abbreviated AVRT).

## ATRIAL FIBRILLATION (OR FLUTTER) WITH WPW PREEXCITATION

AVRT is the arrhythmia most commonly associated with WPW. However, patients with WPW are also more prone to developing atrial fibrillation, although the mechanism of this association is not entirely clear. Most important clinically is that if AF (or atrial flutter) develops in a patient with the WPW substrate, a wide complex tachycardia may result from conduction down the bypass tract into the ventricles at very high rates, much higher than seen through the AV node. Fortunately this occurrence is quite rare, although it appears that younger patients with WPW are more prone to AF than those with normal AV conduction. This kind of WCT is easily confused for VT. An example of WPW syndrome with AF is shown in Fig. 19.12.

WPW syndrome with AF should be strongly suspected if you encounter a WCT (prior to therapy) that shows the following constellation: (1) the QRS cadence is quite irregular and (2) a very high rate (i.e., intermittently showing very short RR intervals). In particular, RR intervals of 200 msec or less are rarely seen with conventional AF. In contrast, very rapid VT (sometimes called ventricular flutter) is usually quite regular when it becomes very rapid. The very short RR intervals in WPW with AF are related to the ability of the bypass tract (in contrast to the AV node) to conduct impulses in extremely rapid, erratic succession (see Fig. 18.7A).

Recognition of WPW syndrome with AF is of considerable clinical importance for a number of reasons. (1) Digitalis, a drug used in rate control of conventional AF, may enhance conduction down the bypass by directly shortening the refractoriness of the accessory pathway, as well as decreasing conduction down the AV node via its vagotonic effects. As a result, the ventricular response may increase to the point where myocardial ischemia occurs, precipitating ventricular fibrillation and sudden cardiac arrest. (2) A similar hazardous effect has been reported with intravenous verapamil, which may cause vasodilation and a reflex increase in sympathetic tone. (3) Emergency direct current (DC) cardioversion may be required. (4) In more stable patients with this phenomenon, intravenous therapy with drugs (e.g., procainamide) that slow or block conduction in the accessory pathway may be considered (see Chapter 11).

## SUMMARY: CLINICAL SIGNIFICANCE OF WPW

The classic WPW appearance on ECG has been reported in roughly 1–2 per 1000 individuals. In some instances, familial occurrence is observed. On rare occasions, finding a right ventricular bypass tract may be the first clue to a specific form of congenital heart disease, namely Ebstein's anomaly of the tricuspid valve. Left-sided bypass tracts usually are not associated with any distinct type of structural heart disease.

The major importance of WPW preexcitation for clinicians is threefold:
1. Individuals with WPW are prone to a specific type of regular PSVT, termed AVRT.
2. Patients with WPW are also more likely to develop atrial fibrillation (Fig. 18.7). Furthermore, if atrial fibrillation develops in conjunction with a manifest accessory pathway (i.e., one that can conduct from atria to ventricles), the ventricular rate may become extremely fast (300/min or more). Indeed, "preexcited atrial fibrillation" at this rate may lead to ventricular fibrillation, associated with increased catecholamines and ischemia, and even sudden cardiac arrest. Fortunately, as discussed, this occurrence is very rare.
3. The WPW ECG is often mistaken for either a bundle branch block, due to the wide QRS, or an MI, due to negative delta waves that may simulate pathologic Q waves (see Fig. 18.3).

### Other Preexcitation Variants and Simulators

WPW is the most commonly recognized preexcitation variant, but not the only one. An even less common preexcitation variant is related to a slowly conducting bypass tract that typically connects the right atrium with the right bundle branch or right ventricle. These "atriofascicular" or "atrioventricular" fibers are sometimes referred to as Mahaim fibers. The 12-lead ECG in sinus rhythm may be normal or may show a normal PR interval with a subtle delta wave. If PSVT develops, the impulse goes down the bypass tract, stimulates the right ventricle before the left, and then reenters up the AV node. This sequence will produce LBBB pattern during the tachycardia. In general, the topic of Mahaim fibers and other preexcitation variants is most appropriate for more advanced discussions.

## Atrial Fibrillation and Wolff–Parkinson–White Syndrome

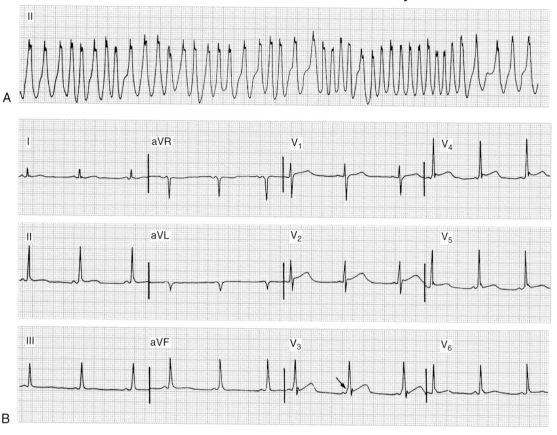

**Fig. 18.7** (A) Atrial fibrillation with the Wolff-Parkinson-White (WPW) preexcitation syndrome may lead to a wide complex tachycardia with a very rapid rate. Notice that some of the RR intervals (due to conduction down the bypass tract) are extremely short (<200 msec), much shorter than those seen with conduction down the atrioventricular node. The irregularity is due to the underlying atrial fibrillation. (B) After the arrhythmia has converted to sinus rhythm, the classic triad of the WPW pattern is visible, albeit subtly, with a relatively short PR interval, wide QRS complex, and delta wave (*arrow* in lead V₃).

As a general guideline, clinicians should be careful not to "over-interpret" an ECG in which the only noteworthy finding is a relatively short PR interval (e.g., 0.10–0.12 sec) as a "preexcitation variant," especially in an asymptomatic person. Such ECGs can be read as: "A relatively short PR interval is noted without other evidence of preexcitation," or as: "A relatively short PR interval is noted which may be seen as a physiologic variant (accelerated AV conduction), without evidence of preexcitation." A physiologically short PR interval is most likely to occur at relatively faster heart rates, and is often seen in

young adults due to increased sympathetic and decreased cardiac vagal tone modulation.

## TREATMENT PRINCIPLES

Patients with WPW syndrome (especially who have symptomatic, recurrent tachycardias) can usually be cured by an invasive procedure during which the bypass tract is ablated using *radiofrequency* (RF) current. This highly successful and permanent treatment requires a cardiac electrophysiologic (EP) procedure in which special catheters are inserted into the heart through the femoral vein; the bypass tract is located by means of ECG recordings inside the heart (*intracardiac electrograms*). Patients who are not candidates for RF catheter ablation therapy can usually be treated with drug therapy (AV nodal blockers or certain antiarrhythmic agents).

Not all individuals with the WPW pattern have associated arrhythmias. Occasionally, the WPW pattern will be discovered in asymptomatic subjects who have an ECG ordered as part of a medical evaluation or for other indications (e.g., preoperative assessment). The major concern is the risk of the sudden onset of atrial fibrillation with a very rapid ventricular response leading, in turn, to ventricular fibrillation. Fortunately, as mentioned, the risk of sudden death from this mechanism is extremely low in completely asymptomatic subjects with the WPW patterns. Individuals in whom a WPW pattern is discovered as an incidental finding, therefore, usually do not require specific intervention. Disappearance of the WPW pattern during exercise (with the appearance of a normal QRS during sinus tachycardia), or intermittent WPW, is particularly reassuring. Electrophysiologic evaluation and prophylactic ablation therapy in asymptomatic subjects are strongly considered in special circumstances, for example, with competitive athletes, pilots, bus drivers, and those with a family history of sudden death.

## BRIEF OVERVIEW: DIFFERENTIAL DIAGNOSIS OF WIDE QRS COMPLEX PATTERNS

A wide QRS complex pattern is of importance because it is often indicative of an important abnormality with clinical implications. The major

ECG patterns that produce a widened QRS complex can be divided into four major categories:

1. Bundle branch blocks (intrinsic intraventricular conduction delays; IVCDs) including the classic RBBB and LBBB patterns, as well as nonspecific IVCDs
2. "Toxic" conduction delays caused by some extrinsic factor, such as hyperkalemia or drugs (e.g., quinidine, propafenone, flecainide, and other related antiarrhythmics, as well as phenothiazines, and tricyclic antidepressants)
3. Beats arising in the ventricles, including premature ventricular beats (complexes), ventricular escape beats, or electronic ventricular pacemaker beats (Chapters 8, 16 and 22)
4. WPW-type preexcitation patterns

Differentiation among these four possibilities is usually straightforward. The ECG effects of RBBB and LBBB have already been described in Chapter 8. Hyperkalemia produces widening of the QRS complex, often with loss of P waves (Chapter 12). Widening of the QRS complex in any patient who is taking an antiarrhythmic or a psychotropic agent should always suggest possible drug toxicity. Conventional pacemakers generally produce LBBB pattern with a pacemaker spike before each QRS complex. An important exception is biventricular pacing used in the treatment of chronic heart failure (CHF) in which RBBB pattern may be seen if the left ventricular impulse is delivered slightly in advance of the right; see Chapter 22. Finally, the WPW pattern is recognized by the triad of a short PR interval, a wide QRS complex, and a delta wave, as discussed in this chapter.

# PART III

# Special Topics and Reviews

# CHAPTER 19

# Bradycardias and Tachycardias: Review and Differential Diagnosis

Preceding chapters have described the major arrhythmias and atrioventricular (AV) conduction disturbances. These abnormalities can be classified in multiple ways. This review/overview chapter categorizes arrhythmias into two major groups: *bradycardias* and *tachycardias*. The tachycardia group is then subdivided into narrow and wide (broad) QRS complex variants, which are a major focus of ECG differential diagnosis in acute care medicine and in referrals to cardiologists.

## BRADYCARDIAS (BRADYARRHYTHMIAS)

The term *bradycardia* (or *bradyarrhythmia*) refers to arrhythmias and conduction abnormalities that produce a heart rate <60 beats/min. Fortunately, their differential diagnosis is usually straightforward in that only a few classes must be considered. For most clinical purposes, we can classify bradyarrhythmias into five major groups (Box 19.1), recognizing that sometimes more than one rhythm is present (e.g., sinus bradycardia with complete heart block and an idioventricular escape rhythm).

### Sinus Bradycardia and Related Rhythms

Sinus bradycardia is simply sinus rhythm with a rate <60 beats/min (Fig. 19.1). When 1:1 (normal) AV conduction is present, each QRS complex is preceded by a P wave that is positive in lead II and negative in lead aVR. Some individuals, especially trained athletes at rest and adults during deep sleep, may have sinus bradycardia with rates as low as 30–40 beats/min.

Sinus bradycardia may be related to a decreased firing rate of the sinus node pacemaker cells (as with athletes who have high cardiac vagal tone at

rest) or to actual SA block (see Chapter 13). Inappropriate sinus bradycardia may be seen with the sick sinus syndrome (discussed below). The most extreme example of sinus node dysfunction is SA node arrest (see Chapters 13 and 21). As now described, sinus bradycardia may also be associated with *wandering atrial pacemaker* (WAP). In addition, sinus rhythm with atrial bigeminy—where each premature atrial complex (PAC) is blocked (nonconducted)—may mimic sinus bradycardia.

### Wandering Atrial Pacemaker

Wandering atrial (supraventricular) pacemaker (WAP) is an "electrophysiologic cousin" of sinus bradycardia. As shown in Fig. 19.2, WAP is characterized by multiple P waves of varying configuration with a relatively normal or slow heart rate. The P wave variations reflect shifting of the intrinsic pacemaker between the sinus node (and likely regions within the SA node, itself), and different atrial sites. WAP may be seen in a variety of settings. Often it appears in normal persons (particularly during sleep or states of high vagal tone), as a physiologic variant. It may also occur with certain drug toxicities, sick sinus syndrome, and different types of organic heart disease.

*Clinicians should be aware that WAP is quite distinct from multifocal atrial tachycardia (MAT), a tachyarrhythmia with multiple different P waves. In WAP the rate is normal or slow. In MAT, the rate is rapid.* For rhythms that resemble MAT, but with rates between 60 and 100 beats/min, the more general term "multifocal atrial rhythm" can be used. MAT is most likely to be mistaken for atrial fibrillation, with both producing a rapid irregular rate; conversely, AF is sometimes misinterpreted as MAT.

### Sinus Rhythm with Frequent Blocked PACs

Clinicians should also be aware that when sinus rhythm is present with frequent blocked PACs

---

Please go to expertconsult.inkling.com for additional online material for this chapter.

**194**

(Fig. 19.3), the rhythm will mimic sinus bradycardia. The early cycle PACs are not conducted because of refractoriness of the AV node from the previous sinus beat and the premature P wave may be partly or fully hidden in the T wave. The slow pulse (QRS) rate is due to the post-atrial ectopic pauses.

## AV Junctional (Nodal) and Related Rhythms

With a slow AV junctional escape rhythm (Fig. 19.4) either the P waves (seen immediately before or just after the QRS complexes) are *retrograde* (inverted in lead II and upright in lead aVR), or not apparent if the atria and ventricles are stimulated simultaneously. Slow heart rates may also be associated with ectopic atrial rhythms, including WAP (see previous discussion). One type of ectopic atrial rhythm—termed low atrial rhythm—was discussed in Chapter 13.

## AV Heart Block (Second- or Third-Degree)/AV Dissociation

A slow, regular ventricular rate of 60 beats/min or less (even as low as 20 beats/min) is the rule with complete heart block because of the slow intrinsic rate of the nodal (junctional) or idioventricular pacemaker (Fig. 19.5). In addition, patients with second-degree block (nodal or infranodal) often have

### Sinus Bradycardia

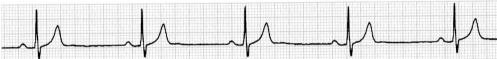

**Fig. 19.1** Marked sinus bradycardia at about 40/min. Sinus arrhythmia is also present. Sinus bradycardia (like sinus tachycardia) always needs to be interpreted in clinical context because it may be a normal variant (due to increased vagal tone in a resting athlete or in a healthy person during sleep) or may be due to drug effect/toxicity, sinus node dysfunction, etc., as discussed in Chapter 13. The PR interval here is also slightly prolonged (0.24 sec), also consistent with increased vagal tone, intrinsic atrioventricular (AV) nodal conduction slowing, or with certain drugs that depress activity in the sinoatrial (SA) and AV nodes (e.g., beta blockers).

Lead II (continuous)
### Wandering Atrial Pacemaker

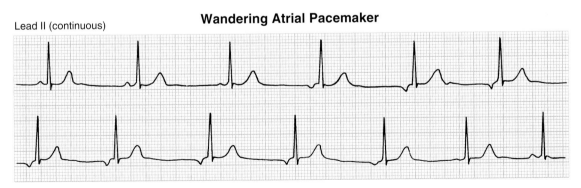

**Fig. 19.2** The variability of the P wave configuration in this lead II rhythm strip is caused by shifting of the pacemaker site between the sinus node and ectopic atrial locations.

### Atrial Bigeminy with Blocked PACs

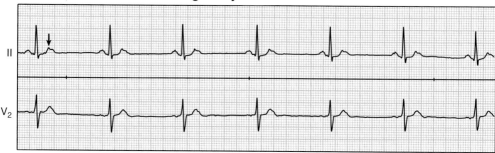

**Fig. 19.3** Superficially, this rhythm looks like sinus bradycardia. However, careful inspection reveals subtle blocked premature atrial complexes (PACs), superimposed on the T waves of each beat (*arrow*). These ectopic P waves are so premature that they do not conduct to the ventricles because of refractoriness of the atrioventricular node. The effective pulse rate will be about 50/min. Shown are modified leads II and $V_2$ from a Holter recording.

### AV Junctional Escape Rhythm

Monitor lead

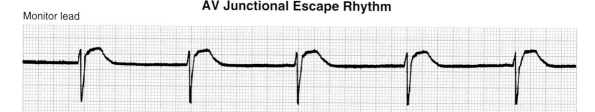

**Fig. 19.4** The heart rate is about 43 beats/min, consistent with an atrioventricular (AV) junctional escape rhythm. Note that the ECG baseline between the QRS complexes is perfectly flat, i.e., no P waves or other atrial activity is evident, This pattern is due to simultaneous activation of the atria and ventricles by the junctional (nodal) pacemaker, such that the P waves are masked by the QRS complexes.

### Sinus Rhythm with Complete Heart Block

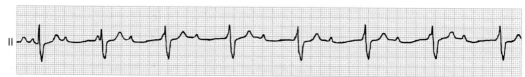

**Fig. 19.5** The sinus (P wave) rate is about 80 beats/min. The ventricular (QRS complex) rate is about 43 beats/min. Because the atria and ventricles are beating independently, the PR intervals are variable. The QRS complex is wide because the ventricles are being paced by an idioventricular pacemaker or by an infranodal pacemaker with a concomitant intraventricular conduction delay.

a bradycardia because of the nonconducted P waves (see Chapter 17). Isorhythmic AV dissociation and related arrhythmias, which may be confused with complete AV heart block, are also frequently associated with a heart rate of less than 60 beats/min (see Chapter 17). This rhythm must be distinguished from sinus rhythm with frequent blocked PACs in a bigeminal pattern (Fig. 19.3), as described above.

### Atrial Fibrillation or Flutter with a Slow Ventricular Rate

New onset atrial fibrillation (AF), prior to treatment, is generally associated with a rapid ventricular rate. However, the rate may become quite slow (less than 50-60 beats/min) because of: (1) drug effects or actual drug toxicity (e.g., with beta blockers, certain calcium channel blockers, or digoxin), or due to (2)

## Atrial Fibrillation with a Slow, Regularized Ventricular Rate

Monitor lead

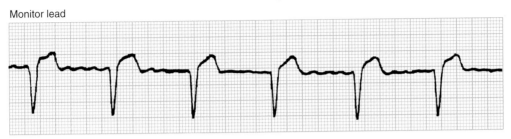

**Fig. 19.6** Regularization and excessive slowing of the ventricular rate with atrial fibrillation are usually due to intrinsic atrioventricular disease or drugs such as beta blockers or digoxin (see Chapters 15 and 20).

underlying disease of the AV junction (Fig. 19.6 and see Fig. 15.8). In some cases, both sets of factors are contributory. In either circumstance, the ECG shows characteristic atrial fibrillatory ( *f* ) waves with a slow, sometimes regularized ventricular (QRS) rate. The *f* waves may be very fast and low amplitude ( *fine AF*) and, thus, easily overlooked. A very slow, regularized ventricular response in AF suggests the presence of underlying complete AV heart block (see Chapters 15 and 17).

### Idioventricular Escape Rhythm

When the SA nodal and AV junctional escape pacemakers fail to function, a very slow back-up pacemaker in the ventricular conduction (His–Purkinje–myocardial) system may take over. This rhythm is referred to as an *idioventricular escape rhythm* (see Fig. 21.4B). The rate is usually less than 40–45 beats/min and the QRS complexes are wide without any preceding P waves. *In such cases of "pure" idioventricular rhythm, hyperkalemia should always be excluded.* In certain cases of complete AV heart block, you may see the combination of sinus rhythm with an idioventricular escape rhythm (see Chapter 17). Idioventricular rhythm, usually without P waves, is a common end-stage finding in irreversible cardiac arrest, preceding a "flat-line" pattern (see also Chapter 21).

### TACHYCARDIAS (TACHYARRHYTHMIAS)

At the opposite end of the rate spectrum are the tachycardias, rhythms with an atrial and/or ventricular rate faster than 100 beats/min. From a clinician's perspective, the tachyarrhythmias can be

| TABLE 19.1 | Major Tachyarrhythmias: Simplified Classification | |
|---|---|
| **Narrow QRS Complexes (NCT)** | **Wide QRS Complexes (WCT)** |
| Sinus tachycardia | Ventricular tachycardia |
| (Paroxysmal) supraventricular tachycardias (PSVTs)* | Supraventricular tachycardia with aberration/anomalous conduction caused by: (a) bundle branch block-type pattern (b) Wolff–Parkinson–White preexcitation with (antegrade) conduction down the bypass tract |
| Atrial flutter | |
| Atrial fibrillation | |

*The three most common types of PSVTs are atrioventricular nodal reentrant tachycardia (AVNRT), atrioventricular reentrant tachycardia (AVRT; which involves a bypass tract), and atrial tachycardia (AT) including unifocal and multifocal variants (see Chapters 14 and 18). Other nonparoxysmal supraventricular tachycardias also may occur, including types of so-called *incessant* atrial, junctional, and bypass tract tachycardias. (For further details of these more advanced topics, see selected references cited in the Bibliography.)

usefully divided into two general groups: those with a "narrow" (normal) QRS duration and those with a "wide" (also called broad) QRS duration (Table 19.1), abbreviated, respectively, as NCTs and WCTs.

NCTs are almost invariably *supra*ventricular (i.e., the focus of stimulation is within or *above* the AV junction). WCTs, by contrast, are either: (a) ventricular, or (b) supraventricular with aberrant (or anomalous) ventricular conduction.

The four major classes of supraventricular tachyarrhythmia (SVTs)[a] are: (1) sinus tachycardia; (2) (paroxysmal) supraventricular tachycardia (PSVT); (3) atrial flutter; and (4) atrial fibrillation (AF). With each class, cardiac activation occurs at one or more sites in the atria or AV junction (node), anatomically located above the ventricles (hence, *supra*ventricular). This activation sequence is in contrast to ventricular tachycardia (VT), defined as a run of three or more consecutive premature ventricular complexes (see Chapter 16). With VT, the QRS complexes are always wide because the ventricles are activated in a non-synchronous way. The rate of monomorphic VT is usually between 100 and 225 beats/min. Polymorphic VT (e.g., torsades de pointes) may be even faster with rates up to 250–300. By contrast, with supraventricular arrhythmias the ventricles are stimulated normally (simultaneously), and the QRS complexes are therefore narrow (unless a bundle branch block or other cause of aberrant conduction is also present).

---
**Key Point**
---

The first step in analyzing a tachyarrhythmia is to look at the width of the QRS complex in all 12 leads, if possible. If the QRS complex is narrow (0.10–0.11 sec or less), you are dealing with some type of supraventricular arrhythmia and not VT. If the QRS complex is wide (0.12 sec or more), you should consider the rhythm to be VT unless it can be proved otherwise.

---

## Differential Diagnosis of Narrow Complex Tachycardias (NCTs)

The characteristics of sinus tachycardia, PSVTs, AF, and atrial flutter have been described in previous

---
[a]*Remember:* supraventricular tachycardia is a source of common confusion in terminology (see Chapters 13–15). Clinicians use the term *supraventricular tachycardia* (SVT) in several related, but different, ways. First, SVT is used by some clinicians to refer to any rapid rhythm originating in the SA node, atria, or AV junction, literally above (*supra* = "above" in Latin) the ventricular conduction system. Second, others use the term in a similar way, but specifically exclude sinus tachycardia. Third, SVT is used by still others in an even more restricted way to be synonymous with the triad of paroxysmal supraventricular tachycardias (PSVTs): atrial tachycardia (AT), AV nodal reentrant tachycardia (AVNRT), and AV reentrant tachycardia (AVRT). The latter (AVRT) may involve a *concealed* or *manifest* (WPW-type) bypass tract (Chapter 18). These three members of the PSVT family are entirely distinct from sinus tachycardia, AF, or atrial flutter (see Chapters 13–15, and 18). Make sure when you hear or say "supraventricular tachycardia (SVT)" you and your audience are clear about the meaning intended.

chapters. *Sinus tachycardia* in adults generally produces a heart rate between 100 and 180 beats/min, with the higher rates (150–180 beats/min) generally occurring in association with exercise.

> **Important Clinical Clue**
>
> If you are called to evaluate an elderly patient (>70–75 years) with a narrow (normal QRS duration) complex tachycardia having a resting QRS rate of 150 beats/min or more, you are most likely dealing with one of three types of non-sinus arrhythmias mentioned previously: paroxysmal supraventricular tachycardia, atrial flutter, or atrial fibrillation.

*PSVT* and *AF* can generally be distinguished on the basis of their regularity. PSVT resulting from AV nodal reentry or a concealed bypass tract is usually almost a perfectly regular tachycardia with a ventricular rate between 140 and 250 beats/min (see Chapters 14 and 15). AF, on the other hand, is distinguished by its irregularity. Remember that with a rapid ventricular response (Fig. 19.7) the *f* waves may not be clearly visible, but the diagnosis can be made in almost every case by noting the absence of true P waves and the haphazardly irregular QRS complexes.

*Atrial flutter* is characterized by "sawtooth" flutter (F) waves between QRS complexes (Fig. 19.8). However, when atrial flutter is present with 2:1 AV block (e.g., the atrial rate is 300 beats/min and the ventricular response is 150 beats/min), the F waves are often hidden or obscured in one or more leads. Therefore, atrial flutter with a regular ventricular rate of 150 beats/min can be confused with sinus tachycardia, PSVT, or AF (Figs. 19.8 and 19.9). AF can be most readily excluded because atrial flutter with 2:1 conduction is very regular.

Nevertheless, the differential diagnosis of sinus tachycardia, PSVT, AF, and atrial flutter can be challenging (see Fig. 19.9). One clinical test used to help separate these arrhythmias is *carotid sinus massage* (CSM)[b] or other vagal maneuvers (e.g., Valsalva maneuver). Pressure on the carotid sinus produces

---
[b]*Note:* CSM is not without risks, particularly in elderly patients or in those with cerebrovascular disease. Interested readers should consult relevant references in the Bibliography for details on this and other vagal maneuvers, as well as on the use of adenosine in the differential diagnosis of narrow complex tachycardias.

## Atrial Fibrillation with a Rapid Ventricular Rate

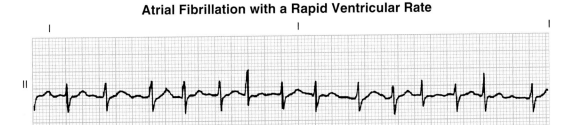

**Fig. 19.7** The ventricular rate is about 130 beats/min (13 QRS cycles in 6 sec). Notice the characteristic haphazardly irregular rhythm.

## Atrial Flutter with 2:1 AV Block (Conduction)

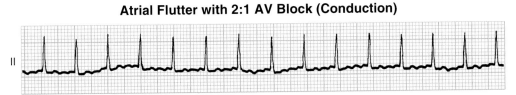

**Fig. 19.8** Atrial flutter with 2:1 atrioventricular (AV) conduction (block). The flutter waves are subtle.

## Four Look-Alike Narrow Complex Tachycardias

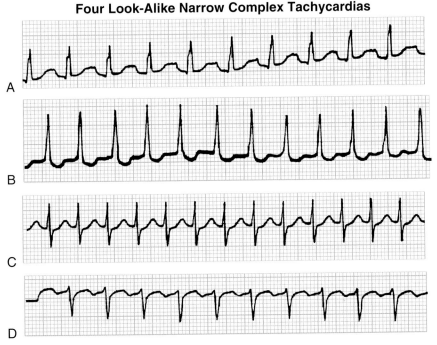

**Fig. 19.9** Four "look-alike" narrow complex tachycardias recorded in lead II. (A) Sinus tachycardia. (B) Atrial fibrillation. (C) Paroxysmal supraventricular tachycardia (PSVT) resulting from atrioventricular nodal reentrant tachycardia (AVNRT). (D) Atrial flutter with 2:1 AV block (conduction). When the ventricular rate is about 150 beats/min, these four arrhythmias may be difficult, if not impossible, to tell apart on the standard ECG, particularly from a single lead. In the example of sinus tachycardia the P waves can barely be seen in this case. Next, notice that the irregularity of the atrial fibrillation here is very subtle. In the example of PSVT, the rate is quite regular without evident P waves. In the atrial flutter tracing, the flutter waves cannot be seen clearly in this lead.

a reflex increase in vagal tone. The effects of CSM (and other vagal maneuvers) on sinus tachycardia, reentrant types of PSVT, and atrial flutter are briefly reviewed next (see also Chapter 14).

## Sinus Tachycardia and CSM

Sinus tachycardia generally slows slightly with CSM. However, no abrupt change in heart rate usually occurs. Slowing of sinus tachycardia may make the P waves more evident. Furthermore, sinus tachycardia almost invariably speeds up and slows down in a graduated way, and ends gradually, not abruptly. (Healthy people can test this assertion out by monitoring their heart rate at rest, with climbing stairs, and after resting.)

## Paroxysmal Supraventricular Tachycardias and CSM

PSVT resulting from AV nodal reentrant tachycardia (AVNRT) or AV reentrant tachycardia (AVRT) involving a concealed or manifest bypass tract usually has an *all-or-none* response to CSM or other maneuvers (e.g. Valsalva) used to rapidly increase vagal tone. In successful cases, the tachycardia breaks suddenly, and sinus rhythm resumes (see Chapter 14). At other times CSM has no effect, and the tachycardia continues at the same rate. In cases of PSVT caused by atrial tachycardia (AT), CSM may increase the degree of block, resulting in a rapid sequence of one or more nonconducted P waves.

## Atrial Flutter and CSM

CSM also often increases the degree of AV block in atrial flutter, converting flutter with a 2:1 response to 3:1 or 4:1 flutter with a ventricular rate of 100 or 75 beats/min, respectively, or to flutter with variable block. Slowing of the ventricular rate may unmask the characteristic F waves (and thereby clarify the diagnosis of the NCT). But CSM or other vagal maneuvers will not convert atrial flutter to sinus (see Chapter 15). *Therefore, if you already know your patient has atrial flutter or fibrillation, there is no justification for CSM (or for giving adenosine).*

## *RACE:* Simple Algorithm for Diagnosing Narrow Complex Tachycardias (NCTs)

Trainees may find the following algorithm helpful in thinking about the differential diagnosis of narrow complex tachycardias:

*R*: *R*ates (atrial and ventricular)
*A*: *A*trial activity

*CE*: Cad*E*nce: regular (or group beating) vs. very irregular

For the most accurate assessment of ventricular rate when the tachycardia is regular, count the number of small boxes between consecutive QRS complexes. Atrial activity (if visible) will be seen as discrete P waves (with sinus tachycardia, atrial tachycardia, AVNRT or AVRT). In the latter two cases, the P waves, if visible, are generally retrograde (negative in lead II). Be careful not to confuse true discrete P waves with continuous atrial activity due to atrial flutter (F waves) or fibrillation (f waves). An NCT with an irregular ventricular response raises consideration of three major possibilities: atrial fibrillation vs. MAT vs. sinus tachycardia with frequent atrial ectopy. A perfectly regular NCT raises consideration of sinus tachycardia vs. PSVT (atrial tachycardia, AVNRT or AVRT). Recall that very fast rates (especially greater than 140/min) are rarely if ever seen in elderly adults in sinus rhythm. An NCT with "group beating" (periodic clusters of QRS complexes) raises consideration of atrial flutter with variable block/conduction vs. atrial tachycardia with variable block.

## Differential Diagnosis of Wide Complex Tachycardias (WCTs)

A tachycardia with widened (broad) QRS complexes (i.e., 120 msec or more in duration) raises two major diagnostic considerations:

1. The first, and most clinically important, is VT, a potentially life-threatening arrhythmia. As noted, VT is a consecutive run of three or more ventricular premature complexes (PVCs) at a rate generally between 100 and 225 beats/min or more. It is usually, but not always, very regular, especially sustained monomorphic VT at higher rates.
2. The second possible cause of a tachycardia with widened QRS complexes is termed *SVT with aberration* or *aberrancy* (sometimes termed *anomalous conduction*). The term *aberration* simply means that some abnormality in ventricular activation is present, causing widened QRS complexes due to asynchronous activation (e.g., bundle branch block). Another term with similar meaning is *anomalous conduction* and includes preexcitation.

## Differentiation of SVT with Aberrancy from VT

Ventricular aberrancy with an SVT, in turn, has two major, general mechanisms: (1) a bundle branch block or related intraventricular conduction delay (which may be transient) and, much more rarely, (2) conduction down a bypass tract in conjunction with the Wolff–Parkinson–White (WPW) preexcitation syndrome (Chapter 18). (Some authors, as noted, prefer the term *anomalous conduction* rather than *aberrancy*, for the latter.)

### SVT with Aberrancy

If any of the SVTs just discussed occurs in association with a bundle branch block or related intraventricular conduction delay (IVCD), the ECG will show a WCT that may be mistaken for VT. For example, a patient with sinus tachycardia (or AF, atrial flutter, or PSVT) and concomitant right bundle branch block (RBBB) or left bundle branch block (LBBB) will have a WCT.

Fig. 19.10A shows AF with a rapid ventricular response occurring in conjunction with LBBB. For comparison, Fig. 19.10B shows an example of VT. Because the arrhythmias look similar, it can be difficult to tell them apart. The major distinguishing feature is the irregularity of the AF as opposed to the regularity of the VT. However, VT sometimes may be irregular. Another example of AF with aberrancy (due to LBBB) is shown in Fig. 19.11.

You need to remember that in some cases of SVT with aberration, the bundle branch block or IVCD is seen only during the episodes of tachycardia. This class of *rate-related bundle branch blocks* are said to be *tachycardia-* (or *acceleration-*) *dependent.*

SVT with aberrancy (IVCD) may also occur in the presence of hyperkalemia or with drugs such as flecainide (Chapter 11), factors that decrease conduction velocity in the ventricles.

### SVT with the Wolff–Parkinson–White Preexcitation Syndrome

The second general mechanism responsible for a WCT is SVT with the Wolff–Parkinson–White syndrome. As noted in Chapter 18, individuals with WPW preexcitation have an accessory pathway (or pathways) connecting the atria and ventricles, thus bypassing the AV junction. Such patients are especially prone to a reentrant type of PSVT with narrow (normal) QRS complexes. This distinct type of PSVT is called (*orthodromic*) *AV reentrant tachycardia* (AVRT).

Sometimes, however, particularly if AF or atrial flutter develops, a WCT may result from conduction down the bypass tract at very high rates. This kind of WCT obviously mimics VT. An example of WPW syndrome with AF is shown in Fig. 19.12.

WPW syndrome with AF should be strongly suspected if you encounter a WCT that (1) is irregular and (2) has a *very* high rate (i.e., very short RR intervals). In particular, RR intervals of 180 msec (4.5 small boxes in duration) or less are rarely seen with conventional AF and very rapid VT is usually quite regular. These very short RR intervals are related to the ability of the bypass tract (in contrast to the AV node) to conduct impulses in extremely rapid succession (see Figs. 19.12 and 19.13).

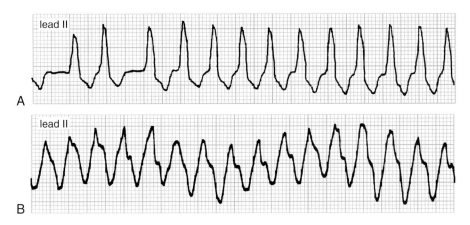

**Fig. 19.10** (A) Atrial fibrillation with a left bundle branch block pattern. (B) Ventricular tachycardia. Based on their ECG appearances, differentiating a supraventricular tachycardia with bundle branch block (or a wide QRS due to WPW or to drug effects) from ventricular tachycardia may be difficult and sometimes impossible.

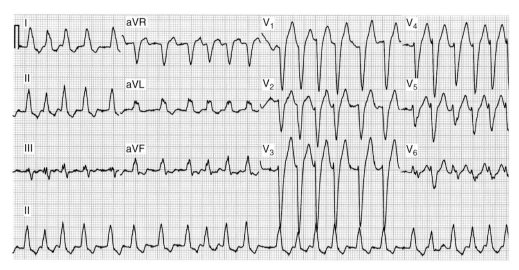

**Fig. 19.11** This wide complex tachycardia is due to atrial fibrillation with a left bundle branch block (LBBB), and not to monomorphic ventricular tachycardia. Note the irregularity of the rate and the typical LBBB pattern. See also Fig. 19.9.

The recognition of WPW syndrome with AF is of considerable clinical importance because digitalis may paradoxically enhance conduction down the bypass tract. As a result, the ventricular response may increase, leading to possible myocardial ischemia and in some cases to ventricular fibrillation. A similar hazardous effect has been reported with intravenous verapamil. Emergency direct current (DC) cardioversion may be required.

WPW syndrome with a wide QRS complex may also occur in two other pathophysiologic contexts: (1) PSVT with a reentrant circuit that goes down the bypass tract and reenters the atria through the ventricular conductions system and AV node is a very rare variant called *antidromic AV reentrant tachycardia* (AVRT). An example is given in Fig. 19.14. (2) The somewhat more common variant, namely, conduction down the AV node–His–Purkinje system and up the bypass tract, can occur in association with a bundle branch block. For more information on these advanced topics, please see Chapter 18 and the Bibliography.

## VT vs. SVT with Aberration: Important Diagnostic Clues
### Clinical Considerations
Discriminating VT from SVT with aberration (aberrancy) is a very frequent problem encountered in emergency departments, cardiac care units (CCUs), and intensive care units (ICUs). This challenge constitutes an important source of urgent consultations with cardiologists. A number of algorithms have been proposed to guide in differential diagnosis. However, before applying any ECG-based diagnostic algorithms to WCT differential diagnosis, clinicians should take into account the following clinical clues:

- Over 80% of WCTs presenting to medical attention in adults in the United States are VTs. In patients with known major structural heart disease (e.g., prior infarcts, cardiomyopathies, after cardiac surgery), this percentage increases to over 90%.
- Treating an SVT as VT will most likely cure the arrhythmia, but treating VT as an SVT can precipitate hemodynamic collapse (see next bullet). *Therefore, when in doubt about managing a WCT, assume the diagnosis of VT until proved otherwise.*
- Intravenously administered verapamil or diltiazem should not be used in undiagnosed WCTs. These calcium channel blocking drugs have both vasodilatory and negative inotropic effects that can cause hemodynamic collapse in patients with VT (or with AF with WPW preexcitation syndrome).

### ECG Considerations
As noted, differentiating VT from SVT (e.g., PSVT, atrial flutter, or AF) with a bundle branch block or

## Atrial Fibrillation and Wolff–Parkinson–White Syndrome

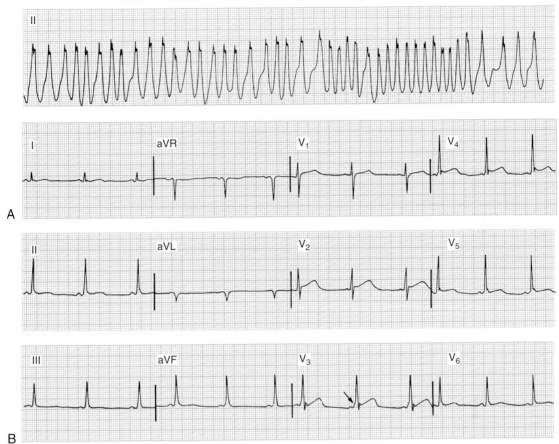

**Fig. 19.12** (A) Atrial fibrillation with the Wolff-Parkinson-White (WPW) preexcitation syndrome may lead to a wide complex tachycardia that has a very rapid rate. Notice that some of the RR intervals are extremely short (about 240 msec). Irregularity is due to the underlying atrial fibrillation. Occasionally, normally conducted (narrow) beats occur because of refractoriness in the accessory pathway. The QRS polarity (predominantly positive in $V_1$ to $V_3$ and negative in the inferolateral leads) is consistent with a left posterior lateral bypass tract. (B) After the arrhythmia has converted to sinus rhythm, the classic triad of the WPW pattern is visible, albeit subtly, with a relatively short PR interval, wide QRS complex, and delta wave (*arrow* in lead $V_3$). The patient underwent successful radiofrequency ablation therapy of the bypass tract.

other causes of aberrancy can be very challenging. *Even the most experienced cardiologists may not be able to make this differential diagnosis with certainty from the standard 12-lead ECG and available rhythm strip data.*

Five sets of ECG clues have been found to be especially helpful in favoring VT over SVT with aberrancy:

1. AV dissociation. Recall from Chapter 17 that with AV dissociation (not due to complete heart block) the atria and ventricles are paced from separate sites, with the ventricular rate equal to or faster than the atrial rate. Some patients with VT also have a variant of AV dissociation in which the ventricles are paced from an ectopic ventricular site at a rapid rate, while the atria continue to be paced independently by the SA node. In such cases, you may, with careful inspection, be able to see sinus P waves occurring at a slower rate than the rapid wide QRS complexes (Fig. 19.15). Some of the P waves may be buried in the QRS

complexes and, therefore, difficult or impossible to discern.

· Unfortunately, only a minority of patients with VT show clear ECG evidence of AV dissociation. Therefore, the absence of overt AV dissociation does not exclude VT. However, the presence of AV dissociation in a patient with a WCT is virtually diagnostic of VT. In other words, AV dissociation with a WCT has very high specificity but limited sensitivity for VT.

### Atrial Fibrillation with WPW

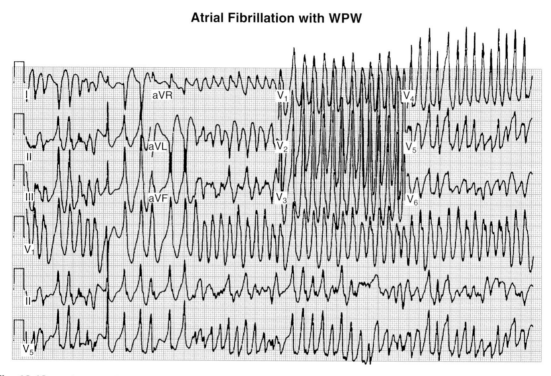

**Fig. 19.13** Another example of atrial fibrillation with Wolff–Parkinson–White (WPW) preexcitation syndrome. The ventricular rate here is extremely rapid (up to 300/min at times) and very irregular. The QRS vector (rightward and inferior) is consistent with a left lateral bypass tract, which was ablated. This rhythm constitutes a medical emergency since it may lead to ischemia and degenerate in ventricular fibrillation with cardiac arrest. In contrast, usually when ventricular tachycardia (monomorphic or polymorphic reaches this rate), the rhythm becomes regular.

**Fig. 19.14** (A) ECG from a young adult man with recurrent palpitations since childhood. The recording shows sinus tachycardia with a wide complex tachycardia and classic Wolff–Parkinson–White (WPW) morphology. The polarity of the delta waves (entirely negative in aVL and QRS axis are consistent with a left lateral bypass tract. Bottom panel, (B), shows the ECG during a run of very rapid PSVT (about 220/min), with identical morphology of the QRS during sinus rhythm. No P waves are visible. The recording mimics ventricular tachycardia because of the side complexes. However, in this case, the wide complexes are due to a large circuit that takes the impulse down the bypass tract and then back up the bundle branch–His system where it reenters the atria and goes back down the bypass tract. This rare form of reentry with WPW is termed *antidromic PSVT*. Give yourself extra credit if you noticed the QRS alternans pattern (most evident in leads III, $V_3$, $V_4$ and some other leads). QRS alternans with non-sinus tachycardia is not due to pericardial tamponade and the "swinging heart" phenomenon (Chapter 12), but to altered ventricular conduction on a beat-to-beat basis. QRS alternans with PSVTs is most common with bypass tract-mediated tachycardias (atrioventricular reentrant tachycardias, AVRTs), but may occur with atrioventricular nodal reentrant tachycardia (AVNRT) and ventricular tachycardias as well.

## Sinus Rhythm with WPW

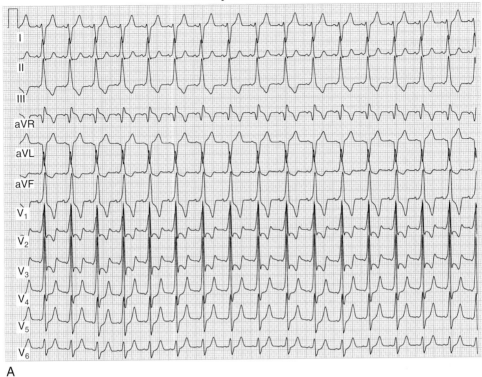

A

## Wide Complex Tachycardia: AV Reentrant Tachycardia with WPW

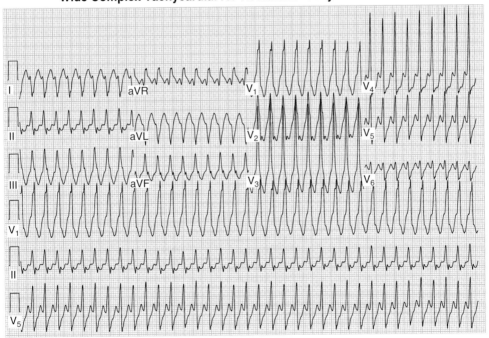

B

### Ventricular Tachycardia: AV Dissociation

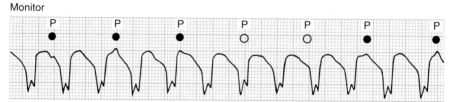

**Fig. 19.15** Sustained monomorphic ventricular tachycardia with atrioventricular (AV) dissociation. Note the independence of the atrial (sinus) rate (75 beats/min) and ventricular (QRS) rate (140 beats/min). The visible sinus P waves are indicated by black circles, and the hidden P waves are indicated by open circles.

### Ventricular Tachycardia: Fusion and Capture Beats

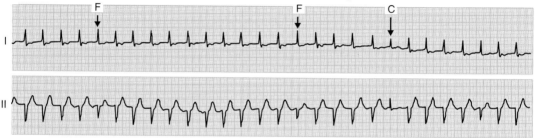

**Fig. 19.16** Sustained monomorphic ventricular tachycardia (VT) with atrioventricular dissociation (sinus node continues to pace in presence of VT) producing fusion (*F*) and capture (*C*) beats. Leads I and II were recorded simultaneously. See text.

· Furthermore, in some cases of VT with AV dissociation the SA node may transiently entrain (take "control of") the ventricles, producing a *capture beat,* which has a normal QRS duration. The same mechanism may sometimes produce a *fusion beat,* in which a sinus beat from above and a ventricular beat from below collide to produce a hybrid complex. Fig. 19.16 illustrates capture and fusion beats due to AV dissociation occurring with VT.

2. Morphology refers to the shape of the QRS complex in selected leads, especially $V_1/V_2$. The morphology of the QRS in selected leads may help provide important clues about whether the WCT is (monomorphic) VT or not. When the QRS shape during a tachycardia resembles RBBB patterns, a typical rSR′ shape in lead $V_1$ suggests SVT while a single broad R wave or a qR, QR, or RS complex in that lead strongly suggests VT (Fig. 19.17). When the QRS shape during a tachycardia resembles LBBB patterns, a broad (≥0.04 sec) initial R wave in lead $V_1$ or $V_2$

or a QR complex in lead $V_6$ strongly suggests VT (Box 19.2).

=== Key Point ===

When cardiologists classify monomorphic VT as having LBBB or RBBB configurations they are speaking only about the appearance of the QRS, especially in leads $V_1$ and $V_6$. This descriptive usage should not be taken to mean that an actual LBBB or RBBB is present. Rather, the bundle branch-like appearance is an indication of asynchronous (right before left or left before right) activation of the ventricles during VT.

3. *QRS duration (width).* A QRS width of interval greater than 0.14 sec with RBBB morphology or greater than 0.16 sec with LBBB morphology suggests VT. However, these criteria are not reliable if the patient is on a drug (e.g., flecainide) that widens the QRS complex, or in the presence of hyperkalemia. Also, remember to look at all

## Sustained Ventricular Tachycardia

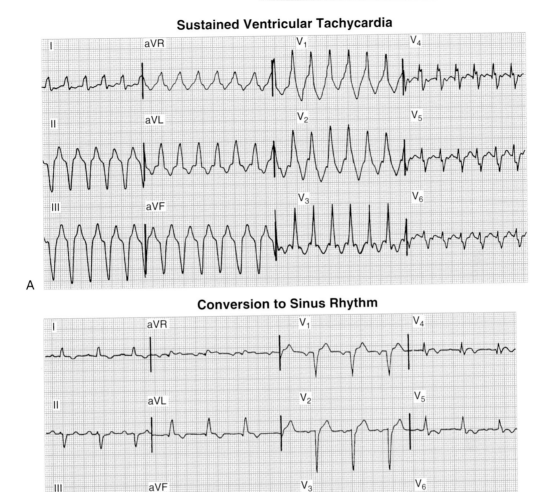

## Conversion to Sinus Rhythm

**Fig. 19.17** (A) Sustained monomorphic ventricular tachycardia at a rate of about 180 beats/min. Note the wide QRS complexes with a right bundle branch block morphology. The QRS complexes in leads $V_1$ and $V_2$ show a broad R wave. (B) Following conversion to sinus rhythm, the pattern of an underlying anterior wall myocardial infarction and ventricular aneurysm becomes evident. Q waves and ST segment elevations are seen in leads in $V_1$, $V_2$, and $V_3$; ischemic T wave inversions are present in leads $V_4$ to $V_6$. Note also that the QRS complex is wide (0.12 sec) because of an intraventricular conduction delay with left axis deviation (left anterior fascicular block). The prominent negative P waves in lead $V_1$ are due to left atrial abnormality.

12 leads and make this measurement in the lead with the widest QRS.[c]

[c]Clinicians should also be aware that even though most cases of VT are associated with a very wide QRS complex, VT may occur with a QRS complex that is only mildly prolonged, particularly if the arrhythmia originates in the upper part of the ventricular septum or in the proximal part of the fascicles.

4. *QRS concordance* means that the QRS waveform has identical or near identical polarity in all six chest leads ($V_1$ to $V_6$). Positive concordance (Fig. 19.18) is defined by wide R waves in leads $V_1$ to $V_6$; negative concordance by wide QS waves (Fig. 19.19) in these leads. Either positive or negative concordance is a specific, but not very sensitive,

| BOX 19.2 | Wide Complex Tachycardia (WCT): Selected Criteria Favoring Ventricular Tachycardia |

1. Atrioventricular (AV) dissociation
2. QRS width:
   0.14 sec with right bundle branch block (RBBB) configuration*
   0.16 sec with left bundle branch block (LBBB) configuration*
3. Shape (morphology) of the QRS complex:
   RBBB: Mono- or biphasic complex in $V_1$
   LBBB: Broad R waves in $V_1$ or $V_2 \geq 0.04$ sec
     Onset of QRS to tip of S wave in $V_1$ or $V_2 \geq$
     0.07 sec
   QR complex in $V_6$

*QRS duration may also be increased in supraventricular tachycardias in the presence of drugs that prolong QRS interval or with hyperkalemia.
Adapted from Josephson ME, Zimetbaum P. The tachyarrhythmias. In Kasper DL, Braunwald E, Fauci A, et al., editors. Harrison's principles of internal medicine. 16th ed. New York: McGraw-Hill; 2005.

### Ventricular Tachycardia: Negative QRS Concordance

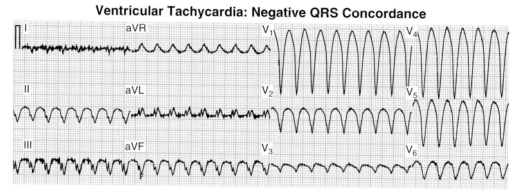

**Fig. 19.18** Monomorphic ventricular tachycardia with left bundle branch block morphology and with superior (marked right) axis. There is *negative QRS concordance*, meaning that all the precordial leads show negative QRS deflections. This pattern is incompatible with aberration. The origin of the tachycardia was in the right ventricular inferior wall. Baseline "noise" here is from electrical interference in this ECG obtained under emergency conditions.

### Ventricular Tachycardia: Positive QRS Concordance

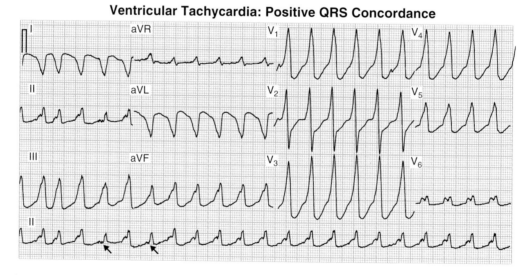

**Fig. 19.19** Positive concordance with monomorphic right bundle branch block morphology ventricular tachycardia originating in the lateral wall of the left ventricle. All precordial leads show positive QRS deflections. *Arrows* in the lead II rhythm strip point to probable fusion beats (see text).

indicator of VT. Thus, this it is helpful when you see these patterns, but most cases of VT show variable polarity of the QRS across the precordium.

5. *Prior sinus rhythm ECGs.* A comparison using any prior ECGs during sinus rhythm (or other supraventricular rhythms) may be very helpful, especially if the previous ECG is relatively recent. First, finding that the QRS configuration (morphology and axis) in sinus rhythm remains identical during the WCT strongly suggests a supraventricular mechanism. Second, if the QRS configuration during the WCT is identical to any PVC during sinus rhythm in a prior ECG, this finding strongly points to VT as the cause of a longer run of wide complex beats.

Box 19.2 summarizes some aspects of the differential diagnosis of VT versus SVT with aberration.

## Tachycardias: Additional Clinical Perspectives

As mentioned previously, the first question to ask when called to see a patient with a tachyarrhythmia is whether the rhythm is VT. If sustained VT is present, emergency treatment is required (see Chapter 16). The treatment of NCTs depends on the clinical setting. In patients with sinus tachycardia (see Chapter 13), treatment is directed at the underlying cause (e.g., fever, sepsis, congestive heart failure, volume loss, alcohol intoxication or withdrawal, or severe pulmonary disease, hyperthyroidism, and so forth).

Similarly, the treatment of MAT should be directed at the underlying problem (usually decompensated chronic pulmonary disease). DC cardioversion should *not* be used with MAT because it is unlikely to be helpful and it may induce serious ventricular arrhythmias. A calcium channel blocker (verapamil or diltiazem) can be used to slow the ventricular response in MAT, unless contraindicated. Most important is treating pulmonary decompensation.

=============== Key Clinical Points ===============

In assessing any patient with an NCT, always ask the following three questions about the effects of the tachycardia on the heart and circulation related to how the patient (not just the ECG) looks!
- Is the patient's blood pressure abnormally low? In particular, is the patient hypotensive or actually in shock?
- Is the patient having an acute myocardial infarction or is there clinical evidence of severe ischemia?
- Is the patient in severe congestive heart failure (pulmonary edema)?

Patients in any one of these categories who have AF or atrial flutter with a rapid ventricular response or a PSVT require emergency therapy. If they do not respond very promptly to initial drug therapy, electrical cardioversion should be considered.

Another major question to ask about any patient with a tachyarrhythmia (or any arrhythmia for that matter) is whether digitalis or other drugs are part of the therapeutic regimen. Some arrhythmias (e.g., AT with block) may be digitalis toxic rhythms, disturbances for which electrical cardioversion is contraindicated (see Chapter 20). Drug-induced QT prolongation is an important substrate for torsades

## Tachy-brady Syndrome

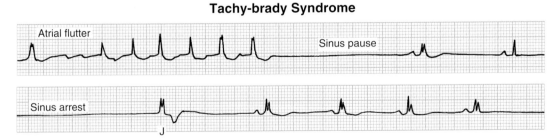

**Fig. 19.20** Tachy-brady variant of sick sinus syndrome. Rhythm strip shows a narrow complex tachycardia (probably atrial flutter) followed by a prominent sinus pause, two sinus beats, an atrioventricular junctional escape beat (*J*), and resumption of sinus rhythm.

de pointes-type of polymorphic VT, as discussed in Chapter 16.

## SLOW AND FAST: SICK SINUS SYNDROME AND TACHY-BRADY VARIANTS

The term *sick sinus syndrome* was coined to describe patients with SA node dysfunction that causes marked sinus bradycardia or sinus arrest, sometimes with junctional escape rhythms, which may lead to symptoms of lightheadedness and even syncope.

In some patients with sick sinus syndrome, bradycardia episodes are interspersed with paroxysms of tachycardia (usually AF, atrial flutter, or some type of PSVT). Sometimes the bradycardia occurs immediately after spontaneous termination of the tachycardia (Fig. 13.8). An important subset includes patients with paroxysmal AF who have marked sinus bradycardia and even sinus arrest after spontaneous conversion of AF (see Chapters 13 and 15). The term *tachy-brady syndrome* has been used to describe patients with sick sinus syndrome who have both slow and fast arrhythmias (Fig. 19.20).

The diagnosis of sick sinus syndrome and, in particular, the tachy-brady variants, often requires ambulatory monitoring of the patient's heartbeat over several hours or even days to weeks (Chapter 4). A single ECG strip may be normal or may reveal only the bradycardia or tachycardia episode. Treatment of symptomatic patients generally requires a permanent pacemaker to prevent sinus arrest and radiofrequency ablation therapy or antiarrhythmic drugs to control the tachycardias after the pacemaker has been implanted.

# CHAPTER 20
# Digitalis Toxicity

This specialized topic is included in an introductory text because it concerns a class of drugs which (1) is still among the most commonly prescribed, and (2) is a major cause of arrhythmias and conduction disturbances. Digitalis preparations (most commonly digoxin) have been used in the treatment of heart failure and of certain supraventricular arrhythmias for over 200 years since their first description in the English scientific literature. The topic is highlighted here, however, not for historic reasons. Digitalis excess continues to cause or contribute to major complications, and even sudden cardiac arrest/death (see also Chapter 21). In addition, since digoxin toxicity may lead to a broad range of brady- and tachycardias, the topic serves as a useful review of abnormalities of impulse control and conduction discussed throughout this text. Early recognition and prevention of digoxin and other drug toxicities (see also Chapters 11 and 16) are paramount concerns to all frontline clinicians.

## MECHANISM OF ACTION AND INDICATIONS

*Digitalis* refers to a class of cardioactive drugs called *glycosides*, which exert both mechanical and electrical effects on the heart. The most frequently used digitalis preparation is digoxin. (Digitoxin is now rarely used in the United States.)

The mechanical action of digitalis glycosides is to increase the strength of myocardial contraction (positive inotropic effect) in carefully selected patients with dilated hearts and systolic heart failure (HF), also referred to as *heart failure with reduced ejection fraction*. The electrical effects relate primarily to decreasing automaticity and conductivity in the sinoatrial (SA) and atrioventricular (AV) nodes, in large part by increasing cardiac parasympathetic (vagal) tone. Consequently, digitalis is sometimes used to help to control the ventricular response in atrial fibrillation (AF) and atrial flutter (Chapter 15), both associated with excessive frequency of electrical stimuli impinging on the AV node.

Since a number of more efficacious and safer medications have become available for this purpose,

along with ablational procedures, digoxin use is mostly limited to the patients with atrial fibrillation or flutter who cannot tolerate beta blockers (due to bronchospasm or hypotension) or certain calcium channel blockers because of low left ventricular ejection fraction or hypotension. When used in AF or HF, digoxin is most often employed adjunctively with other drugs. More rarely, digoxin is still used in the treatment of certain reentrant types of paroxysmal supraventricular tachycardias (PSVT), for example, during pregnancy, when other drugs might be contraindicated.

Although digitalis has indications in the treatment of certain forms of chronic systolic heart failure and selected (non-sinus) supraventricular arrhythmias, it also has a relatively *narrow therapeutic margin of safety*. This term means that the difference (gradient) between therapeutic and toxic serum concentrations of digoxin is low.

## DIGITALIS TOXICITY VS. DIGITALIS EFFECT

Confusion among trainees sometimes arises between the terms digitalis toxicity and digitalis effect. *Digitalis toxicity* refers to the arrhythmias and conduction disturbances, as well as the toxic systemic effects described later, produced by this class of drug. *Digitalis effect* (Figs. 20.1 and 20.2) refers to the distinct scooping (sometimes called the "thumbprint" sign) of the ST-T complex, associated with shortening of the QT interval, typically seen in patients taking digitalis glycosides.

*Note:* The presence of digitalis effect, by itself, does not imply digitalis toxicity and may be seen with therapeutic drug concentrations. However, most patients with digitalis toxicity manifest ST-T changes of digitalis effect on their ECG.

## DIGITALIS TOXICITY: SIGNS AND SYMPTOMS

Digitalis toxicity can produce general systemic symptoms as well as specific cardiac arrhythmias and conduction disturbances. Common non-cardiac symptoms include weakness, lethargy, anorexia, nausea, and vomiting. Visual effects with altered color perception, including yellowish vision (xanthopsia), and mental status changes may occur.

As a general clinical rule *virtually any arrhythmia and all degrees of AV heart block can be produced by digitalis excess.* However, certain arrhythmias and conduction disturbances are particularly suggestive of digitalis toxicity (Box 20.1). In some cases, combinations of arrhythmias will occur, such as AF with (1) a slow, often regularized ventricular response and/or (2) increased ventricular ectopy (Fig. 20.3).

Two distinctive arrhythmias, when encountered, should raise heightened concern for digitalis toxicity.

### Digitalis Effect

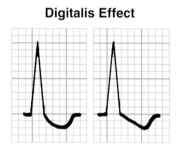

**Fig. 20.1** Characteristic scooping or downsloping of the ST-T complex produced by digitalis.

---

| **BOX 20.1** | Arrhythmias and Conduction Disturbances Caused by Digitalis Toxicity |
|---|---|

**Bradycardias**
Sinus, including sinoatrial (SA) block
Junctional rhythms*
Atrial fibrillation (or flutter) with a slow/regularized response

**Tachycardias**
Accelerated junctional rhythms
Atrial tachycardia with block
Frequent ventricular ectopy, including ventricular bigeminy and multiform premature ventricular premature complexes (PVCs)
Ventricular tachycardia/ventricular fibrillation

**AV Conduction Delays and Related Disturbances**
Prolonged PR interval (first-degree atrioventricular [AV] block)
Second-degree AV block (AV Wenckebach, but *not* Mobitz II block)
Third-degree AV block/AV dissociation

---

*Two classes of junctional (nodal) rhythms may occur: (1) a typical junctional escape rhythm with a rate of 60 beats/min or less, and (2) an accelerated junctional rhythm (also called *nonparoxysmal junctional tachycardia*) at a rate of about 60–130 beats/min.

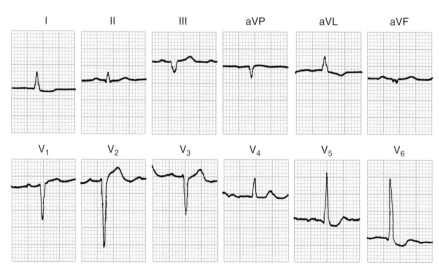

**Fig. 20.2** The characteristic scooping of the ST-T complex produced by digitalis is best seen in leads $V_5$ and $V_6$. (Low voltage is also present, with total QRS amplitude of 5 mm or less, in all six limb leads.)

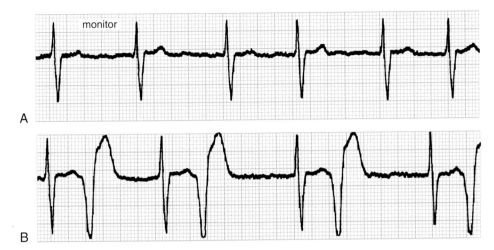

**Fig. 20.3** Ventricular bigeminy caused by digitalis toxicity. Ventricular ectopy is one of the most common signs of digitalis toxicity. (A) The underlying rhythm is atrial fibrillation. (B) Each normal QRS complex is followed by a premature ventricular complex.

### Bidirectional Ventricular Tachycardia

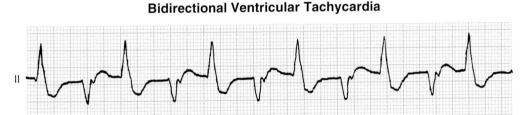

**Fig. 20.4** This digitalis toxic arrhythmia is a special type of ventricular tachycardia with QRS complexes that alternate in direction from beat to beat. No P waves are present.

### Atrial Tachycardia with AV Block

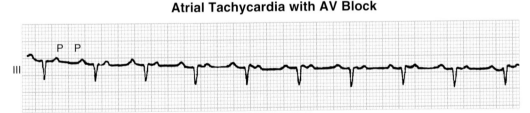

**Fig. 20.5** This rhythm strip shows atrial tachycardia (about 200 beats/min) with 2:1 AV block producing a ventricular rate of about 100 beats/min.

The first is *bidirectional ventricular tachycardia* (VT) (Fig. 20.4), a rare type of VT in which each successive beat in any lead alternates in direction. However, this rare arrhythmia may also be seen in the absence of digitalis excess (e.g., with catecholaminergic polymorphic VT; see Chapters 16 and 21).

The second arrhythmia suggestive of digitalis toxicity in the appropriate clinical context is *atrial tachycardia (AT) with AV block* (Fig. 20.5). Not uncommonly, 2:1 AV block is present so that the ventricular rate is half the atrial rate. Atrial tachycardia with AV block is usually characterized by regular, rapid P waves occurring at a rate between 150 and 250 beats/min (due to increased automaticity) and a slower ventricular rate (due to AV block). Superficially, AT with block may resemble atrial flutter;

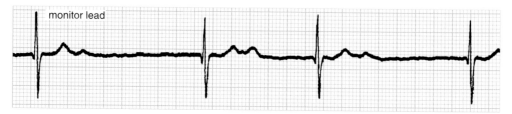

**Fig. 20.6** Atrial fibrillation with an excessively slow ventricular rate because of digitalis toxicity. Atrial fibrillation with a rapid ventricular rate is rarely caused by digitalis toxicity. However, in patients with underlying atrial fibrillation, digitalis toxicity is sometimes manifested by excessive slowing or regularization of the QRS rate.

however, when atrial flutter is present, the atrial rate is faster (usually 250–350 beats/min). Furthermore, in AT with block the baseline between P waves is isoelectric. *Note:* Clinicians should be aware that most cases of AT with block encountered clinically are *not* due to digitalis excess, but it is always worth checking to rule out the possibility that the patient is or might be taking digoxin.

In a related way, the designation of "paroxysmal atrial tachycardia (PAT) with block" may be misleading. Atrial tachycardia due to digoxin excess is more likely to be sustained, not truly paroxysmal, and should be more properly noted as "AT with block." Furthermore, this arrhythmia is both a relatively insensitive and a nonspecific marker of digitalis toxicity.

Digitalis toxicity is *not* a primary cause of AF or of atrial flutter with a rapid ventricular response. However, clinicians should be aware that digitalis toxicity may occur in patients with these arrhythmias. In such cases, as noted above, toxicity may be evidenced by marked slowing of the ventricular rate, e.g., to less than 50 beats/min (Fig. 20.6) or the appearance of frequent premature ventricular complexes (PVCs). In some cases, the earliest sign of digitalis toxicity in a patient with AF may be a subtle *regularization* of the ventricular cadence (Fig. 20.7).

In summary, digitalis toxicity causes a number of important arrhythmias and conduction disturbances. You should suspect digitalis toxicity in any patient taking a digitalis preparation who has an unexplained new arrhythmia until you can prove otherwise.

## DIGITALIS TOXICITY: PREDISPOSING FACTORS

A number of factors significantly increase the hazard of digitalis intoxication (Box 20.2).

---

| BOX 20.2 | Some Factors Predisposing to Digitalis Toxicity* |
|---|---|

Advanced age
Hypokalemia
Hypomagnesemia
Hypercalcemia
Hypoxemia/chronic lung disease
Myocardial infarction (especially acute)
Renal insufficiency
Hypothyroidism
Heart failure caused by amyloidosis
Wolff-Parkinson-White syndrome and atrial fibrillation

*In addition, digoxin is contraindicated with hypertrophic cardiomyopathy, an inherited heart condition associated with excessive cardiac contractility, and sometimes with left ventricular outflow obstruction. Digoxin may worsen the degree of outflow obstruction by increasing contractility.

### Electrolyte Disturbances

A low serum potassium concentration increases the likelihood of certain digitalis-induced arrhythmias, particularly ventricular ectopy and atrial tachycardia (AT) with block. The serum potassium concentration should be checked periodically in any patient taking digitalis and in every patient suspected of having digitalis toxicity. In addition, both hypomagnesemia and hypercalcemia are also predisposing factors for digitalis toxicity. Electrolyte levels should be monitored in patients taking diuretics. In particular, furosemide can cause hypokalemia and hypomagnesemia. Thiazide diuretics can also occasionally cause hypercalcemia.

### Coexisting Conditions

Hypoxemia and chronic lung disease may also increase the risk of digitalis toxicity, probably because they are associated with increased sympathetic tone. Patients with acute myocardial infarction (MI) or

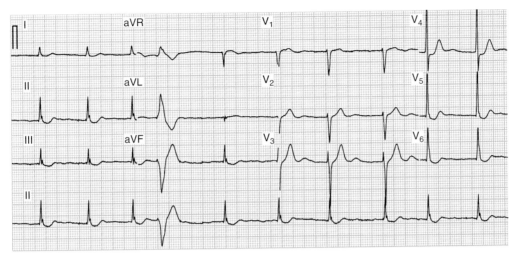

**Fig. 20.7** Digitalis (digoxin) excess in a patient with underlying atrial fibrillation. Note the slow (about 60 beats/min) and relatively regularized ventricular response. A single ventricular premature beat (beat 4) is also present. The "scooping" of the ST-T in lead II and the lateral chest leads is consistent with digitalis effect, although other factors, including ischemia or left ventricular hypertrophy (LVH), cannot be excluded. The borderline prominent chest lead voltage raises consideration of LVH, but is not diagnostic. The relatively vertical QRS axis (about +75°) also raises consideration of biventricular hypertrophy given the possible LVH.

ischemia appear to be more sensitive to digitalis. Digitalis may worsen the symptoms of patients with hypertrophic cardiomyopathy, an inherited heart condition associated with excessive cardiac contractility. Patients with heart failure due to amyloidosis are also extremely sensitive to digitalis. In patients with the Wolff–Parkinson–White (WPW) syndrome and AF (see Chapter 18), digitalis may cause extremely rapid transmission of impulses down the AV bypass tract (see Fig. 19.14), potentially leading to ventricular fibrillation and cardiac arrest. Patients with hypothyroidism appear to be more sensitive to the effects of digitalis. Women also appear to be more sensitive to digitalis. Because digoxin is excreted primarily in the urine, any degree of renal insufficiency, as measured by increased blood urea nitrogen (BUN) and creatinine concentrations, requires a lower maintenance dose of digoxin. Thus, elderly patients may be more susceptible to digitalis toxicity, in part because of decreased renal excretion of the drug. Furthermore, the elderly are more susceptible to abrupt changes in renal function, making digoxin excess more unpredictable despite stable doses of the drug.

**Drug–Drug Interactions**

A number of commonly prescribed medications can raise serum levels of digoxin, including (but not limited to) amiodarone, dronedarone, propafenone, quinidine, and verapamil. This type of effect appears to be at least in part mediated by these drugs' effects in blocking the ability of the *p-glycoprotein* molecular complex that exports digitalis into the intestine and renal tubule, thus lowering its serum concentration. Spironolactone, used in the treatment of heart failure, may also raise digoxin levels owing to decreased renal clearance. In contrast, certain antibiotics (e.g., erythromycin) reduce digoxin concentrations, which may rise when the antibiotics are stopped.

## DIGITALIS TOXICITY: PREVENTION

As noted, the initial step in treatment is always prevention. Before any patient is started on digoxin or a related drug, the indications should be carefully reviewed. Some patients continue to receive digoxin or related drugs for inappropriate reasons, e.g., diastolic heart failure (also referred to as heart failure with preserved left ventricular ejection fraction). Prior to therapy, your patient should have a baseline ECG, serum electrolytes, and blood urea nitrogen (BUN)/creatinine measurements. Serum magnesium blood levels should also be considered, particularly if indicated by diuretic therapy, malabsorption syndromes, etc. Other considerations include the patient's age and pulmonary status, as well as whether the patient is having an acute MI.

Early signs of digitalis toxicity (e.g., increased frequency of PVCs, sinus bradycardia, or increasing AV block) should be carefully checked. Furthermore, digoxin dosages should be preemptively lowered in advance of starting medications that routinely increase digoxin levels.

## DIGITALIS TOXICITY: TREATMENT PRINCIPLES

Definitive treatment of digitalis toxicity depends on the particular arrhythmia. With minor arrhythmias (e.g., isolated PVCs, sinus bradycardia, prolonged PR interval, AV Wenckebach, or accelerated AV junctional rhythms), discontinuation of digitalis and careful observation are usually adequate. More serious arrhythmias (e.g., prolonged runs of VT) may require suppression with an intravenous (IV) drug such as lidocaine. For tachycardias, potassium supplements should be carefully given to raise the serum potassium level to well within normal limits.

Patients with complete heart block from digitalis toxicity may require a temporary pacemaker (Chapter 22) until the effects of the digitalis dissipates, particularly if patients have symptoms of syncope, hypotension, or heart failure related to the bradycardia. In other cases, complete heart block can be managed conservatively with inpatient monitoring while the digitalis wears off.

Occasionally patients present with a large overdose of digitalis taken inadvertently or in a suicide attempt. In such cases the serum digoxin level is markedly elevated, and severe brady- or tachyarrhythmias may develop. In addition, massive digitalis toxicity may cause life-threatening *hyperkalemia* because the drug blocks the cell membrane mechanism that pumps potassium into the cells in exchange for sodium. Patients with a potentially lethal overdose of digitalis can be treated intravenously with the specific digitalis-binding antibody called digoxin immune Fab (antigen-binding fragment). Of note, when hyperkalemia is present in a patient with digitalis toxicity, IV calcium should be avoided.

Finally, clinicians should be aware that direct current electrical cardioversion of arrhythmias in patients who have digitalis toxicity is extremely hazardous and may precipitate fatal VT and fibrillation. Therefore, you should not electrically cardiovert patients suspected of having digitalis toxicity (e.g., those with AF and a slow ventricular response, AT with block, etc.).

## SERUM DIGOXIN CONCENTRATIONS (LEVELS)

The concentration of digoxin in the serum can be measured by means of an immunoassay. "Therapeutic concentrations" are still widely reported in the range from about 0.5 to 2 ng/mL by many laboratories.

However, serum concentrations exceeding 2.0 ng/mL are associated with a high incidence of digitalis toxicity. Therefore, when ordering a test of digoxin level in a patient, you must be aware that "therapeutic levels" do not rule out the possibility of digitalis toxicity. As mentioned, some patients are more sensitive to digitalis and may show signs of toxicity with "therapeutic" levels. In other patients, factors such as hypokalemia or hypomagnesemia may potentiate digitalis toxicity despite an "unremarkable" serum drug level. Although a "high" digoxin level does not necessarily indicate overt toxicity, these patients should be examined for early evidence of digitalis excess, including systemic symptoms (e.g., gastrointestinal symptoms) and all cardiac effects that have been discussed. Efforts should be made to keep the digoxin level well within therapeutic bounds, and lower levels appear to be as efficacious as (and safer than) higher ones in the treatment of heart failure. A spuriously high digoxin level may be obtained if blood is drawn within a few hours of its administration.

For most patients being treated for systolic heart failure, it is safest to maintain the digoxin levels at what was previously considered the low end of the therapeutic range, namely around 0.4-0.8 ng/mL. Recommendations for rate control in AF are less well defined, but the same low therapeutic levels as in heart failure syndromes can be used, pending the availability of more data.

---

### Use of Digoxin: General Principles

- Use only when indicated.
- Use lowest dosage to achieve a therapeutic goal.
- Always reassess the need for the drug and its dosage (especially in context of other medications and renal status) when seeing a new patient or following up from an earlier visit.
- Inform other clinical caregivers, and the patient, of any dosage changes in digoxin or other medications you make (medication reconciliation).

# CHAPTER 21

## Sudden Cardiac Arrest and Sudden Cardiac Death Syndromes

*Cardiac arrest occurs when the heart stops contracting effectively and ceases to pump blood.* The closely related term *sudden cardiac death* describes the situation in which an individual who sustains an unexpected cardiac arrest and who is not resuscitated dies within minutes, or within an hour or so of the development of acute symptoms such as chest discomfort, shortness of breath, lightheadedness or actual syncope.

Sudden cardiac arrest is not a single disease, per se, but a syndrome having multiple causes. Furthermore, sudden cardiac arrest/death, as discussed below, is not synonymous with acute myocardial infarction (MI; "heart attack"). Indeed, acute MI is only responsible for a minority of cases of sudden death.

### CLINICAL ASPECTS OF CARDIAC ARREST

The patient in cardiac arrest loses consciousness within seconds, and irreversible brain damage usually occurs within 4 minutes, sometimes sooner. Furthermore, shortly after the heart stops pumping, spontaneous breathing also ceases (*cardiopulmonary arrest*). In some cases, respirations stop first (primary respiratory arrest) and cardiac activity stops shortly thereafter.

===== Key Point =====

Unresponsiveness, agonal (gasping) or absent respirations, and the lack of a central (e.g., carotid or femoral), palpable pulse are the major diagnostic signs of cardiac arrest.

No heart sounds are audible with a stethoscope placed on the chest, and the blood pressure is unobtainable. The patient in cardiac arrest becomes cyanotic (bluish gray) from lack of circulating oxygenated blood, and the arms and legs become

cool. If the brain becomes severely hypoxic, the pupils are fixed and dilated, and brain death may ensue. Seizure activity may occur.

When cardiac arrest is recognized, *cardiopulmonary resuscitation* (CPR) efforts must be started without delay (Box 21.1). The specific details of CPR and advanced cardiac life support including intubation, drug dosages, the use of automatic external defibrillators (AEDs) and standard defibrillators, along with other matters related to definitive diagnosis and treatment, lie outside the scope of this book but are discussed in selected references cited in the Bibliography and at the websites of major professional societies, including the American Heart Association.

### BASIC ECG PATTERNS IN CARDIAC ARREST

The three basic ECG patterns seen with cardiac arrest were mentioned in earlier chapters, listed in Box 21.2. These patterns are briefly reviewed in the following sections, with emphasis placed on their clinical implications (Figs. 21.1–21.6).

### Ventricular Tachyarrhythmia (Ventricular Fibrillation or Pulseless VT)

With ventricular fibrillation (VF) the ventricles do not contract but instead twitch rapidly and erratically in a completely ineffective way. No cardiac output occurs, and the patient loses consciousness within seconds. The characteristic ECG pattern, with its unmistakable fast oscillatory waves, is illustrated in Fig. 21.1.

VF may appear spontaneously, as noted in Chapter 16, but is often preceded by another ventricular arrhythmia (usually ventricular tachycardia [VT] or frequent premature ventricular beats) or by polymorphic VT. Fig. 21.2 shows a run of VT degenerating into VF during cardiac arrest.

The treatment of VF was described in Chapter 16. The patient should be immediately defibrillated, given a direct current electric shock (360 joules) to

Please go to expertconsult.inkling.com for additional online material for this chapter.

<table>
<tr><td>

**BOX 21.1**

</td><td>

**2015 Updated Cardiopulmonary Resuscitation (CPR) Guidelines**

</td></tr>
</table>

1. Call 911 [emergency services].
2. Begin manual chest compressions at the sternum, at 100–120 compressions per minute.
3. Perform manual compressions at a depth of at least 2 inches (5 centimeters) for an average adult.
4. All lay rescuers should initiate CPR until trained professionals arrive, or the victim becomes responsive.
5. Trained rescuers may consider ventilation in addition to chest compressions, with a 30:2 sternal compression to breath ratio (delivering each breath over approximately one second).

<table>
<tr><td>

**BOX 21.2**

</td><td>

**Three Basic ECG Patterns with Cardiac Arrest**

</td></tr>
</table>

- Ventricular tachyarrhythmia, including ventricular fibrillation (VF) or a sustained type of pulseless ventricular tachycardia (VT)
- Ventricular asystole or a brady-asystolic rhythm with an extremely slow rate

the heart by means of paddles or pads placed on the chest wall (usually in an anterior–posterior position).

*VT and VF are the only "shockable" sudden cardiac arrest rhythms.* An example of successful defibrillation is presented in Fig. 21.6D.

Success in defibrillating any patient depends on a number of factors. The single most important factor in treating VF is haste: the less delay in defibrillation, the greater the chance of succeeding.

Sometimes repeated shocks must be administered before the patient is successfully resuscitated. In other cases, all attempts fail. Finally, external cardiac compression *must* be continued between attempts at defibrillation.

In addition to defibrillation, additional measures include intravenous drugs to support the circulation (e.g., epinephrine) and antiarrhythmic agents such as amiodarone, and magnesium sulfate (in cases of torsades de pointes and when hypomagnesemia is present).

## Ventricular Asystole and Brady-Asystolic Rhythms

The normal pacemaker of the heart is the sinus node, which is located in the high right atrium (Chapters

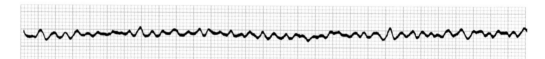

**Fig. 21.1** Ventricular fibrillation inducing cardiac arrest.

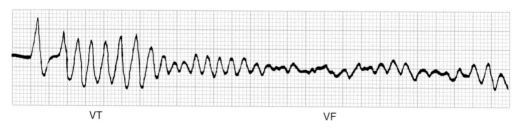

VT                                    VF

**Fig. 21.2** Ventricular tachycardia (VT) and ventricular fibrillation (VF) recorded during cardiac arrest. The rapid sine wave type of ventricular tachycardia seen here is sometimes referred to as *ventricular flutter*.

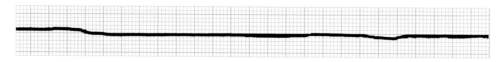

**Fig. 21.3** Complete ventricular standstill (asystole) producing a flat-line or straight-line pattern during cardiac arrest.

**Cardiac Arrest: Brady-Asystolic Patterns**

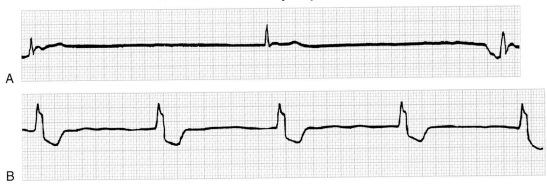

**Fig. 21.4** Escape rhythms with underlying ventricular standstill. (A) Junctional escape rhythm with narrow QRS complexes. (B) Idioventricular escape rhythm with wide QRS complexes. Treatment should include the use of intravenous atropine and, if needed, sympathomimetic drugs in an attempt to speed up these bradycardias, which cannot support the circulation. If hyperkalemia is present, it should be treated.

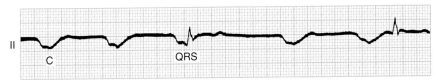

**Fig. 21.5** External cardiac compression artifact. External cardiac compression during resuscitation produces artifactual ECG complexes (C), which may be mistaken for QRS complexes.

4 and 13). Failure of the sinus node to function (sinus arrest) leads to ventricular standstill (asystole) if no other subsidiary pacemaker (e.g., in the atria, atrioventricular [AV] junction, or ventricles) takes over. In such cases the ECG records a so-called *flat-line* or *straight-line pattern* (see Fig. 21.3), indicating asystole. Whenever you encounter a straight-line pattern, you need to confirm this finding in at least two leads (as seen in most conventional monitoring systems) and check to see that all electrodes are connected to the patient (electrodes often become disconnected during a cardiac arrest, leading to the mistaken diagnosis of asystole). Very low amplitude VF (so-called "fine VF") may also mimic a straight-line pattern. Increasing the gain on the monitor may reveal this "hidden" VF pattern.

The treatment of asystole also requires continued external cardiac compression; *however, unlike VT or VF, defibrillation is not appropriate, nor is it effective.* Sometimes spontaneous cardiac electrical activity resumes. Drugs such as epinephrine may help

support the circulation or stimulate cardiac electrical activity. Patients with refractory ventricular standstill require a *temporary pacemaker, inserted into the right ventricle through the internal jugular or femoral veins.* Noninvasive, *transcutaneous* pacing uses special electrodes that are pasted on the chest wall. However, transcutaneous pacing may only be effective with bradycardia, not frank asystole, and is usually quite painful in conscious patients.

Not uncommonly with ventricular standstill, you also see occasional QRS complexes appearing at infrequent intervals against the background of the basic straight-line rhythm. These are *escape beats* and represent the attempt of intrinsic cardiac pacemakers to restart the heart's beating (see Chapter 13). Examples of escape rhythms with underlying ventricular standstill are shown in Fig. 21.4. In some cases the escape beats are narrow, indicating their origin from either the atria or the AV junction (see Fig. 21.4A). In others they come from a lower focus in the ventricles, producing a slow *idioventricular*

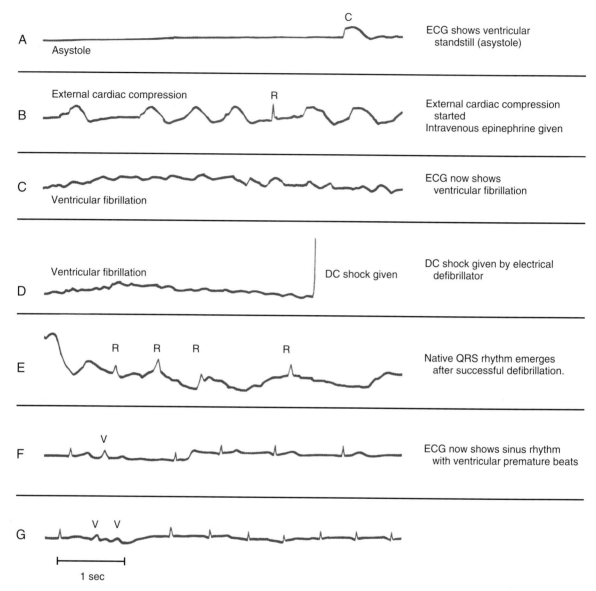

**Fig. 21.6** ECG "history" of cardiac arrest and successful resuscitation. The left panel shows the ECG sequence during an actual cardiac arrest. The right panel shows sequential therapy used in this case for the different ECG patterns. (A,B) Initially the ECG showed ventricular asystole with a straight-line pattern, which was treated by external cardiac compression, along with intravenous medications. (C,D) Next ventricular fibrillation was seen. Intravenous amiodarone and other medications may also be used in this setting (see text and Bibliography). (E–G) Sinus rhythm appeared after defibrillation with a direct current electric shock. C, external cardiac compression artifact; R, R wave from the spontaneous QRS complex; DC, direct current; V, ventricular premature beat.

rhythm with wide QRS complexes (see Fig. 21.4B). The term *brady-asystolic pattern* is used to describe this type of cardiac arrest ECG.

*Hyperkalemia, as well as other potentially reversible causes, such as drugs or ischemia, should always be excluded as causes of brady-asystolic rhythms.*

Escape beats should not be confused with *artifacts* produced by external cardiac compression. Artifacts are large, wide deflections that occur with each compression (see Fig. 21.5). Their size varies with the strength of the compression, and their direction varies with the lead in which they appear (i.e., usually negative in leads II, III, and aVF, positive in leads aVR and aVL).

## Pulseless Electrical Activity (Electromechanical Dissociation)

In occasional patients with cardiac arrest, the person is unconscious and does not have a palpable pulse or blood pressure despite the presence of recurring QRS complexes and even P waves on the ECG. In other words, the patient has cardiac electrical activity but insufficient mechanical heart contractions to pump blood effectively. This syndrome is called *pulseless electrical activity* (PEA) or *electromechanical dissociation* (EMD). Similar to asystole, defibrillation is not appropriate therapy for PEA.

PEA with a physiologic rate can arise in a number of settings. When assessing a patient with PEA, you must consider potentially *reversible* causes first. Box 21.3 presents an adaptation of the classic "5 Hs and the 5 Ts" that may lead to PEA.

| BOX 21.3 | "Hs and Ts" of Pulseless Electrical Activity* |
| --- | --- |

**Hs**
- Hypovolemia
- Hypoxemia
- Hyperkalemia
- Hypothermia
- Hydrogen ions (acidemia)

**Ts**
Thrombosis myocardial infarction
Thromboembolism (pulmonary embolism)
Tamponade (cardiac/pericardial)
Tension pneumothorax
Tablets (drugs)/Toxins

*Pulseless electrical activity (PEA), also referred to as electromechanical dissociation (EMD).

One of the most common settings in which PEA occurs is when the myocardium has sustained severe generalized injury that may not be reversible, such as with extensive myocardial infarction (MI). In such cases, even though the heart's conduction system may be intact enough to generate a relatively normal rhythm, the amount of functional ventricular muscle is insufficient to respond to this electrical signal with an adequate contraction. Sometimes the myocardial depression is temporary and reversible ("stunned myocardium"), and the patient may respond to resuscitative efforts.

In summary, the main ECG patterns seen with cardiac arrest are a sustained ventricular tachyarrhythmia or VF, ventricular asystole (including brady-asystolic patterns), and PEA. During the course of resuscitating any patient, you may see two or even all three of these ECG patterns at different times during the arrest. Fig. 21.6 shows the "ECG history" of a cardiac arrest.

## SUDDEN CARDIAC DEATH/ARREST

As noted in the introduction, the term *sudden cardiac death* describes situations in which an individual sustains an unexpected cardiac arrest, is not resuscitated and dies instantly or within an hour or so of the development of acute symptoms. The term applies to cases in which CPR may not be available or initiated, or in those in which it is unsuccessful. Over 400,000 sudden cardiac deaths occur each year in the United States, striking individuals both with and without known cardiovascular disease. Unexpected sudden cardiac death is most often initiated by a sustained ventricular tachyarrhythmia, less commonly by a brady-asystolic mechanism or PEA.

Most individuals with unexpected cardiac arrest have underlying structural heart disease. An estimated 20% of individuals in the United States with acute MI die suddenly before reaching the hospital. Another important substrate for sudden death is severe left ventricular scarring from previous (chronic) MI.

## CLINICAL CAUSES OF CARDIAC ARREST

During and after successful resuscitation of the patient in cardiac arrest, an intensive search for the cause(s) must be started. Serial 12-lead ECGs and serum cardiac enzyme levels are essential in diagnosing acute MI. A complete blood count, serum electrolyte concentrations, and arterial blood–gas measurements should be obtained. A portable chest X-ray unit and, if needed, an echocardiograph machine can be brought to the bedside. In addition, a careful physical examination (signs of congestive heart failure, pneumothorax, etc.) should be performed in concert with a pertinent medical history with particular attention to drug use (e.g., digitalis, drugs used to treat arrhythmias, psychotropic agents, "recreational" drugs, etc.) and previous cardiac problems (see also Chapters 10, 15, and 19).

Cardiac arrest may be due to any type of organic heart disease. For example, a patient with an acute or prior MI (Box 21.4) may have cardiac arrest for at least five reasons. Cardiac arrest may also occur when severe electrical instability is associated with other types of chronic heart disease resulting from valvular abnormalities, hypertension, or cardiomyopathy.

An electric shock (including a lightning strike) may produce cardiac arrest in the normal heart. Cardiac arrest may also occur during surgical procedures, particularly in patients with underlying heart disease.

Drugs such as epinephrine can produce VF. Quinidine, disopyramide, procainamide, ibutilide, sotalol, dofetilide, and related "antiarrhythmic" drugs may lead to long QT(U) syndrome culminating in sustained torsades de pointes (see Chapter 16).

Digitalis toxicity can also lead to fatal ventricular arrhythmias (see Chapter 20). Other cardiac drugs may also precipitate sustained ventricular tachyarrhythmias through their so-called *proarrhythmic effects* (see Chapter 16). The "recreational" use of *cocaine* or *amphetamines* may also induce fatal arrhythmias.

Hypokalemia and hypomagnesemia may potentiate arrhythmias associated with a variety of antiarrhythmic drugs and with digitalis glycosides.

Other patients with unexpected sudden cardiac arrest have structural heart disease with valvular abnormalities or myocardial disease associated, for example, with severe aortic stenosis, dilated or hypertrophic cardiomyopathies, acute or chronic myocarditis, arrhythmogenic right ventricular cardiomyopathy/dysplasia (ARVC/D), or anomalous origin of a coronary artery. Cardiac sarcoidosis is a relatively rare but important cause of sudden cardiac arrest/death due to ventricular tachyarrhythmia or complete AV heart block.

*QT prolongation*, a marker of risk for torsades de pointes type of VT, was discussed in Chapter 16. QT prolongation syndromes may be divided into acquired and hereditary (congenital) subsets. The major acquired causes include drugs, electrolyte abnormalities, and bradyarrhythmias, especially high-degree AV blocks. Fig. 21.7 shows an example of marked QT prolongation due to quinidine that was followed by torsades de pointes and cardiac arrest. Hereditary long QT syndromes (Fig. 21.8) are due to a number of different abnormalities of cardiac ion channel function ("channelopathies"). A detailed list of factors causing long QT syndrome and risk of torsades de pointes is summarized in Chapter 25.

Some individuals with sudden cardiac death do not have mechanical cardiac dysfunction, but they may have intrinsic electrical instability as a result of the long QT syndromes (predisposing to torsades de pointes), Wolff–Parkinson–White (WPW) preexcitation syndrome, particularly when associated with atrial fibrillation with a very rapid ventricular response (Chapter 18), the Brugada syndrome, and severe sinoatrial (SA) or AV conduction system disease causing prolonged sinus arrest or high-grade heart block, respectively.

The *Brugada syndrome* refers to the association of a characteristic ECG pattern with risk of ventricular tachyarrhythmias. The Brugada pattern consists of unusual ST segment elevations in the right chest leads ($V_1$ to $V_3$) with a QRS pattern somewhat

---

**BOX 21.4** | **Major Causes of Cardiac Arrest in Coronary Artery Disease Syndromes**

- Acute myocardial ischemia and increased ventricular electrical instability, precipitating ventricular fibrillation (VF) or polymorphic ventricular tachycardia (VT) leading to VF
- Damage to the specialized conduction system resulting in high-degree atrioventricular (AV) block. Cardiac arrest may be due to bradycardia/asystole or to torsades de pointes
- Sinus node dysfunction leading to marked sinus bradycardia or even asystole
- Pulseless electrical activity (PEA) related to extensive myocardial injury
- Rupture of the infarcted ventricular wall, leading to pericardial (cardiac) tamponade
- Chronic myocardial infarction (MI) with ventricular scarring, leading to monomorphic VT degenerating into VF

## Quinidine-Induced Long QT and Torsades de Pointes

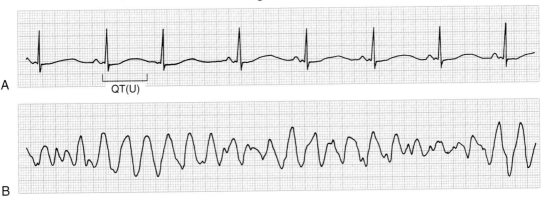

**Fig. 21.7** Patient on quinidine developed marked prolongation of repolarization with low amplitude T-U waves (panel A) followed (panel B) by cardiac arrest with torsades de pointes ventricular tachycardia. (Note that the third beat in panel A is a premature atrial complex.)

## Hereditary Long QT Syndrome

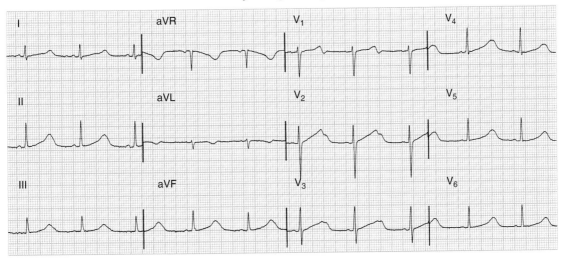

**Fig. 21.8** Hereditary long QT syndrome. ECG from 21-year-old woman with history of recurrent syncope, initially mistaken for a primary seizure disorder. The ECG demonstrates a prolonged QT interval of 0.6 sec. Note the broad T waves with notching (or possibly U waves) in the precordial leads. Syncope, with risk of sudden cardiac death, is due to episodes of torsades de pointes type of ventricular tachycardia (Chapter 16).

resembling a right bundle branch block (Fig. 21.9). The basis of the Brugada pattern and associated arrhythmias is a topic of active study. Abnormal repolarization of right ventricular muscle related to sodium channel dysfunction appears to play an important role.

An important, but fortunately rare cause of recurrent syncope and sometimes sudden cardiac arrest and death is *catecholaminergic polymorphic ventricular tachycardia* (CPVT), typically induced by exercise or stress. Some cases are familial (autosomal dominant), related to a genetic mutation that alters

## Brugada Pattern

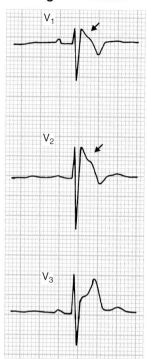

**Fig. 21.9** Brugada pattern showing characteristic ST elevations in the right chest leads. The ECG superficially resembles a right bundle branch block (RBBB) pattern. However, typical RBBB produces an rSR′ pattern in right precordial leads and is *not* associated with ST segment elevation (*arrows*) in this distribution. The Brugada pattern appears to be a marker of abnormal right ventricular repolarization and in some individuals (Brugada syndrome) is associated with an increased risk of life-threatening ventricular arrhythmias and sudden cardiac arrest.

## Catecholaminergic Polymorphic Ventricular Tachycardia (CPVT)

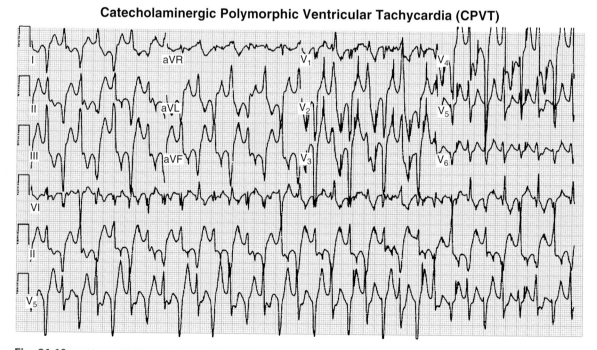

**Fig. 21.10** Rapid run of bidirectional ventricular tachycardia in a 6-year-old child with exertional syncope and a hereditable form of catecholaminergic polymorphic ventricular tachycardia (CPVT). A number of genetic defects have been identified with this syndrome, which is associated with abnormal myocyte calcium ion dynamics. He was treated with an ICD and with beta blockers.

calcium dynamics in myocytes. Subjects with CPVT may show a distinct type of VT where the premature complexes alternate in direction on a beat-to-beat basis (bidirectional VT) (Fig. 21.10). Digoxin toxicity (see Chapter 20) is a separate cause of bidirectional VT.

A very rare cause of cardiac arrest from ventricular tachyarrhythmias (and sometimes atrial fibrillation) in young individuals is the so-called "short QT syndrome." As implied by the name, these individuals usually have an ECG showing an abbreviated ST segment and a very short QTc (usually <330 msec). This abnormal repolarization (the opposite of long QT in its appearance) is likely due to abnormal function of one or more cardiac ion channels. However, the link between very short QT in certain individuals and ventricular arrhythmogenesis remains unresolved.

As noted, "recreational" drugs, such as *cocaine* or *amphetamines*, may induce lethal ventricular arrhythmias, as may dietary supplements containing *ephedra alkaloids*.

The term *commotio cordis* (Latin for "cardiac concussion") refers to the syndrome of sudden cardiac arrest in healthy individuals who sustain nonpenetrating chest trauma that triggers VF. This syndrome has been reported after chest wall impact during sports, but may occur during other activities, such as car or motorcycle accidents. The possibility of mechanical trauma to the chest inducing VF appears to be highest when the impact has sufficient force and occurs just before the peak of the T wave (vulnerable period; see also Chapter 16).

Patients with advanced chronic lung disease are also at increased risk for sudden cardiac arrest/death. Multiple factors may play a role, including hypoxemia and therapeutic exposure to cardiac stimulants (short and longer-acting beta-2 agonists), concomitant coronary disease, and so forth.

*Sudden death with epilepsy* (SUDEP) is a syndromic term used to describe the finding that unexplained cardiac arrest occurs in about 1/1000 patients with epilepsy and an even higher percentage (estimated 1/150) whose seizures are refractory to treatment. Most cases have been reported during sleep. The variety of proposed mechanisms for this syndrome include post-ictal bradycardias due to excessive vagal activation or ventricular tachyarrhythmias provoked directly by the seizure or cardiac arrhythmias induced by respiratory dysfunction.

Finally, when the cause of a cardiac arrest due to ventricular tachyarrhythmia in a previously healthy individual remains undiscovered, the term *idiopathic VT/VF* is applied.

The identification and management of patients at high risk for sudden arrest/death are active areas of investigation in cardiology today. The important role of *implantable cardioverter–defibrillator* (ICD) devices in preventing sudden death in carefully selected, high-risk patients is discussed in the next chapter.

# CHAPTER 22

# Pacemakers and Implantable Cardioverter–Defibrillators: Essentials for Clinicians

This chapter provides a brief introduction to an important aspect of everyday ECG analysis related to the two major types of electronic cardiac devices: *pacemakers* and *implantable cardioverter–defibrillators* (ICDs). Additional material is provided in the online supplement and Bibliography.

## PACEMAKERS: DEFINITIONS AND TYPES

━━━━━━━━━━━━━━ Key Point ━━━━━━━━━━━━━━

Pacemakers are electronic devices primarily designed to correct or compensate for symptomatic abnormalities of cardiac impulse formation (e.g., sinus node dysfunction) or conduction (e.g., severe atrioventricular [AV] heart block).

An electronic pacemaker consists of two primary components: (1) a pulse generator (battery and microcomputer) and (2) one or more electrodes (also called leads). The electrodes can be attached to the skin (in the case of emergency transcutaneous pacing), but more often are attached directly to the inside of the heart (Fig. 22.1).

Pacemaker therapy can be *temporary* or *permanent*. Temporary pacing is used when the electrical abnormality is expected to resolve within a relatively short time. Temporary pacing electrodes are inserted transvenously and connected to a generator located outside the body. Less commonly, these leads are placed via a transcutaneous approach. For example, temporary pacing is used in severe, symptomatic bradycardias associated with cardiac surgery, inferior wall myocardial infarction (MI), Lyme disease, or drug toxicity. When normal cardiac electrical function returns, the temporary pacing electrode can be easily removed.

Permanent pacemakers have both the generator and electrode(s), also called *leads*, implanted inside the body (see Fig. 22.1). Electronic pacemakers are used for three major purposes:

- To restore properly timed atrial impulse formation in severe sinus node dysfunction
- To restore properly timed ventricular contractions during atrioventricular block (AV synchrony[a])
- To compensate for left bundle branch block (LBBB) conduction abnormalities, especially with heart failure, by providing synchronization[a] of right and left ventricular contraction. This use is called *resynchronization therapy* or *biventricular pacing*.

Depending on the indication, pacemakers have from one to three leads.

Most often the pacemaker leads are implanted transvenously (through cephalic or subclavian veins) with the generator unit (consisting of the power supply and a microcomputer) positioned subcutaneously in the anterior shoulder area. In some instances the leads are implanted on the epicardial (outer) surface of the heart, using a surgical approach (for example, to avoid intravascular exposure in patients with a high risk of endocarditis).

All contemporary pacemakers are capable of sensing intrinsic electrical activity of the heart and are externally *programmable* (adjustable) using special computer devices provided by the manufacturers. Pacemakers are usually set to operate in an *on-demand*

---

[a]The terms *synchrony* and *synchronization* refer to a harmonization of chamber activation and contraction. Specifically, the terms describe events occurring (1) at a fixed interval (lag or delay), or (2) simultaneously. The first is exemplified by *AV synchrony* in which the ventricles are stimulated to contract by the initiation of atrial depolarization after a physiologic delay (native PR interval) or the electronic (pacemaker) interval. The second is exemplified by *intraventricular synchrony* in which the pacemaker electrodes stimulate the RV and LV to contract in a coordinated way, simulating the normal activation process.

Please go to expertconsult.inkling.com for additional online material for this chapter.

mode, providing electronic pacing support only when the patient's own electrical system fails to generate impulses in a timely fashion. Modern pacemaker batteries last on average between about 8 and 12 years, depending on usage.[b]

---

[b]Leadless pacemakers are now approved for use in the United States. These devices (currently about 2 grams in weight and about the length of AAA batteries) combine the pulse generator and lead system in a compact cylinder implanted into the right ventricle via the femoral vein. Advantages of leadless pacemakers are that they do not require a subcutaneous battery insertion in a surgical chest pocket, and they can be readily retrieved (for example, in the case of infection). However, current leadless devices are single (right) chamber systems, limiting their universal applicability.

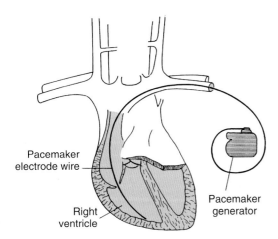

**Fig. 22.1** Schematic of an implanted pacemaker consisting of a generator (battery with microcomputer) connected to a single wire electrode (lead) inserted through the left subclavian vein into the right ventricle. This is the simplest type of pacemaker. Dual-chamber pacemakers have electrodes in both the right atrium and right ventricle. Biventricular pacemakers can pace both ventricles and the right atrium.

## Single- and Dual-Chamber Pacemakers

Single-lead (or single-chamber) pacemakers (see Fig. 22.1), as their name indicates, are used to stimulate only the right atrium or right ventricle. Atrial single-lead pacemakers (with the lead positioned in the right atrium) can be used to treat isolated sinus node dysfunction with normal AV conduction (Fig. 22.2). In the United States, single-lead atrial pacemakers are rarely implanted. Even patients with isolated sinus node dysfunction usually receive dual-chamber devices because AV conduction abnormalities often develop as the patient ages (thus requiring the additional ventricular lead).

Ventricular single-lead pacemakers (with the lead positioned in the right ventricle) are primarily used to generate a reliable heartbeat in patients with chronic atrial fibrillation with an excessively slow ventricular response. The atrial fibrillation precludes effective atrial stimulation such that there is no reason to insert an atrial lead (Fig. 22.3).

In *dual-chamber pacemakers*, electrodes are inserted into both the right atrium and right ventricle (Figs. 22.4 and 22.5). The circuitry is designed to allow for a physiologic delay (normal synchrony) between atrial and ventricular stimulation. This *AV delay* (interval between the atrial and ventricular pacemaker stimuli) is analogous to the PR interval under physiologic conditions.

## ECG Morphology of Paced Beats

Paced beats are characterized by the pacing stimulus (often called a "pacing spike"), which is seen as a sharp vertical deflection. If the pacing threshold is low, the amplitude of pacing stimuli can be very small and easily overlooked on the standard ECG.

## Atrial Pacemaker

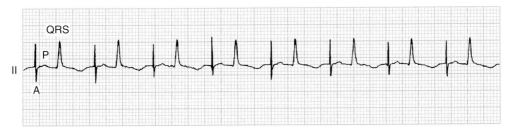

**Fig. 22.2** With the pacemaker electrode placed in the right atrium, a pacemaker stimulus (*A*) is seen before each P wave. The QRS complex is normal because the ventricle is depolarized by the atrioventricular conduction system.

## Atrial Fibrillation with Ventricular Pacing

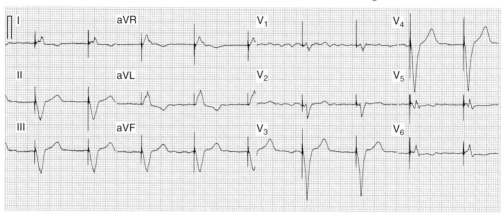

**Fig. 22.3** The ventricular (QRS) rhythm is completely regular because of ventricular pacing. However, the underlying rhythm is atrial fibrillation. Fibrillatory waves are small in amplitude in most leads and best seen in lead $V_1$. Most computer ECG interpretations will read this as "ventricular pacing" without noting atrial fibrillation. Unless the reader specifies "atrial fibrillation" in the report, this important diagnosis, which carries risk of stroke, will go unnoticed. Furthermore, on physical examination, the clinician may overlook the underlying atrial fibrillation because of the regular rate.

## Dual-Chamber (DDD) Pacemaker Functions

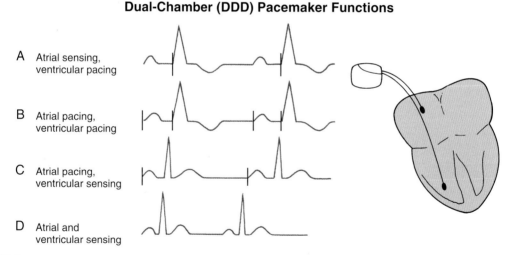

**A**  Atrial sensing, ventricular pacing

**B**  Atrial pacing, ventricular pacing

**C**  Atrial pacing, ventricular sensing

**D**  Atrial and ventricular sensing

**Fig. 22.4** Dual-chamber pacemakers sense and pace in both atria and ventricles. The pacemaker emits a stimulus (spike) whenever a native P wave or QRS complex is not sensed within some programmed time interval.

A paced P wave demonstrates a pacing stimulus followed by a P wave (see Fig. 22.2).

A paced QRS beat also starts with a pacing stimulus, followed by a wide QRS complex (see Figs. 22.3 and 22.6). The wide QRS is due to the fact that activation of the ventricles starts at the tip of the lead and spreads to the other ventricle through slowly conducting myocardium, similar to what occurs with bundle branch blocks, premature ventricular complexes (PVCs), or ventricular escape beats. The QRS morphology depends on the lead (electrode) position. The most commonly used ventricular electrode site is the right ventricular apex. Pacing at this location produces a wide QRS (usually

## Dual-Chamber Pacing

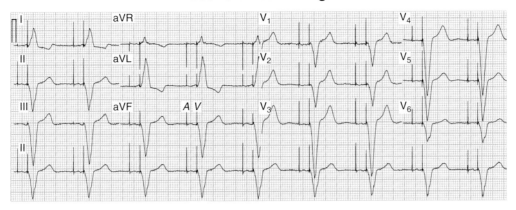

**Fig. 22.5** Paced beat morphology in dual-chamber pacemaking. Both atrial and ventricular pacing stimuli are present. The atrial (*A*) pacing stimulus is followed by a P wave with very low amplitude. The ventricular (*V*) pacing stimulus is followed by a wide QRS complex with T wave pointing in the opposite direction (discordant). The QRS after the pacing stimulus resembles a left bundle branch block, with a leftward axis, consistent with pacing from the right ventricular apex.

## Ventricular Pacing with Retrograde P Waves

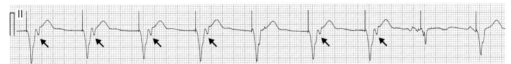

**Fig. 22.6** Note the negative P wave (*arrows*) after the ventricular demand (VVI) paced beats due to activation of the atria from bottom to top following the paced ventricular beats.

resembling a LBBB pattern; see Chapter 8) with a leftward axis (QRS deflections are typically negative in leads II, III, and aVF and positive in leads I and aVL).

As with PVCs, the T waves in paced beats normally are *discordant*—directed opposite to the main QRS direction (see Figs. 22.3 and 22.5). Concordant T waves (i.e., pointing in the same direction as the QRS complexes during ventricular pacing) may indicate acute myocardial ischemia (see following discussion).

Ventricular paced beats, similar to PVCs, can also sometimes conduct in a retrograde manner to the atria, producing near simultaneous atrial and ventricular depolarization and contraction (Fig. 22.6). When this occurs repeatedly, atrial contraction against the closed AV valves produces recurrent, sudden increases in jugular (and pulmonary) vein pressures, which may be seen as intermittent, large ("cannon") A waves in the neck examination. These

abrupt pressure changes, in turn, may activate autonomic reflexes and cause severe symptoms (palpitations, pulsation in the neck, dizziness, and blood pressure drop), often referred to as the *pacemaker syndrome*. Therefore, patients in sinus rhythm with AV block are usually implanted with dual-chamber pacemakers so that ventricular pacing will be timed to occur after atrial pacing, maintaining physiologic AV synchrony.

### Electronic Pacemaker Programming: Shorthand Code

Historically, pacemaker programming has been described by a standard three- or four-letter code, usually followed by a number indicating the lower rate limit. Although many new pacing enhancements have been introduced since the inception of this code, it is still widely used (Table 22.1). Depending on the atrial rate and the status of intrinsic AV conduction, dual-chamber pacemaker function can

| TABLE 22.1 | | Standard Four-Letter Pacemaker Code | | | | | |
|---|---|---|---|---|---|---|---|
| **I: Chamber Paced** | | **II: Chamber Sensed** | | **III: Response to Sensing** | | **IV: Rate Modulation** | |
| A | Atrium | A | Atrium | I | Inhibit | R | Rate-responsive |
| V | Ventricle | V | Ventricle | T | Trigger | | |
| D | Both (A and V) | D | Both (A and V) | D | Both (I and T) | | |
| O | None | O | None | O | None | | |

### VVI Pacing: Intrinsic, Fusion and Fully Paced Beats

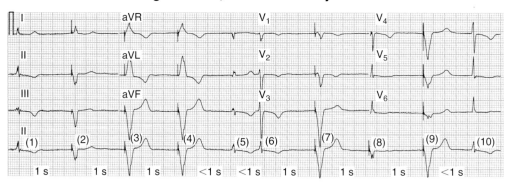

**Fig. 22.7** VVI pacing cycle (10 beats). Sensing of intrinsic activity in the ventricles inhibits pacemaker output. Once the pause after the last QRS complex reaches 1 sec, the pacemaker produces a pacing stimulus resulting in a paced beat (wide QRS). Beats 2 and 8 are fusion beats (coinciding conducted and paced beats). Note also that the normally conducted beats (narrow QRS complexes) have inverted T waves, probably due to "cardiac memory" associated with intermittent pacing, not to ischemia.

produce four different combinations of pacing/sensing ECG patterns (Figs. 22.4, 22.7, and 22.8):
- A sense, V sense
- A sense, V pace
- A pace, V sense
- A pace, V pace

This programming corresponds to the code in Table 22.1.

### Single-Chamber Pacemaker Programming

As noted, modern pacemakers are programmed in the *on-demand mode* providing pacing support only when needed. In the case of a single-chamber pacemaker, usually VVI, this function is accomplished by specifying the *lower rate limit* (for example 60 beats/min). The pacemaker constantly monitors the patient's heart rate in the implanted chamber on a beat-to-beat basis. Any time the rate drops below the lower rate limit (in the case of 60 beats/min, the critical pause after a spontaneous QRS complex will

be >1 sec), the pacemaker will deliver a pacing stimulus (Fig. 22.7). This corresponds to the code: VVI 60.

To simulate the heart rate increase that normally occurs with exertion, pacemakers can be programmed in a *rate-responsive or adaptive mode*. The purpose of this mode is to increase the lower rate limit dynamically, depending on the level of physical activity as detected by a sensor incorporated in the generator unit. For example, one of your patients may have rate-responsive ventricular single-chamber pacemaker programming, referred to as VVIR 60–110, in which the R indicates "rate-responsive" and the second number (110 in this case) represents the upper pacing limit, which is the maximum rate that the device will pace the ventricles in response to its activity sensor.

### Dual-Chamber Pacemaker Programming

Dual-chamber (DDD) pacemakers have two leads (one in the right atrium, one in the right ventricle), each capable of sensing intrinsic electrical activity

## DDD Pacemaker Patterns
### Sinus Rate

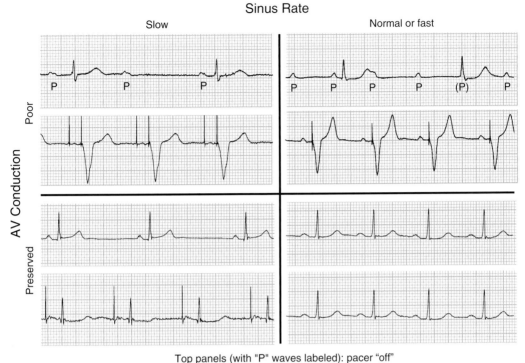

**Fig. 22.8** DDD pacing. Four different pacing/sensing combinations can be present depending on the sinus rate and atrioventricular (AV) conduction. See also Fig. 22.4.

to determine the need for pacing in each chamber. For "on-demand" dual-chamber pacemakers—the most common types—atrial pacing is determined by the *lower rate limit* while ventricular pacing is determined by the separately programmed *maximum AV delay*.

DDD pacing and sensing occur in both chambers (the first and second D). The response to sensing is also dual (D): inhibition if intrinsic activity in the chamber is sensed (A sense, V sense) or triggering V pacing when there is sensing in the A but no AV conduction at maximum AV delay (A sense, V pace). As with single-chamber pacemakers, dual-chamber devices can be programmed in a rate-responsive mode.

DDD and DDDR are the most commonly used pacing modes in dual-chamber pacemakers. Dual-chamber pacemakers can be reprogrammed in a single-chamber mode as well; for example, if the patient develops permanent atrial fibrillation.

On-demand programming has significant advantages, including prolonging battery life and avoiding unnecessary pacing especially in the ventricle. The downside of demand pacing is the possibility that the pacemaker algorithms will mistake external electrical signals for the patient's own electrical activity. This "false positive" detection will result in pacemaker inhibition and inappropriate withholding of pacing. This scenario can occur, for example, with the use of electrosurgical equipment or exposure to strong electromagnetic fields, such as created by magnetic resonance imaging (MRI) machines. In these cases, pacemakers will automatically be reset to the *asynchronous mode* (DOO or VOO) and will provide pacing at the lower rate limit regardless of ambient electrical activity. DOO mode is used in MRI-compatible pacemakers for the duration of the scan.

Clinicians should also be familiar with two additional programming features in dual-chamber pacemakers designed to optimize device function during atrial arrhythmias: *maximal tracking rate* and *automatic mode switching*.

1. The *maximal tracking rate* is the highest ventricular pacing rate allowed in response to atrial sensing and is typically set at 110–150 beats/min. This cut-off feature is designed to prevent excessively rapid ventricular pacing during supraventricular arrhythmias. (Note the distinction between the maximum activity-related rate, the highest rate the pacemaker will fire during exercise as part of its rate-responsiveness, and the maximal tracking rate, the absolute highest the pacemaker will fire in response to atrial sensing.)

2. *Automatic mode switching* changes the pacing mode from DDD to VVIR in response to sensing high atrial rates most often associated with atrial flutter or fibrillation. This functionality prevents ventricular tracking of very high atrial rates, thereby slowing and regularizing the ventricular pacing rhythm. A high number of mode-switch episodes recorded during pacemaker "interrogation" can be a clue that the patient may have developed atrial fibrillation. This finding is very important since the development of atrial fibrillation may have gone unnoticed due to regular heart rate during ventricular pacing.

## Managing Adverse Effects of Right Ventricular Pacing

Right ventricular pacing produces a wide QRS similar to that seen in LBBB and delayed activation/contraction of the left ventricular lateral wall (*ventricular dyssynchrony*). Accumulating evidence suggests that pacing-induced ventricular dyssynchrony over time can lead to worsening of left ventricular function and development or worsening of heart failure especially in patients with impaired baseline ventricular fraction.

Contemporary dual-chamber pacemakers have sophisticated algorithms aimed to minimize the amount of right ventricular pacing by automatically adjusting the maximum AV delay to take full physiologic AV conduction. This protective function can result in very long PR or "AR" intervals (in case of A-paced rhythms) to allow for conducted QRS complexes and does not necessarily imply pacemaker malfunction. Some of these algorithms even permit single nonconducted P waves (second-degree AV block). In such cases, once the P wave blocks, V pacing is initiated.

## Biventricular Pacemakers: Cardiac Resynchronization Therapy

Similar to right ventricular pacing, LBBB causes late activation/contraction of the left ventricular lateral wall (*ventricular dyssynchrony*). Often present in patients with cardiomyopathy and heart failure, LBBB further reduces the effectiveness of ventricular contraction and exacerbates cardiac dysfunction. Restoring appropriate timing of left ventricular lateral wall activation (*resynchronization*) usually results in improvement in the left ventricular function as well as *reverse remodeling* of the left ventricle over time with progressive recovery (and sometimes complete normalization) of the left ventricular function.

This positive effect is accomplished by *biventricular pacing*. In addition to the usual right ventricular pacing lead, another electrode is placed to stimulate the left ventricle. Usually this second lead is advanced transvenously through a branch of the coronary sinus on the posterolateral wall of the left ventricle (Fig. 22.9) because this is the area last activated with intrinsic LBBB or with right ventricular pacing.

Both ventricles are then paced simultaneously, producing *fusion-type* QRS complexes (Figs. 22.10 and 22.11) that represent a "hybrid" between those seen with pure right and left ventricular pacing. The QRS morphology can be quite variable depending on the position of the left ventricular electrode, but usually the QRS has prominent R waves in leads $V_1$ to $V_2$ (RBBB-type morphology) due to posterior left ventricular wall activation from back to front as well as Q waves in leads I and aVL (left ventricular electrode activating the heart from left to right). The QRS duration during biventricular pacing is usually slightly shorter than with right ventricular pacing or with an intrinsic LBBB.

## Major ECG Diagnoses in the Presence of Paced Rhythms

Ventricular paced rhythms regularize the ventricular rate and distort QRS and T wave shapes in a manner similar to LBBB. This makes definitive analysis of the QRS, ST segment, and T wave difficult and at times virtually impossible. However, clinicians should be aware of a number of distinct ECG patterns that should not be missed even in paced rhythms or in ECGs obtained after ventricular pacing.

### Atrial Fibrillation

The usual pacing mode in atrial fibrillation is VVI(R). Paced QRS complexes occur at regular intervals

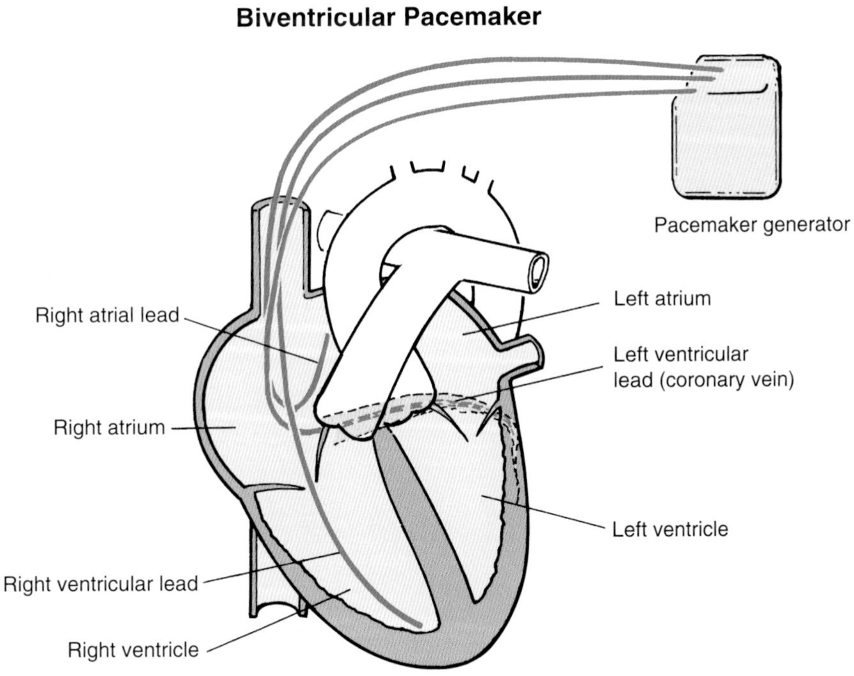

## Biventricular Pacemaker

**Fig. 22.9** Biventricular (BiV) pacemaker. Note the pacemaker lead in the coronary sinus vein that allows pacing of the left ventricle simultaneously with the right ventricle. BiV pacing is used in selected patients with congestive heart failure with left ventricular conduction delays to help "resynchronize" cardiac activation and thereby improve cardiac function.

masking the irregular heart rate, characteristic of atrial fibrillation. If only V-paced beats are present, most computer ECG interpretation algorithms will read this as "ventricular paced rhythm" without commenting on the atrial activity. Unless you specifically mention atrial fibrillation in the report, it will go unnoticed and the patient might be exposed to the risk of a stroke if not properly anticoagulated. The best single lead to evaluate atrial activity is $V_1$ because it usually shows the highest amplitude fibrillatory signals (see Fig. 22.3). However, all leads should be examined.

### Acute Myocardial Ischemia

Although ischemic ST-T wave changes are often obscured by pacing (similar to LBBB), sometimes severe ischemia can still be visible as disappearance of the normal QRS-T discordance during ventricular pacing. Similar to the signs of ischemia in LBBB, concordant ST segment depressions or prominent T wave inversions in leads $V_1$ to $V_3$ point to severe

myocardial ischemia during ventricular pacing with a negative QRS in those leads (Fig. 22.12). In contrast, ST elevations in paced beats showing a positive QRS complex (i.e., R or Rs type) raise consideration of acute ischemia.

### Cardiac "Memory" T Wave Inversions

Ventricular pacing produces electrical changes in the heart that last a long time after the pacing stops (a phenomenon called *cardiac memory*). In patients who are paced intermittently, these changes can be seen in nonpaced beats, appearing as T wave inversions in the leads that showed predominantly negative QRS during ventricular pacing (usually precordial and inferior leads) (see Fig. 22.7). These changes look very much like T wave inversions due to myocardial ischemia (Wellens' pattern: see Chapter 10). However, after a period of ventricular pacing, leads I and aVL usually show upright T waves in normally conducted beats. In contrast, anterior ischemia is often (but not always) associated with T wave inversions in these leads (Fig. 10.12).

## Biventricular Pacing Effects

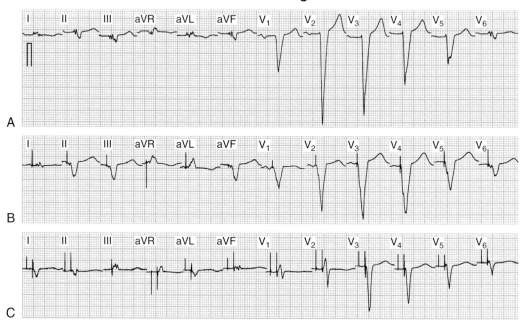

**Fig. 22.10** Effect of biventricular pacing on QRS width and shape. (A) Baseline ECG shows a typical left bundle branch block pattern with QRS duration of 160 msec. (B) Right ventricular apical pacing. QRS duration has increased to 182 msec. (C) Biventricular pacing. Note change in QRS morphology with prominent Q waves in leads I and aVL, and R waves in leads $V_1$ and $V_2$ as the result of early left ventricular activation. Of note, the QRS duration has decreased to 136 msec due to resynchronization effects.

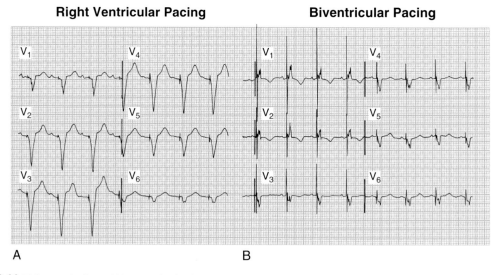

**Fig. 22.11** Right ventricular and biventricular (BiV) pacing. (A) Patient with heart failure who had a standard dual-chamber (right atrial and right ventricular) pacemaker. (B) To improve cardiac function, the pacemaker was upgraded to a biventricular device. Note that during right ventricular pacing (A), the ECG shows a left bundle branch block morphology. The preceding sinus P waves are sensed by the atrial lead. In contrast, during biventricular pacing (BiV), the QRS complexes show a right bundle branch block morphology. Also, the QRS duration is somewhat shorter during BiV pacing, due to the cardiac resynchronization effects of pacing the ventricles in a nearly simultaneous fashion.

## Acute ST Elevation Inferior Wall MI with Ventricular Pacemaker

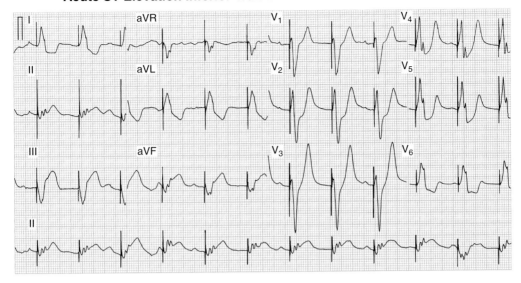

**Fig. 22.12** Temporary transvenous pacing in a patient with acute inferior (posterior) wall ST segment elevation myocardial infarction. Concordant QRS-ST-T pattern in lead II and reciprocal ST segment depressions in leads $V_2$ to $V_6$ during ventricular pacing suggest acute myocardial ischemia (similar to ischemic changes in left bundle branch block). The rhythm strip demonstrates sinus bradycardia with heart block and atrioventricular (AV) dissociation (most likely due to complete AV heart block; see Chapter 17).

## IMPLANTABLE CARDIOVERTER–DEFIBRILLATORS

═══════════════ Key Point ═══════════════

Implantable cardioverter–defibrillators (ICDs) are electronic devices designed to terminate life-threatening ventricular arrhythmias by delivering bursts of antitachycardia pacing (ATP) or internal direct current shocks if needed.

Modern ICD systems resemble pacemakers in appearance, but with slightly larger generators and thicker right ventricular leads (Fig. 22.13). They are both implanted in a similar fashion. ICDs differ from the usual external defibrillation paddles or patches because in ICDs electrical current passes between one or two special coils on the ventricular lead and the generator.

All current ICDs are capable of pacing and can be single-chamber, dual-chamber, or biventricular.

Arrhythmia detection is based primarily on the heart rate and can be programmed in up to several different heart rate zones (for example, slow VT, fast VT, and VF zones at 160, 180, 200 beats/min, respectively). Arrhythmia treatments then can be set up separately in each of the zones (Fig. 22.14) as part of automatic "tiered" (ramped) therapy.

ICDs provide two programmable modalities of treatment for ventricular tachyarrhythmias: antitachycardia pacing (ATP) and direct current (DC) shocks. ATP works by pacing the heart faster than the rate of VT. This mechanism allows penetration of the signal into the reentrant arrhythmia circuit, "breaking" the loop and restoring normal rhythm. ATP terminates approximately 50% of ventricular arrhythmias, avoiding the need for ICD shocks. Unlike shock delivery, ATP is completely painless and usually goes unnoticed by the patient.

If ATP fails to convert the arrhythmia, then up to six consecutive synchronized or unsynchronized shocks can be delivered by the device (see Fig. 12.14). Modern ICD batteries have the capacity to deliver more than 100 shocks and usually last 5–7 years.

Because tachyarrhythmia detection is based on the heart rate, a risk of inappropriate therapies exists for supraventricular tachyarrhythmias with rapid ventricular responses (for example, atrial fibrillation).

## Single-Chamber Implantable Cardioverter-Defibrillator

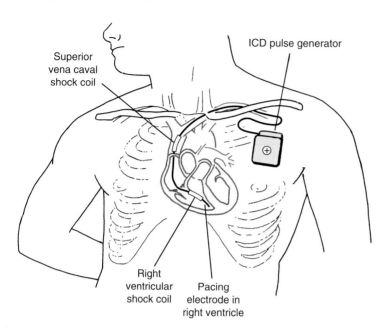

Superior
vena caval
shock coil

ICD pulse generator

Right
ventricular
shock coil

Pacing
electrode in
right ventricle

**Fig. 22.13** An implantable cardioverter-defibrillator (ICD) device resembles a pacemaker with a pulse generator and a lead system. The device can sense potentially lethal ventricular arrhythmias and deliver appropriate electrical therapy, including defibrillatory shocks.

## ICD: Tiered Therapy

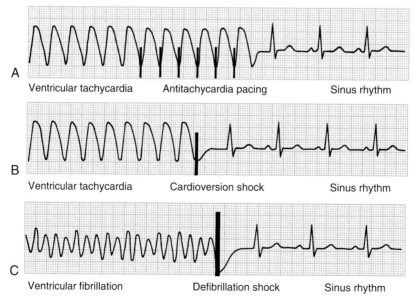

A Ventricular tachycardia     Antitachycardia pacing     Sinus rhythm

B Ventricular tachycardia     Cardioversion shock     Sinus rhythm

C Ventricular fibrillation     Defibrillation shock     Sinus rhythm

**Fig. 22.14** Tiered (staged) arrhythmia therapy and implantable cardioverter–defibrillators (ICDs). These devices are capable of automatically delivering staged therapy in treating ventricular tachycardia (VT) or ventricular fibrillation (VF), including antitachycardia pacing (A) or cardioversion shocks (B) for VT and defibrillation shocks (C) for VF.

## Dual-Chamber Pacemaker Malfunction

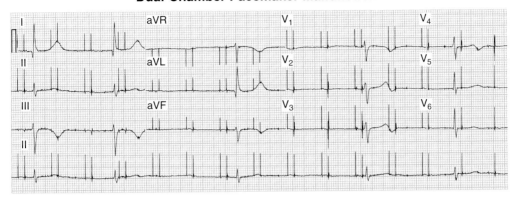

**Fig. 22.15** ECG in magnet mode (DOO) obtained shortly after pacemaker implant shows pairs of atrial and ventricular pacing spikes at the magnet rate. Small P waves following A pacing spikes (stimuli) indicate appropriate atrial capture. In contrast, there is no ventricular response after the V pacing spikes (failure to capture the ventricle). The likely cause here is pacemaker lead dislodgment. Of note is an underlying slow junctional escape rhythm with a markedly prolonged QT interval. LVH is also present.

## Pacemaker Malfunction: Failure to Pace

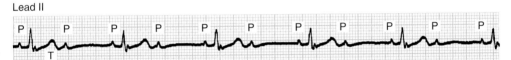

**Fig. 22.16** The underlying rhythm is second-degree (2:1) atrioventricular (AV) block. Despite the very slow QRS, the pacemaker fails to function.

ICDs use sophisticated algorithms to discriminate VT from supraventricular tachycardias (SVTs). However, limited information about arrhythmia mechanism and distinction is obtainable from a single ventricular lead—as such, inappropriate shocks due to SVT occur in approximately 15% of patients.[c] Inappropriate shocks can be very painful and lead to emotional distress.

## RECOGNIZING PACEMAKER AND ICD MALFUNCTION

Pacemakers are very reliable devices and pacemaker malfunctions are rare, especially after the acute post-implant phase. The three most commonly

encountered electrical problems are: failure to capture, failure to sense, and failure to pace.

*Failure to capture* is characterized by appropriately timed pacing stimuli that are not followed by electrical activity of the heart (Fig. 22.15). The most common causes are lead dislodgment, leakage in the pacing circuit, inappropriately set pacing outputs, and an increased pacing threshold due to ischemia, fibrosis, or electrolyte abnormalities (e.g., hyperkalemia).

*Failure to sense* is characterized by excessive and inappropriately timed pacing activity. It can be due to lead dislodgment, inappropriately set sensitivity, or changes in intrinsic signal amplitude due to ischemia, electrolyte abnormalities, or fibrosis. Similar pacemaker behavior can be seen during magnet application (see Fig. 22.17).

*Failure to pace* (Fig. 22.16) is usually due to the pacemaker inhibition by non-cardiac electrical signals, such as from skeletal muscle, the diaphragm, external electromagnetic sources (electrocautery, lithotripsy, MRI machines), or electrical interference

[c]A new advance is the development of a subcutaneous ICD. Instead of using intravenous leads, this device has a single lead implanted subcutaneously in an L-shaped fashion from a generator unit inserted in the left axillary area, parallel to the sternum. The lack of intravascular components minimizes the risk of infectious complications and the need for invasive lead removal. However, current subcutaneous ICDs are *not* capable of providing long-term pacing. Therefore, they are only indicated for selected patients who do not have this requirement.

("noise") created by fractured pacemaker leads. In general, clinicians should be mindful that: (1) oversensing leads to underpacing and (2) undersensing leads to overpacing.

ICDs are much more complex devices and their malfunctions occur more often than with pacemakers. In addition to the pacing malfunctions similar to those described previously, the most important tachyarrhythmia malfunctions include inappropriate therapies (ATP and shocks) for SVT or for oversensing of extracardiac electrical activity (from fractured leads or electromagnetic interference).

Once a device malfunction is suspected, a magnet can be applied over the generator if indicated for emergency management, and a full device interrogation needs to be performed by qualified personnel.

## MAGNET RESPONSE OF PACEMAKERS AND ICDs

Programming and interrogation of pacemakers and ICDs requires vendor-specific equipment and their follow-up is usually carried out by specialized device clinics or specially trained personnel. The majority of the new generation heart rhythm devices are equipped with "home monitors" and can automatically transmit information (including self-checks and arrhythmia reports) to secure websites where they can be viewed by designated healthcare professionals. Pacemakers and ICDs also respond to magnet application, which allows direct interaction with these devices in urgent settings.

The response of pacemakers to magnet application is different from that of ICDs, and varies slightly based on the specific model. In general, magnet application over the pacemaker generator switches the current mode to an "asynchronous" mode (DDD → DOO; VVI → VOO) at a preset *magnet rate* (Fig. 22.17), which varies between manufacturers and indicates the battery status. As the battery is depleted, the magnet rate usually slows.

Thus, the magnet application provides key information about the following "troubleshooting" questions for evaluating an electronic pacemaker:
1. Is there appropriate sensing on both atrial and ventricular channels?
2. Is there appropriate capture on both channels?
3. Is the magnet pacing rate consistent with full battery life or partial depletion? (In the example shown in Fig. 22.17, the magnet rate of 85 beats/min was indicative of full battery life for this manufacturer.)

The magnet response persists as long as the magnet remains close to the generator device header. In contrast, magnet application over an ICD header *does not change its pacing mode*. Instead, the magnet mode, by design, *disables arrhythmia detection*. This response is useful, for example, to prevent further shocks in a patient receiving multiple inappropriate shocks for atrial fibrillation with a rapid ventricular

### Magnet Application in a Dual-Chamber Pacemaker

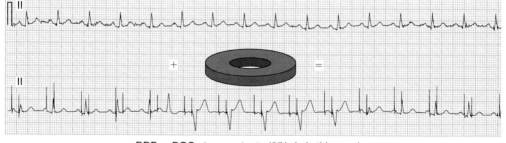

DDD → DOO at magnet rate (85/min in this case)

**Fig. 22.17** Dual-chamber pacemaker response to external magnet application, which switches it from DDD to DOO mode at the "magnet" rate (in this case 85 beats/min). The top tracing shows normal sinus rhythm with preserved atrioventricular (AV) conduction. As the result, pacemaker activity is appropriately inhibited. Switching to DOO mode by magnet application produces a continuous output on both atrial and ventricular pacemaker channels, regardless of intrinsic cardiac activity (bottom tracing). When timed appropriately, both atria and ventricles are captured by the pacemaker as evidenced by different P and QRS morphology (beats #7–11). The other pacemaker stimuli fall into the refractory periods of both atria and ventricles, resulting in stimuli with appropriate non-capture. This scenario is identical to the inappropriate pacing seen in the "failure to sense" situation.

response or because of ICD lead fracture. Of course, while the device is disabled, the patient has to be continuously monitored.

## PACEMAKER AND ICD IMPLANTATION: SPECIFIC USES

Specific clinical indications for device implantation are subject to review and updates by the cardiac specialty societies that operate nationally and internationally.

In general, pacemakers are commonly implanted in three major settings:

- Symptomatic bradycardia or pauses (especially due to sinus node dysfunction or AV heart block) at rest or during exercise. This category also includes abnormalities induced by medications that are essential (e.g., tachy-brady syndrome exacerbated by beta blockers). *Note: Pacemaker implantation is not indicated in asymptomatic sinus bradycardia.*
- Symptomatic conduction abnormalities with high risk of abrupt progression to a life-threatening condition (e.g., Mobitz II second-degree heart block; major conduction abnormalities associated with certain neuromuscular diseases, such as myotonic dystrophy).
- Syncope when causes other than bradycardia (especially sustained VT) have been ruled out.

ICD implantation is indicated for secondary and primary prevention of sudden cardiac death due to ventricular tachyarrhythmias. *Secondary prevention* refers to therapy of patients who have already survived an episode of life-threatening ventricular arrhythmia and, therefore, are at high risk of its recurrence. This group includes:

- Resuscitated victims of cardiac arrest due to VT or VF due to non-reversible causes (for example, *not* associated with acute infarction or metabolic abnormality).
- Patients with sustained VT and structural heart disease (ischemic or nonischemic cardiomyopathy).

*Primary prevention* refers to prophylactic ICD implantation in patients who have never had a cardiac arrest or had documented sustained ventricular arrhythmias but who are considered to be at sufficiently high risk for arrhythmic cardiac death to warrant intervention. This population is comprised primarily of selected patients with symptomatic heart failure and a left ventricular ejection fraction ≤35%. This indication is usually in the context of a prior myocardial infarction (ischemic cardiomyopathy). Patients with symptomatic heart failure due to nonischemic causes may also be candidates for primary (prophylactic) prevention with an ICD. Readers are strongly encouraged to visit the websites of the major cardiology specialty societies for specific indications and evolving recommendations for ICD use.

Finally, we note that a *wearable cardioverter–defibrillator* has been developed for use in selected patients, usually as a temporizing measure in those at high risk of sudden cardiac death who are not (yet) candidates for an implantable unit. This vest-type device is capable of automated detection of ventricular tachycardia and ventricular fibrillation and of shock delivery. Discussion of the uses and limitations of current vest-type devices is outside the scope of this introductory chapter.

---

 Key Point

---

Cardiac resynchronization with biventricular pacing is currently indicated in patients with a wide QRS (LBBB or related intraventricular conduction delay [IVCD]), reduced left ventricular ejection fraction, and heart failure. Often, these patients also qualify for primary prevention of sudden cardiac arrest and receive biventricular ICDs.

---

# CHAPTER 23

# Interpreting ECGs: An Integrative Approach

## ECG READING: GENERAL PRINCIPLES

This review chapter details a systematic approach to ECG analysis. Accurate interpretation of ECGs requires thoroughness and care. Trainees should be encouraged to cultivate a comprehensive disciplined method of reading ECGs that can be applied in every case.

Many of the most common mistakes are errors of omission, specifically the failure to note subtle but critical findings. For example, overlooking a short PR interval may cause you to miss the Wolff–Parkinson–White (WPW) pattern. Marked prolongation of the QT interval and/or prominent U waves, a potential precursor of sudden cardiac arrest due to torsades de pointes (see Chapters 16 and 21), may go unnoticed until a *code blue* is called. Atrial fibrillation is mistaken for other supraventricular tachycardias (e.g., flutter, paroxysmal supraventricular tachycardia [PSVT] or even sinus tachycardia with atrial ectopy) with surprising frequency. Sometimes the diagnosis is missed, with underlying ventricular pacing due to the regularized ventricular response. These and other major, and avoidable, pitfalls in ECG diagnosis are reviewed in Chapter 24.

The most experienced readers approach an ECG in several "takes," much like your expert colleagues examine medical imaging studies. First, get an overall *gestalt*, a "big picture" scan to survey the "lay of the land." Next home in on each of the 14 features below, looking at single leads, usually beginning with the rhythm strip, and then at various sets of leads. This process should be repeated in an iterative way several times before you formulate an integrative interpretation. The final step is writing out a concise summary.

Trainees can more quickly refine their ECG skills if they get into the mode of *testing hypotheses* in the context of working through a differential diagnosis. Take for instance the general finding of sinus rhythm

with *group beating patterns* that are formed by clusters of normal duration QRS complexes. The general differential diagnosis of group beating includes two pathophysiologic mechanisms: prematurity and/or block. Thus, you can address the key question of whether the group beating pattern represents: (1) sinus rhythm with premature atrial complexes, which could be blocked or conducted, vs. (2) sinus rhythm with intermittent block in the atrioventricular (AV) (more rarely sinoatrial [SA]) node. If the nonconducted P waves "march out" with "missing" QRS complexes suggesting second-degree AV block, you should then ask: is the second-degree AV block nodal (Mobitz I) or infranodal (Mobitz II), or is it indeterminate in location (see Chapter 17)?

Also get in the habit of doing your reading with the computer (electronic) analysis, if one is available, covered up. This way you will not be biased or misled. Computer interpretations are frequently incomplete and sometimes partly or fully wrong. Once you have committed to your own reading, take a careful look at the computer interpretation. It may point out something you missed. Conversely, it may miss something you found. Be aware that even computer-measured intervals, which should be the most reliable part of electronic assessments, may need to be amended. This important caveat is discussed further below.

### The Importance of Being Systematic: 14 Points

On every ECG, 14 features (parameters) should be analyzed. These "must-check" items are listed in Box 23.1 and discussed in the next section. Note that items 2–4 are best considered as a group, since they are interrelated. An example is given in Fig. 23.1.

### 1. Standardization (Calibration and Technical Quality)

As a "reading reflex," make sure that the electrocardiograph has been properly calibrated so that the

Please go to expertconsult.inkling.com for additional online material for this chapter.

| BOX 23.1 | Be Systematic: 14 Features to Analyze on Every ECG |
| --- | --- |

1. Standardization (calibration) and technical quality
2. Heart rates(s): atrial and ventricular if not the same
3. Rhythm/AV conduction
4. PR (AV) interval
5. QRS interval (width)
6. QT/QTc intervals
7. QRS axis
8. P waves (width, amplitude, shape)
9. QRS voltages: normal, high or low
10. R wave progression in chest leads
11. Q waves (normal vs. abnormal)
12. ST segments
13. T waves
14. U waves

*Analyzed as a group* (items 2, 3, 4)

standardization mark is 10 mm tall (1 mV = 10 mm) (see Chapter 3). In special cases the ECG may be intentionally recorded at one-half standardization (1 mV = 5 mm) or two times normal standardization (1 mV = 20 mm). However, overlooking this change in gain may lead to the mistaken diagnosis of low or high voltage. The paper speed of 25 mm/sec may also be changed in some situations. Finally, check for limb lead reversal (see Chapter 24) and ECG artifacts (discussed later in this chapter).

## 2. Heart Rate(s): Atrial and Ventricular

Calculate the heart rate(s)—atrial and ventricular (see Chapter 3). Normally, the atrial (P) and ventricular (QRS) rates are the same (sinus rhythm with 1:1 AV conduction), as implied in the term "normal sinus rhythm." If the P or QRS rate is faster than 100 beats/min, a tachycardia is present. A rate slower than 60 beats/min means that a bradycardia is present.

Remember: You can see a combination of both fast and slow rates with certain arrhythmias and

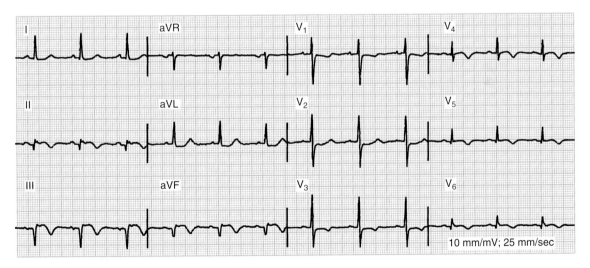

**Fig. 23.1** Twelve-lead ECG for interpretation using the 14 points (see text). (1) Calibration (electronic): 10 mm/mV; 25 mm/sec. (2) Rhythm: sinus (with 1:1 AV conduction). (3) Heart rate: 75 beats/min. (4) PR interval: 0.16 sec. (5) QRS interval: 0.08 sec (normal). (6) QT/QTc intervals: 0.40 sec/0.43 sec (normal). (7) P waves: normal size and morphology. (8) QRS voltages: normal. (9) Mean QRS axis: about 30°. (10) R wave progression in chest leads: early precordial transition with relatively tall R wave in lead $V_2$. (11) Abnormal Q waves: leads II, III, and aVF. (12) ST segments: slightly elevated in leads II, III, aVF, $V_4$, $V_5$, and $V_6$; slightly depressed in leads $V_1$ and $V_2$. (13) T waves: inverted (negative) in leads II, III, aVF, and $V_3$ through $V_6$. (14) U waves: not prominent.
*Summary: Sinus rhythm. Multiple abnormalities consistent with an inferolateral (or infero-postero-lateral) ST elevation/Q wave MI of indeterminate age, possibly recent or evolving. No prior ECG for comparison.*
Additional comments: The relatively tall R wave in lead $V_2$ could reflect loss of lateral potentials or true posterior wall involvement. QTc calculated using Hodges formula (see Chapter 3).

conduction disturbances, e.g., atrial flutter with a slow ventricular rate. If second- or third-degree (complete) heart block is present with underlying sinus rhythm, there will be more P than QRS complexes.

### 3. Rhythm/AV Conduction

The basic heart rhythm(s) and rate(s) are usually summarized together (e.g., sinus bradycardia at a rate of 40 beats/min; atrial fibrillation with a mean ventricular response of 80/min at rest). The cardiac rhythm can almost always be described in one of five categories:

- Sinus rhythm (including sinus bradycardia and sinus tachycardia).
- Sinus rhythm with extra (ectopic) beats, usually premature atrial complexes (PACs) or premature ventricular complexes (PVCs), or sometimes escape beats.
- Ectopic (non-sinus) mechanism, such as paroxysmal supraventricular tachycardia (PSVT; actually a group of arrhythmias), atrial fibrillation or flutter, monomorphic ventricular tachycardia, accelerated idioventricular rhythm (AIVR), or a slow ventricular escape rhythm.
- Sinus rhythm or an ectopic rhythm (e.g., atrial tachycardia) with second- or third-degree AV block. When complete AV heart block is present, you need to specify both the atrial and ventricular components (e.g., sinus rhythm at 70/min with complete AV block and a narrow complex ventricular escape rhythm at 30/min).
- Paced rhythm (single or dual chamber). Note: the rhythm may be fully or partly paced as described in Chapter 22.

If you are unsure of the atrial or ventricular mechanism, give a differential diagnosis if possible. For example, you might say or write: "the rhythm appears to be atrial fibrillation with a noisy baseline, but MAT [multifocal atrial tachycardia] is not excluded." If artifact precludes determining the rhythm with certainty, you should also state that and suggest a repeat ECG if indicated.

### 4. PR (AV) Interval

The normal PR interval (measured from the beginning of the P wave to the beginning of the QRS complex) is 0.12 to 0.2 sec. A uniformly prolonged PR interval is referred to as *first-degree AV block* or preferably, as *PR prolongation* (see Chapter 17). A short PR interval with sinus rhythm and with a wide QRS complex and a delta wave is seen in Wolff–Parkinson–White (WPW) patterns. By contrast, a short PR interval with retrograde P waves (negative in lead II) generally indicates an ectopic (atrial or AV junctional) pacemaker. With atrial fibrillation there is no PR interval. With atrial flutter the "FR" interval is usually not reported as such. With other rhythms, the PR interval is variable, as in second- or third-degree AV blocks or with MAT or wandering atrial pacemaker (WAP).

### 5. QRS Interval (Width or Duration)

Normally the QRS interval is 0.1 sec (100 msec) or less, measured by eye, in all leads (or 110 msec if measured electronically by computer algorithm). The general differential diagnosis of a wide QRS complex is described in Chapter 11. The specific differential diagnosis of wide complex tachycardias is described in Chapter 19.

### 6. QT/QTc Intervals

A prolonged QT/QTc interval, with or without prominent U waves, may be a major clue to electrolyte disturbances (hypocalcemia or hypokalemia) or drug effects/toxicities (e.g., dofetilide, quinidine, procainamide, amiodarone, sotalol, etc.). Shortened QT intervals are most commonly seen with hypercalcemia and digitalis effect, but may be due to a "channelopathy." The finding of a prolonged (or shortened) QT/QTc interval as determined by computer interpretation should always be rechecked manually. Conversely, computers sometimes miss prolonged QT intervals that are actually present. Formulas for computing the calculation of a rate-corrected QT interval (QTc), with physiologic values, are discussed in Chapter 3.

### 7. Mean QRS Electrical Axis

Estimate the mean QRS axis in the frontal plane, usually termed the "QRS axis" or sometimes just "axis." Decide by inspection whether the axis is normal (between −30° and +90-100°) or whether left or right axis deviation is present (see Fig. 6.13), or whether the axis is indeterminate.

### 8. P Waves (Width, Amplitude, and Shape)

Normally the P wave does not exceed 2.5 mm in amplitude and is less than 3 mm (120 msec) wide in all leads. Tall, peaked P waves may be a sign of right atrial overload (formerly called "P pulmonale"). Wide (and sometimes notched P) waves are seen with left atrial abnormality/enlargement (formerly called "P mitrale"). A biphasic P wave with a broad negative component (>40 msec side and 1 mm deep) is also a sign of left atrial abnormality.

## 9. QRS Voltages

Look for signs of right or left ventricular hypertrophy (see Chapter 7). Remember that thin people, athletes, and young adults frequently show tall voltage without left ventricular hypertrophy (LVH).

In contrast, low QRS voltages may result from multiple causes including: anasarca (generalized edema), larger pericardial effusion or pleural effusions, hypothyroidism, emphysema, obesity, diffuse myocardial disease, among others (see Chapter 25).

## 10. R Wave Progression in Chest Leads

Inspect leads $V_1$ to $V_6$ to see if the normal increase in the R/S ratio occurs as you move across the chest (see Chapter 5). The term "slow" (preferable to older designation of "poor") R wave progression (small or absent R waves in leads $V_1$ to $V_3$) refers to a finding that may be a sign of anterior myocardial infarction (MI), but may also be seen in many other settings, including: improper/altered lead placement, LVH, chronic lung disease, left bundle branch block (LBBB), and many other conditions in the absence of infarction.

*Reversed R wave progression* describes abnormally tall R waves in lead $V_1$ that progressively decrease in amplitude. This pattern may occur with a number of conditions, including right ventricular hypertrophy, posterior (or posterolateral) infarction, and (in concert with a pattern simulating a limb lead reversal) with dextrocardia (as part of mirror image *situs inversus*).

## 11. Abnormal Q Waves

Prominent Q waves in leads II, III, and aVF may indicate inferior wall infarction. Prominent Q waves in the anterior leads (I, aVL, and $V_1$ to $V_6$) may indicate anterior wall infarction (see Chapter 9).

## 12. ST Segments

Look for abnormal ST segment elevations or depressions. The J (junction) point is simply the point where the QRS complex meets the ST segment. Recall that J point elevations or depressions are not specific for any abnormality, and may be seen as physiologic variants as part of the benign early repolarization pattern (Chapter 10) or with ischemia or pericarditis.

## 13. T Waves

Inspect the T waves. Normally they are positive in leads with a positive QRS complex. They are also normally positive in leads $V_3$ to $V_6$ in adults, negative in lead aVR, and positive in lead II. The polarity of the T waves in the other extremity leads depends on the QRS electrical axis. (T waves may be normally negative in lead III even in the presence of a vertical QRS axis.) Remember that one of the P waves (with blocked PACs or atrial tachycardia [AT] with block) can "hide" in the T waves, giving it a slightly different appearance from the other T waves.

## 14. U Waves

Look for prominent U waves. These waves, usually most apparent in chest leads $V_2$ to $V_4$, may be a sign of hypokalemia or drug effect or toxicity (e.g., amiodarone, dofetilide, quinidine, or sotalol). Inverted U waves can be seen with myocardial ischemia. Rarely, prominent U waves are related to an inherited long QT syndrome (see Chapter 16).

---

### "IR-WAX" Memory Aid

Students looking for a mnemonic to help recall key features of the ECG can try using "IR-WAX." *I* stands for the four basic groups of *intervals* (heart rate based on RR, PR, QRS, QT/QTc); *R* for *rhythm* (sinus or other); *W* for the five alphabetically named *waves* (P, QRS, ST, T, and U); and *AX* for the mean QRS electrical *axis* in the frontal plane.

---

## Formulating an Interpretation

After you have analyzed the 14 ECG features, you should formulate an overall interpretation based on these details and the integration of these findings in the specific clinical context. The final ECG report usually consists of the following five elements:

- Rate/PR-QRS-QT/QTc intervals/QRS axis (Note: electronic analyses usually include P and T wave axes)
- Rhythm/AV conduction (latter if abnormal)
- Key waveform findings
- Clinical inferences/implications, if appropriate
- Comparison with any prior ECGs; if none, this should be stated. *This comparative assessment is of major importance in clinical ECG assessment and no ECG reading is complete without it.*

For example, your ECG reading for a patient's ECG might state: *"Sinus rhythm with a markedly prolonged QT/QTc interval and prominent U waves. Repolarization prolongation raises consideration of drug effect/toxicity or hypokalemia. These findings are new since the previous ECG of [give date]."*

Another ECG might show: sinus rhythm with very wide P waves, right axis deviation, and a tall R wave in lead $V_1$ (see Fig. 24.1). The clinical inference could be: *"Findings consistent with left atrial abnormality (enlargement) and right ventricular hypertrophy. This constellation raises consideration of mitral stenosis. Findings are more apparent than on the previous ECG of [give date]."*

In yet a third case the overall interpretation might simply state: *"Sinus rhythm. Within normal limits. No previous ECG available for comparison."*

Every ECG abnormality you identify should summon a list of differential diagnostic possibilities (see Chapter 25). *As a clinician responsible for a patient's care, you should search for an explanation of every abnormality found.* For example, if the ECG shows resting sinus tachycardia at 125/min in a 50-year-old woman, you need to find the cause of the very rapid rate. Is it a result of infection/fever, hyperthyroidism, chronic heart failure, hypovolemia, sympathomimetic or other drugs, alcohol withdrawal, or some other cause? If you see signs of marked LVH, is the likely cause valvular heart disease (e.g., severe aortic stenosis or regurgitation), hypertensive heart disease, or cardiomyopathy?

Finally, as a clinician you should also adopt an anticipatory, scientific posture by asking the following questions before and after looking at the ECG: (1) "Based on the history and physical, what ECG findings might be predicted?" For example, you would anticipate signs of right ventricular hypertrophy/right atrial abnormality in a patient with severe primary pulmonary hypertension. (2) As a follow-up, you should ask: "What findings are unexpected?" If the patient just described showed ECG evidence of LVH, that finding would be highly unexpected. Such "outlier" findings may be important clues to a mistaken diagnosis, to an unsuspected abnormality, to an ECG from a different patient, etc. Making predictions and looking for the unexplained and the surprising will help improve your ECG skills and also enhance clinical management. In this way the interpretation of an ECG, more than just "another lab test," becomes an integral part of clinical diagnosis and patient care.

---

> ### ECG Triads (Relatively Specific, but Not Necessarily Sensitive)
>
> A number of ECG findings may come in groups of threes:
> - Renal failure: LVH (hypertension), peaked T waves (hyperkalemia), long QT (ST segment part from hypocalcemia)
> - Wolff-Parkinson-White pattern (in sinus rhythm): short PR, delta wave, and wide QRS
> - Tricyclic antidepressant overdose: sinus tachycardia, wide QRS (often with S wave in lead I) and long QT
> - RVH from pressure overload: tall R in V (often as R or qR complex), right axis QRS deviation and right-mid precordial T wave inversions (right ventricular overload)
> - Pericardial effusion/tamponade: sinus tachycardia, low voltage QRS complexes, and beat-to-beat QRS alternans
> - CHF (dilated cardiomyopathy with reduced left ventricular ejection fraction): LVH by voltage in chest leads, relatively low precordial voltage and slow $r$ wave progression ($V_1$ to $V_4$)

---

## CAUTION: COMPUTERIZED ECG INTERPRETATIONS

Computerized ECG systems are now widely, if not ubiquitously, available. These digital systems provide not only for acquisition and storage of ECG records, but also algorithms for analysis. The computer programs (software) for ECG analysis have become more sophisticated and accurate.

Despite advances, computer ECG analyses still have important limitations and not infrequently are subject to error. Diagnostic errors are most likely with arrhythmias and more complex waveform abnormalities.

*Therefore, computerized interpretations (including measurements of basic ECG intervals and electrical axes) must never be accepted without careful review.*

## ECG ARTIFACTS

The ECG, like any other electronic recording, is subject to numerous artifacts that may interfere with accurate interpretation. Some of the most common of these are described here.

Monitor lead

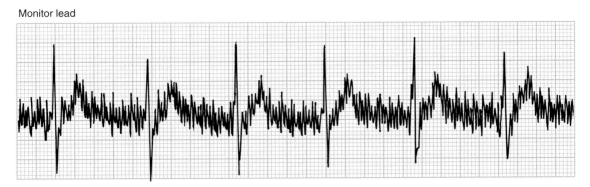

**Fig. 23.2** Magnified view highlights rapid oscillations of the baseline due to 60 cycle/sec (Hertz) alternating current (AC) electrical interference.

Monitor lead

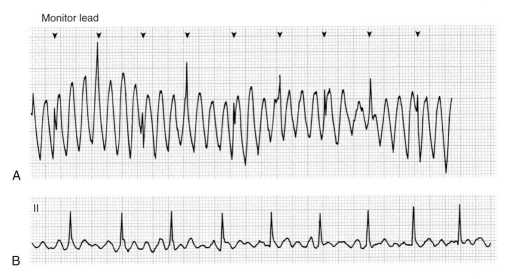

A

II

B

**Fig. 23.3** Artifacts simulating major arrhythmias. (A) Motion artifact mimicking a rapid ventricular tachycardia. The normal QRS complexes (*arrows*) (and largely obscured by the artifact) can be seen at a rate of about 100 beats/min. (B) Parkinsonian tremor causing oscillations of the baseline in lead II that mimic atrial fibrillation. Note the regularity of the QRS complexes, which provides a clue that atrial fibrillation is not present. (Reproduced with permission from Mirvis DM, Goldberger AL. Electrocardiography. In Bonow RO, Mann DL, Zipes DP, Libby P, editors. Braunwald's heart disease. 9th ed. Philadelphia: WB Saunders, 2012; p 163.)

## 60-Hertz (Cycle) and Related Electrical Interference

Interference from alternating current generators produces the characteristic pattern shown in Fig. 23.2. Notice the characteristic "fine-tooth comb" 60-Hertz (Hz) artifacts.[a] You can usually eliminate 60-Hz interference by switching the electrocardio-graph plug to a different outlet or turning off other electrical appliances in the room.

## Muscle Tremor

Involuntary muscle tremor (e.g., Parkinsonism) or voluntary movements (e.g., due to teeth brushing) can produce undulations in the baseline that may be mistaken for atrial flutter or fibrillation or sometimes even ventricular tachycardia (Fig. 23.3).

[a] In Europe and much of Asia this power line interference is at 50 Hz vs. 60 Hz in North America.

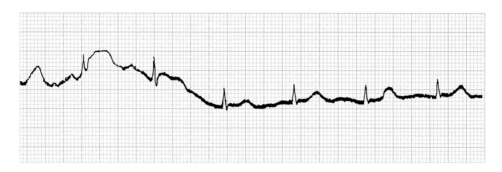

**Fig. 23.4** Wandering baseline resulting from patient movement or loose electrode contact.

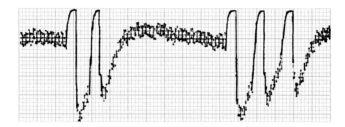

**Fig. 23.5** Deflections simulating ventricular premature beats, produced by patient movement. An artifact produced by 60-Hz interference is also present.

## Poor Electrode Contact or Patient Movement

Upward or downward movement of the baseline may produce spurious ST segment elevations or depressions (Fig. 23.4). Poor electrode contact or patient movement (Figs. 23.4 and 23.5) can also produce artifactual deflections in the baseline that may obscure the underlying pattern or be mistaken for abnormal beats.

## Improper Standardization

The electrocardiograph, as mentioned, should be standardized before each tracing so that a 1-mV pulse produces a square wave 10 mm high (see Fig. 3.1). Failure to standardize properly results in complexes that appear spuriously low or high. Most ECG machines are left in their default mode of 10 mm/mV. However, be aware that electrocardiographs are usually equipped with half-standardization and double-standardization settings.

## Limb Lead Reversal

A common source of error is reversal of ECG leads, which is discussed in Chapter 24.

# CHAPTER 24

# Limitations and Uses of the ECG

We have focused most of our attention on the major clinical uses of the ECG. This review and overview chapter: (1) underscores some important *limitations* of the ECG; (2) reemphasizes its *utility*; and (3) discusses some common *pitfalls* to help clinicians avoid preventable errors.

## IMPORTANT LIMITATIONS OF THE ECG

The diagnostic accuracy of any test is determined by the percentages of false-positive and false-negative results it generates. The *sensitivity* of a test is a measure of the percentage of patients with a particular abnormality that can be identified by an abnormal test result. For example, a test with 100% sensitivity has no false-negative results. The more false-negative results, the less sensitive is the test. The *specificity* of a test is a measure of the percentage of false-positive results. The more false-positive test results, the less specific is the test.

Like most clinical tests, the ECG yields both *false-positive* and *false-negative* results, as previously defined. A false-positive result is exemplified by an apparently abnormal ECG in a normal subject. Prominent precordial voltage may occur in the absence of left ventricular hypertrophy (LVH) (see Chapter 7); Q waves may occur as a normal variant and are not necessarily abnormal (see Chapters 9 and 10). In other cases, Q waves may be abnormal (e.g., due to hypertrophic cardiomyopathy) but lead to a mistaken diagnosis of myocardial infarction (MI).

False-negative results, on the other hand, occur when the ECG fails to show evidence of some cardiac abnormality. Some patients with acute MI may not show diagnostic ST-T changes, and patients with severe coronary artery disease may not show ST segment depressions during stress testing (see Chapters 9 and 10). Furthermore, while the ECG may be strongly *suggestive* of ventricular hypertrophy (LVH) or other chamber enlargement, cardiomyopa-

thy or pericardial effusion, the gold standard for these structural abnormalities is the echocardiogram.

Clinicians need to be aware of these and other major diagnostic limitations. The following are some important problems that *cannot* be excluded simply because the 12-lead ECG is normal or shows only nondiagnostic abnormalities:

- Prior MI
- Acute MI[a]
- Severe coronary artery disease
- LVH
- Right ventricular hypertrophy (RVH)
- Intermittent major arrhythmias such as paroxysmal atrial fibrillation (AF), paroxysmal supraventricular tachycardia (PSVT), ventricular tachycardia (VT), and bradycardias, including complete atrioventricular (AV) block
- Acute pulmonary embolism or chronic pulmonary thromboembolic disease
- Pericarditis, acute or chronic
- Arrhythmogenic right ventricular cardiomyopathy
- Hypertrophic cardiomyopathy

## UTILITY OF THE ECG IN SPECIAL SETTINGS

Although the ECG has definite limitations, it often helps in the diagnosis of specific cardiac conditions and sometimes is an essential aid in the evaluation and management of general medical problems such as life-threatening electrolyte disorders (Box 24.1). Some particular areas in which the ECG may be helpful are described here.

### Myocardial Infarction (MI)

The ECG is pivotal in the diagnosis of ST elevation myocardial infarction (STEMI). Most patients with acute MI show diagnostic or suggestive ECG changes (i.e., ST segment elevations, hyperacute T waves, ST

---

[a]The pattern of acute MI may also be masked in patients with left bundle branch block (LBBB), Wolff–Parkinson–White (WPW) preexcitation patterns, or with electronic ventricular pacemaking.

depressions, or T wave inversions, and sometimes new Q waves). However, in the weeks and months after an acute MI these changes may become less apparent and in some cases may even disappear.

ST segment elevation in right chest precordial leads (e.g., $V_3R$ to $V_6R$ and occasionally $V_1$ and $V_2$) in a patient with acute inferior infarction points to associated right ventricular ischemia or infarction (see Chapter 9).

Persistent ST elevations several weeks after a Q-wave MI should suggest a ventricular aneurysm.

The pattern of acute STEMI can be exactly mimicked by takotsubo (stress) cardiomyopathy and other conditions (Chapter 9).

## Acute Pulmonary Embolism

A new $S_1Q_3T_3$ pattern or right bundle branch block (RBBB) pattern, particularly in association with sinus tachycardia and tall P waves, should suggest the possibility of acute right heart overload (acute cor pulmonale) resulting from acute pulmonary embolism (see Chapter 12). However, this constellation of findings is not specific and may occur with other causes, including acute pneumonitis or severe asthma. Also the sensitivity of the ECG is limited in pulmonary embolism—acute or chronic.

## Pericardial Tamponade

Low QRS voltage in a patient with elevated central venous pressure (distended neck veins) and sinus tachycardia suggests possible pericardial tamponade. The triad of sinus tachycardia with electrical alternans, and relatively low voltage is virtually diagnostic of pericardial effusion with tamponade (see Chapter 12).

## Aortic Valve Disease

LVH is seen in most patients with severe aortic stenosis or severe aortic regurgitation.

## Mitral Valve Disease

ECG signs of left atrial enlargement (abnormality) with concomitant RVH suggest mitral stenosis (Fig. 24.1). Frequent premature ventricular complexes may occur in association with mitral valve prolapse, especially with severe mitral regurgitation.

## Atrial Septal Defect

Most patients with a moderate to large atrial (ostium secundum) septal defect (ASD) have RBBB patterns with right axis deviation. Patients with an ostium primum ASD (less common, and often with other associated congenital defects) are likely to have RBBB patterns with left axis deviation. However, even with relatively large ASDs, the ECG may fail to show classic changes.

## Hyperkalemia

Severe hyperkalemia, a life-threatening electrolyte abnormality, virtually always produces ECG changes, beginning with T wave peaking, loss of P waves, QRS widening, and finally asystole (see Chapter 11).

## Renal Failure

The triad of LVH (caused by hypertension), peaked T waves (caused by hyperkalemia), and a prolonged QT interval (caused by hypocalcemia) should suggest chronic renal failure.

## Thyroid Disease

The combination of low voltage and sinus bradycardia should suggest possible *hypothyroidism*. ("Low and slow—think hypo.") Nonspecific T wave flattening is usually seen.

Unexplained AF (or sinus tachycardia at rest) should prompt a search for *hyperthyroidism*. However, most patients with atrial fibrillation do not have hyperthyroidism.

## Chronic Lung Disease

The combination of low voltage and slow precordial R wave progression (usually with prominent S waves in $V_4$ to $V_6$) is commonly seen with chronic obstructive lung disease (see Chapter 12). Peaked P waves

**Severe Mitral Stenosis**

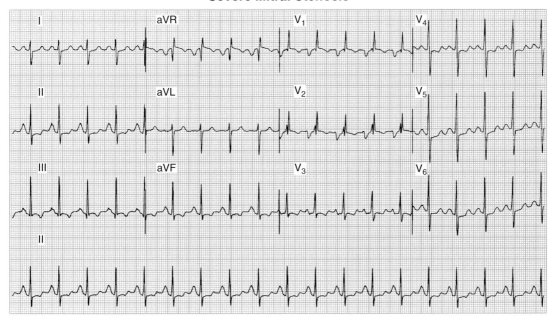

**Fig. 24.1** ECG from a 45-year-old woman with severe mitral stenosis (due to rheumatic heart disease) shows multiple abnormalities. The rhythm is sinus tachycardia. Right axis deviation and a tall R wave (as part of narrow qR) in lead $V_1$ are consistent with right ventricular hypertrophy. The prominent biphasic P wave in lead $V_1$ indicates left atrial abnormality. The tall P wave in lead II may indicate concomitant right atrial enlargement (i.e., biatrial abnormality). Nonspecific ST-T changes and incomplete right bundle branch block (rSr' in $V_2$) are also present. The combination of right ventricular hypertrophy and prominent left atrial abnormality (or atrial fibrillation) is highly suggestive of mitral stenosis.

(indicating right atrial abnormality) and right-mid precordial T wave inversions (from right ventricular overload) may also be present.

## Dilated Cardiomyopathy

The ECG-CHF (chronic heart failure) triad of relatively low limb lead QRS voltage, prominent precordial voltage, and slow R wave progression ($V_1$ to $V_4$) suggests an underlying heart failure syndrome with low left ventricular ejection fraction (see Chapter 12). The pattern has moderate specificity but low sensitivity. The pattern also does not indicate whether the heart failure syndrome is due to ischemic or nonischemic causes.

## SOME OTHER MEDICAL APPLICATIONS OF THE ECG

The ECG may also provide important and immediately available clues in the evaluation of four major medical problems: syncope, coma, shock, and weakness.

## Syncope

Fainting (transient loss of consciousness) can result from primary cardiac factors (those directly involving the heart and great vessels) and a variety of non-cardiac causes. The primary cardiac causes can be usefully divided into those with (1) mechanical obstructions (e.g., aortic stenosis and other causes of left ventricular outflow tract obstruction, primary pulmonary hypertension, or left atrial myxoma); (2) mechanical insufficiency (markedly low cardiac output); and (3) electrical problems (severe bradyarrhythmias or tachyarrhythmias). Non-cardiac causes of transient loss of consciousness include neurogenic mechanisms (e.g., vasovagal attacks), orthostatic (postural) hypotension, and brain dysfunction from vascular insufficiency, seizures, or metabolic derangements (e.g., acute or chronic alcohol abuse or hypoglycemia).

Patients with syncope possibly as a result of critical aortic stenosis generally show LVH on their resting ECG. Primary pulmonary hypertension is most common in young and middle-aged adult women and the ECG generally shows signs of RVH. The presence of frequent PVCs may be a clue to intermittent sustained VT. Evidence of a previous Q wave MI in a patient presenting with syncope should suggest the possibility of sustained monomorphic VT. Syncope with QT(U) prolongation should suggest torsades de pointes, a potentially lethal ventricular arrhythmia (see Chapter 16). A severe bradycardia (usually from high-degree AV heart block, and sometimes with torsades de pointes) in a patient with syncope constitutes the Stokes–Adams (or Adams–Stokes) syndrome (see Chapter 17).

In some cases serious arrhythmias can be detected only when long-term monitoring is performed (see Chapter 4). Syncope in a patient with ECG evidence of "bifascicular block" (e.g., RBBB with marked left axis deviation) should prompt a search for intermittent second- or third-degree heart block or for ventricular tachyarrhythmias. Syncope in patients taking dofetilide, sotalol, quinidine and other "antiarrhythmic" drugs may occur due to torsades de pointes or other arrhythmias. Syncope in patients with AF may result from long pauses after spontaneous conversion to sinus rhythm, an example of the *tachy-brady* syndrome (see Chapters 13, 15 and 19).

Carefully selected patients with *unexplained syncope* may benefit from invasive electrophysiologic testing. During these studies the placement of intracardiac catheters permits more direct and controlled assessment of atrial activity, AV conduction, and the susceptibility to sustained ventricular or supraventricular tachycardias. Other patients with unexplained syncope and suspected brady- or tachyarrhythmias may require long-term implantable cardiac monitors for definitive diagnosis (Chapter 4).

## Coma

An ECG should be obtained in all comatose patients. If coma is from MI with subsequent cardiac arrest (hypoxic brain damage), diagnostic ECG changes related to the infarct are usually seen. Subarachnoid hemorrhage or certain other types of central nervous system pathology may cause very deep T wave inversions (see Chapter 10), simulating the changes of MI. When coma is associated with severe hypercalcemia, the QT interval is often short. Myxedema coma generally presents with ECG evidence of sinus bradycardia and low voltage, with nonspecific ST-T changes. Widening of the QRS complex in a comatose patient should also always raise the possibility of drug overdose (e.g., tricyclic antidepressant) or of hyperkalemia. The triad of a wide QRS, a prolonged QT interval, and sinus tachycardia, in particular, should suggest tricyclic antidepressant overdose (Chapter 11).

## Shock

An ECG should be obtained promptly in patients with severe hypotension because MI is the major cause of cardiogenic shock. In other cases, hypotension may be caused or worsened by a sustained bradyarrhythmia or tachyarrhythmia. Finally, some patients with shock from non-cardiac causes (e.g., hypovolemia or diabetic ketoacidosis) may have myocardial ischemia and sometimes MI induced by their initial problem.

## Weakness

An ECG may be helpful in evaluating patients with unexplained weakness. Atrial fibrillation may present with weakness or fatigue. Elderly or diabetic patients, in particular, may have relatively "silent" MIs with minimal or atypical symptoms, such as the onset of fatigue or general weakness. Distinctive ECG changes may also occur with certain pharmacologic and metabolic factors (e.g., hypokalemia or hypocalcemia) that cause weakness (see Chapter 11).

## REDUCING MEDICAL ERRORS: COMMON PITFALLS IN ECG INTERPRETATION

Reducing and eliminating preventable medical errors are central preoccupations of contemporary practice. ECG misinterpretations are an important source of such errors, which include under- and over-diagnosis. For example, failing to recognize AF puts a patient at increased risk for stroke and other thromboembolic events. Missing AF with an underlying ventricular pacemaker (the pulse and the QRS will often be regular during pacing) is a common and important diagnostic oversight (see Chapter 22). At the same time, mistaking multifocal atrial tachycardia (MAT) or baseline artifact for AF can lead to inappropriate anticoagulation.

You can help minimize errors in interpreting ECGs by taking care to analyze *all* the points listed in the first section of Chapter 23. Many mistakes result from the failure to be systematic. Other mistakes result from confusing ECG patterns that are "look-alikes." Important reminders are provided in Box 24.2. Some common pitfalls in ECG interpretation are discussed further here.

- Unless recognized and corrected, inadvertent reversal of limb lead electrodes can cause diagnostic confusion. For example, reversal of the left and right arm electrodes usually causes an apparent rightward QRS axis shift as well as an abnormal P wave axis that simulates an ectopic atrial rhythm (Fig. 24.2). As a general rule, *when lead I shows a negative P wave and a negative QRS, reversal of the left and right arm electrodes should be suspected.*
- Voltage can appear abnormal if standardization is not checked. ECGs are sometimes mistakenly thought to show "high" or "low" voltage when the voltage is actually normal but the standardization marker is set at half standardization or two times normal gain.
- Atrial flutter with 2:1 AV block is one of the most commonly missed diagnoses. The rhythm is often incorrectly identified as sinus tachycardia (mistaking part of a flutter wave for a true P wave) or PSVT. *When you see a regular narrow complex tachycardia with a ventricular rate of about 150 beats/ min, you should always consider atrial flutter as well as a PSVT variant* (see Chapters 14 and 15).
- Coarse AF and atrial flutter are sometimes confused. When the fibrillatory (f) waves are prominent (coarse), the rhythm is commonly mistaken for

| BOX 24.2 | Minimizing ECG Misinterpretation: Some Important Reminders |

- Check standardization (calibration).
- Exclude limb lead reversal. (For example, a negative P wave with a negative QRS complex in lead I suggests a left/right arm electrode switch.) Other unexpected patterns may be present with other combinations of limb lead reversal, causing confusion.
- Look for hidden P waves, which may indicate atrioventricular (AV) block, blocked atrial premature beats, or atrial tachycardia with block.
- With a regular narrow complex tachycardia at about 150 beats/min at rest, consider atrial flutter with 2:1 AV block versus paroxysmal supraventricular tachycardia or (less likely, especially in the very elderly) sinus tachycardia.
- With group beating (clusters of QRS complexes), consider Mobitz type I (Wenckebach) or II block or blocked premature atrial complexes.
- With wide QRS complexes and with short PR intervals, consider Wolff-Parkinson–White preexcitation.
- With wide QRS complexes without P waves, or with AV block, think of hyperkalemia.

## Lead Reversal

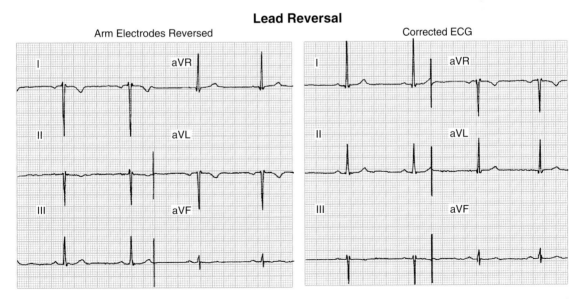

**Fig. 24.2** Whenever the QRS axis is unusual, limb lead reversal may be the culprit. Most commonly, the left and right arm electrodes become switched so that lead I shows a negative P wave and a negative QRS complex.

atrial flutter. However, with AF the ventricular rate is erratic, and the atrial waves are not exactly consistent from one segment to the next. With pure atrial flutter, the atrial waves are identical from one moment to the next, even when the ventricular response is variable. Furthermore, with atrial flutter when the block is variable, the RR intervals will either show a consistent degree of block or as some type of nonrandom patterning. In contrast, with atrial fibrillation, the RR intervals are erratic, without any pattern or predictability (see Chapter 15).

- The Wolff–Parkinson–White (WPW) pattern is sometimes mistaken for bundle branch block, hypertrophy, or infarction because the preexcitation results in a wide QRS complex, sometimes with increased QRS voltage (due to uncancelled forces), secondary T wave inversions, and Q waves (due to negative delta waves), as described in Chapter 18.

- Isorhythmic AV dissociation and complete AV heart block can be confused. With isorhythmic AV dissociation, the SA and AV node pacemakers become "desynchronized," and the QRS rate is the same as or slightly faster than the P wave rate (see Chapter 17). With complete heart block, the atria and ventricles also beat independently, but the ventricular rate is typically much slower than the atrial (sinus) rate. Consequently, there are more P waves than QRS complexes. Isorhythmic AV dissociation is usually a minor arrhythmia and often transient, although it may reflect conduction disease or drug toxicity (e.g., digitalis, diltiazem, verapamil, and beta blockers). Complete AV heart block is always a major arrhythmia and generally requires consideration of pacemaker therapy, unless reversible factors are identified.

- Normal variant and pathologic Q waves require special attention. Remember that Q waves may be a normal variant as part of QS waves in leads aVR, aVL, aVF, III, $V_1$, and occasionally $V_2$ (see Chapter 10). Small "septal" q waves (as part of qR waves), due to normal septal depolarization, may occur in leads I, II, III, aVL, and aVF as well as in the left chest leads ($V_4$ to $V_6$). These septal Q waves are less than 0.04 sec in duration. On the other hand, small pathologic Q waves may be overlooked because they are not always very deep, but are wide (e.g., >0.04 sec). In some cases it may not be possible to state definitively whether or not a Q wave is pathologic. The reading may

indicate this uncertainty by stating that: "*Nondiagnostic Q waves are present in* ... [state the leads]."

- Sinus rhythm with Mobitz type I (Wenckebach) or Mobitz II second-degree AV block are commonly missed diagnoses. "Group beating" is an important clue to these problems (see Chapter 17). With AV Wenckebach, the QRS complexes become grouped in clusters because of the intermittent failure of AV nodal conduction. The PR interval after the nonconducted ("dropped") P wave is shorter than the last one to conduct to the ventricles. Sinus rhythm with Mobitz type II AV block may also cause group beating pattern due to an intermittently nonconducted P wave. While Mobitz II AV block is often misdiagnosed as complete heart block, it is important to remember that, in the latter case, the ventricular rate is almost invariably very slow and regular (i.e., there is no group beating) and the PR intervals will vary throughout.

- Hidden P waves may lead to mistakes in the diagnosis of a number of arrhythmias, including blocked premature atrial complexes (PACs), atrial tachycardia (paroxysmal or sustained) with block, and second- or third-degree (complete) AV block. Therefore, clinicians should make it a routine part of interpretation to actively scan the ST segment and T wave for "buried" P waves (see Chapters 17 and 19).

- LBBB patterns may be mistaken for infarction because they are associated with very slow R wave progression and often ST elevation (including J point) elevation in the right chest leads.

- U waves are sometimes overlooked. Small U waves (≤1 mm or less in amplitude) are a physiologic finding, but large U waves (which may be apparent in only the mid-chest leads) are an important marker of hypokalemia or drug toxicity (e.g., dofetilide, sotalol or quinidine). Large U waves are associated with increased risk of torsades de pointes (see Chapter 16). Inverted (negative) U waves in leads with positive T waves are rare, and have been associated with myocardial ischemia or left ventricular hypertrophy.

- Severe hyperkalemia must be considered immediately in any patient with an unexplained wide QRS complex, particularly if P waves are not apparent. Delay in making this diagnosis can be fatal because severe hyperkalemia may lead to asystole and cardiac arrest while the clinician is waiting for the laboratory report (see Chapter 11).

## ECGs: PAST, PRESENT, AND FUTURE

We conclude with a few thoughts on the past and future of electrocardiography. Less than a handful of technologies—introduced into clinical practice more than 100 years ago—now exist in a form that would be recognizable to their inventors. The ECG, developed by Dutch physicist/physiologist Dr. Willem Einthoven, was introduced in the early 1900s. Einthoven's work was based directly on the seminal contributions of others, notably August T. Waller, the British physiologist whose group reported the recording of a human ECG using a device called a capillary electrometer (1887).

Since that formative era, much has changed with respect to the electronics of the ECG, going beyond the addition of the nine other standard leads (and supplemental ones, such as right and left lateral chest leads, as well as vector leads). But the essence of the original, clinical time-voltage recording as developed by Einthoven, standing on the shoulders of Waller and others, would be fully recognizable by these pioneers and their contemporaries, including the basic P-QRS-T sequence. For his exceptional contributions, Einthoven was awarded the Nobel Prize in Physiology or Medicine in 1924. One of the few comparable examples of a technology with such an enduring impact on modern medicine would be William Conrad Roentgen's discovery of X-rays (Nobel Prize in Physics, 1901).

The further development of wearable technology to allow long-term monitoring of the ECG for detection of intermittent arrhythmias is an area where emerging, imaginative technologies may foster improvements in diagnosis, prevention, and care. Another potentially exciting area of translational ECG research concerns the use of modern signal analysis techniques to extract additional information from the ECG signal. For example, as briefly mentioned in the supplemental material, the information in beat-to-beat heart rate variations may provide a window into the functional status of the control network linking the neuroautonomic system, the lungs, and the heart, in health and disease.

We do anticipate that the ECG in its current and electronically-evolving forms will likely remain a mainstay of clinical diagnosis and therapy for the indefinite future. This prediction is made in light of the ECG's central importance in cardiology and critical care, as well as virtually all other fields of clinical medicine. We anticipate basic advances in ECG diagnosis related to correlative studies with magnetic resonance imaging, intracardiac recordings, and echocardiography, as well as technical advances in data recording, storage, and communication. Computer (electronic) algorithms for interpreting ECGs may improve and become more sophisticated, but over-reading and review by a physician or other trained caregiver will remain essential in optimal, personalized patient care (see Chapter 1).

# CHAPTER 25
# ECG Differential Diagnoses: Instant Replays

This chapter presents a series of boxes that summarize selected aspects of ECG differential diagnosis for easy reference. For the most part, these boxes recap topics covered in this book previously. However, some more advanced topics are briefly mentioned, with additional discussions available in the references cited in the Bibliography.

---

### Low Voltage QRS Complexes

1. Artifactual or spurious, e.g., unrecognized standardization of the ECG at half the usual gain (i.e., 5 mm/mV). Always check both limb and chest leads!
2. Adrenal insufficiency (Addison's disease)
3. Anasarca (i.e., generalized edema, involving upper and lower body)
4. Cardiac infiltration or replacement (especially with amyloid or tumor)
5. Cardiac transplantation, especially with acute or chronic rejection
6. Cardiomyopathies: dilated, hypertrophic, or restrictive types*
7. Chronic obstructive pulmonary disease
8. Constrictive pericarditis
9. Hypothyroidism/myxedema (usually with sinus bradycardia)
10. Left pneumothorax (mid-left chest leads)
11. Myocardial infarction, usually extensive
12. Myocarditis, acute or chronic
13. Normal variant
14. Obesity
15. Pericardial effusion/tamponade (latter usually with sinus tachycardia)
16. Pleural effusion

---

*Dilated cardiomyopathies may be associated with a paradoxical combination of relatively low limb lead voltage and prominent precordial voltage (Chapter 12).

---

### Wide QRS Complex (Normal Rate)

I. Intrinsic intraventricular conduction delays (IVCDs)*
   A. Left bundle branch block and variants
   B. Right bundle branch block and variants
   C. Other (nonspecific) patterns of IVCD
II. Extrinsic ("toxic") intraventricular conduction delay (ICVD)
   A. Hyperkalemia
   B. Drugs: class 1 antiarrhythmic drugs (e.g., flecainide) and other sodium channel blocking agents (e.g., tricyclic antidepressants and phenothiazines)
III. Ventricular beats: premature, escape, or paced
IV. Ventricular preexcitation: Wolff-Parkinson-White (WPW) pattern and variants

---

*Bundle branch block patterns may occur transiently. Note also that a spuriously wide QRS complex occurs if the ECG is unintentionally recorded at fast paper speeds (50 or 100 mm/sec).

---

### Left Axis Deviation (QRS Axis of —30° or More Negative)

I. Left ventricular hypertrophy
II. Left anterior fascicular block/hemiblock (strictly, —45° or more negative, typically with qR waves in lead aVL and sometimes I, and rS complexes in the inferior leads)
III. Inferior wall myocardial infarction (typically with QS or rS waves in two or more of leads II, III, and aVF)
IV. Endocardial cushion defects (congenital), especially ostium primum atrial septal defects

---

## Right Axis Deviation (QRS Axis of +90–100° or More Positive)

I. Spurious (artifactual), most commonly due to left–right arm electrode reversal (look for negative P wave and negative QRS complex in lead I)
II. Normal variant, especially in children and young adults
III. Dextrocardia ("mirror image" type, usually with situs inversus)
IV. Right ventricular overload syndromes
   A. Acute (e.g., pulmonary embolus or severe asthma attack)
   B. Chronic
      1. Chronic obstructive pulmonary disease
      2. Any cause of right ventricular hypertrophy (e.g., pulmonary stenosis, ostium secundum atrial septal defects, chronic thromboembolic pulmonary hypertension, primary pulmonary hypertension, pulmonary sarcoidosis)
V. Lateral wall myocardial infarction (usually with pathologic Q waves in I and aVL)
VI. Left posterior (hemiblock) fascicular block. RS\rS complexes typically present in leads I and aVL. Note: need to exclude all other causes of right axis deviation and rigorously requires marked rightward axis (+110–120° or more) in adults.

## QT(U) Prolongation (Long QT Patterns/Syndromes)

I. Acquired long QT syndrome
   A. Electrolyte abnormalities
      1. Hypocalcemia
      2. Hypokalemia
      3. Hypomagnesemia
   B. Drugs
      1. Class 1A or 3 antiarrhythmic agents (e.g., quinidine, procainamide, disopyramide, dofetilide, ibutilide, sotalol, amiodarone, and dronedarone)
      2. Psychotropic agents (e.g., phenothiazines, tricyclic antidepressants, tetracyclic agents, atypical antipsychotic agents, haloperidol)
      3. Many others: arsenic trioxide, chloroquine, methadone, certain antibiotics (e.g., erythromycin, levofloxacin, and pentamidine), etc.
   C. Myocardial ischemia or infarction (especially, with deep T wave inversions)
   D. Cerebrovascular injury (e.g., intracranial bleeds)
   E. Bradyarrhythmias (especially high-grade AV heart block)
   F. Systemic hypothermia
   G. Miscellaneous conditions
      1. Liquid protein diets
      2. Starvation
      3. Arsenic poisoning
II. Congenital (hereditary) long QT syndromes (LQTS)
   A. Romano-Ward syndrome* (autosomal dominant disorders)
   B. Jervell and Lange-Nielsen syndrome (autosomal recessive disorder, associated with congenital sensorineural deafness)

*The Romano-Ward syndrome is the classic, general term used to designate a growing number of specific, inherited abnormalities in ion channel function ("channelopathies") that are associated with prolongation of ventricular repolarization (long QT-U) and increased risk of torsades de pointes (TdP; see Chapter 16). These hereditary ion channel (potassium, sodium, or calcium) disorders can prolong and increase heterogeneity of ventricular repolarization and promote *early afterdepolarizations* as a prelude to TdP.

### Q Waves

I. Physiologic or positional factors
   A. Lead misplacements, e.g., left–right arm electrodes; chest electrodes
   B. Normal variant septal Q waves (I, $V_5$, $V_6$)
   C. Normal variant QS waves in $V_1$ to $V_2$ (rare), qR complexes in aVL, III, and aVF, $V_5$, $V_6$; also occasionally QS or QR complexes in III, aVF, aVL
   D. Left pneumothorax (loss of lateral R wave progression)
   E. Dextrocardia with situs inversus (loss of R wave progression $V_1$ to $V_6$, with reversal of usual pattern in leads I, aVL, aVR, etc.)
II. Myocardial injury or infiltration
   A. Acute processes
      1. Myocardial ischemia or infarction
      2. Myocarditis
      3. Hyperkalemia
   B. Chronic processes
      1. Myocardial infarction
      2. Idiopathic cardiomyopathy
      3. Myocarditis
      4. Amyloidosis
      5. Tumor
      6. Sarcoidosis
III. Ventricular hypertrophy or enlargement
   A. Left ventricular hypertrophy (slow R wave progression*)
   B. Right ventricular hypertrophy (reversed R wave progression**) or slow R wave progression (particularly with chronic obstructive lung disease)
   C. Hypertrophic cardiomyopathy (may simulate anterior, inferior, posterior, or lateral infarcts)
IV. Conduction abnormalities
   A. Left bundle branch block (slow R wave progression*)
   B. Wolff–Parkinson–White (WPW) patterns (leads with negative delta waves)

### Tall R Wave in Lead $V_1$

I. Physiologic and positional factors
   A. Misplacement of chest leads
   B. Normal variants
   C. Displacement of heart toward right side of chest
II. Myocardial injury
   A. Posterior or lateral myocardial infarction
   B. Duchenne muscular dystrophy (due to posterobasal fibrosis)
III. Ventricular enlargement
   A. Right ventricular hypertrophy (usually with QRS right axis deviation)
   B. Hypertrophic cardiomyopathy
IV. Altered ventricular depolarization
   A. Right ventricular conduction abnormalities
   B. Wolff–Parkinson–White patterns (caused by posterior or lateral wall preexcitation)

*Small or absent R waves are seen in the right to mid-precordial leads.
**The R wave amplitude decreases progressively from lead $V_1$ to the mid-lateral precordial leads.

## ST Segment Elevations

I. Myocardial ischemia/infarction
   A. Transient transmural ischemia without infarction: Prinzmetal's angina pattern and some cases of takotsubo ("stress") cardiomyopathy
   B. Transmural myocardial ischemia with infarction not due to obstructive coronary disease: especially severe takotsubo cardiomyopathy*
   C. Acute myocardial infarction (MI) due to atherosclerotic coronary occlusion
   D. Post-MI (ventricular aneurysm pattern)
II. Acute pericarditis
III. Normal variant (benign "early repolarization" and related patterns)
IV. Left ventricular hypertrophy/left bundle branch block ($V_1$ to $V_2$ or $V_3$ and other leads with QS or rS waves, only)
V. Brugada patterns (right bundle branch block patterns with ST elevations in right precordial leads)
VI. Myocardial injury (noncoronary injury or infarction)
   A. Myocarditis (ECG may resemble myocardial infarction or pericarditis patterns)
   B. Tumor invading the left ventricle
   C. Trauma to the ventricles
   D. Acute right ventricular ischemia (usually $V_1$ to $V_2/V_3$, e.g., with massive pulmonary embolism)
VII. Hypothermia (J waves/Osborn waves)
VIII. Hyperkalemia (usually localized to $V_1$ to $V_2$)
IX. Ventricular paced rhythms

*May exactly simulate ECG sequence of acute ST elevation MI due to atherosclerotic coronary disease.

## ST Segment Depressions

I. Myocardial ischemia or infarction
   A. Acute subendocardial ischemia or non-Q wave myocardial infarction
   B. Reciprocal change with acute ST elevation ischemia (e.g., ST depression in $V_1$ to $V_2$ with acute ST elevation with a posterolateral MI)
II. Abnormal non-coronary patterns
   A. Left or right ventricular hypertrophy ("strain" pattern)
   B. Takotsubo cardiomyopathy
   C. Secondary ST-T changes (in leads with predominant, wide R waves)
      1. Left bundle branch block
      2. Right bundle branch block
      3. Wolff–Parkinson–White preexcitation pattern
   D. Drugs (e.g., digitalis)
   E. Metabolic conditions (e.g., hypokalemia)
   F. Miscellaneous conditions (e.g., cardiomyopathy)
III. Physiologic and normal variants*

*With physiologic and normal variants the very transient ST segment/J point depressions are usually less than 1 mm and are seen especially with exertion or hyperventilation.

## Deep T Wave Inversions

  I. Normal variants
    A. Juvenile T wave pattern
    B. Early repolarization variants
  II. Myocardial ischemia/infarction due to obstructive coronary disease
  III. Takotsubo (stress; apical ballooning) cardiomyopathy
  IV. Cerebrovascular accident (especially intracranial bleeds) and related neurogenic patterns
  V. Left or right ventricular overload
    A. Typical patterns (formerly referred to as "strain" patterns)
    B. Apical hypertrophic cardiomyopathy (Yamaguchi syndrome)
    C. Chronic or acute pulmonary thromboembolism
  VI. Idiopathic global T wave inversion syndrome
  VII. Secondary T wave alterations: bundle branch blocks, Wolff-Parkinson-White patterns
  VIII. Intermittent left bundle branch block, preexcitation, or ventricular pacing (*memory T wave syndrome*)

## Tall, Positive T Waves

  I. Nonischemic causes
    A. Normal variants (early repolarization patterns)
    B. Hyperkalemia
    C. Cerebrovascular hemorrhage (more commonly, T wave inversions)
    D. Left ventricular hypertrophy
    E. Right precordial leads, usually in conjunction with left precordial ST segment depressions and T wave inversions
    F. Left precordial leads, particularly in association with "diastolic overload" conditions (e.g., aortic or mitral regurgitation)
    G. Left bundle branch block (right precordial leads)
    H. Acute pericarditis (occasionally)
  II. Ischemic causes
    A. Hyperacute phase of myocardial infarction
    B. Acute transient transmural ischemia (Prinzmetal's angina)
    C. Chronic (evolving) phase of myocardial infarction (tall positive T waves reciprocal to primary deep T wave inversions)

## Major Bradycardias

  I. Sinus bradycardia and its variants, including sinus arrest/sinus pauses, sinoatrial block and wandering atrial pacemaker (WAP)
  II. Atrioventricular (AV) heart block or dissociation
    A. Second- or third-degree AV block*
    B. Isorhythmic AV dissociation and related variants
  III. Junctional (AV nodal) and slow ectopic atrial escape rhythms
  IV. Atrial fibrillation or flutter with a slow ventricular response
  V. Ventricular escape (idioventricular) rhythms

*AV heart block may occur with sinus rhythm or with other rhythms (e.g., complete heart block with atrial fibrillation or flutter).

## Narrow Complex Tachycardias (NCTs)

I. Sinus tachycardia (physiologic) and rare pathophysiologic variants*

II. Paroxysmal (non-sinus) supraventricular tachycardias (PSVTs)
  A. Atrioventricular (AV) nodal reentrant tachycardia (AVNRT)
  B. Atrioventricular reentrant tachycardia (AVRT) (orthodromic, i.e., with retrograde conduction up the bypass tract); formerly called circus movement tachycardia or AV reciprocating tachycardia
  C. Atrial tachycardias, including unifocal and multifocal (MAT) variants
  D. Accelerated AV junctional rhythms (due to enhanced automaticity)**

III. Atrial flutter with 1:1, 2:1, or variable AV conduction†

IV. Atrial fibrillation with a rapid ventricular response

*Unusual (and rare) variants of physiologic sinus tachycardia include sinus node reentrant tachycardia, sinus tachycardia with idiopathic postural syncope (POTS) syndrome, and other idiopathic types of "inappropriate" sinus tachycardia.
**May be seen in adults after mitral valve surgery, with digoxin toxicity, with acute inferior myocardial infarction, etc.
†1:1 conduction (300 bpm) can occur spontaneously, with increased sympathetic tone, or sometimes as a complication of class 1A or 1C antiarrhythmics administered without concomitant AV nodal blockers.

## Wide QRS Complex Tachycardias (WCTs)

I. Artifactual (e.g., tooth-brushing; Parkinsonian tremor)

II. Ventricular tachycardia (VT): monomorphic or polymorphic (latter including torsades de pointes) and bidirectional (latter may be seen with catecholaminergic VT or digitalis toxicity)

III. Supraventricular tachycardia (including sinus, paroxysmal supraventricular tachycardias [PSVTs], atrial fibrillation [AF] or flutter) with aberrant ventricular conduction ("aberrant" or "anomalous" activation) associated with:
  A. Bundle branch block or other intraventricular conduction delay (IVCD), which may be rate- (tachycardia-) related
  B. Atrioventricular (AV) reentrant tachycardia (AVRT) with conduction down the AV node and up the bypass tract ("orthodromic conduction") with concomitant bundle branch block
  C. AVRT with antegrade conduction over an AV bypass tract ("antidromic conduction")
  D. Drug toxicity, especially class 1 (sodium channel blocking) agents such as flecainide or tricyclic antidepressants
  E. Hyperkalemia (usually associated with normal or slow heart rate)

IV. Pacemaker-associated
  A. Sinus or other supraventricular tachyarrhythmia with appropriate pacemaker tracking to upper rate limit
  B. Pacemaker-mediated tachycardia (PMT)

## Atrial Fibrillation: Some Major Causes and Contributors

1. Alcohol abuse ("holiday heart" syndrome)
2. Autonomic factors
   A. Sympathetic (occurring during exercise or stress)
   B. Vagotonic (occurring during sleep)
3. Cardiothoracic surgery
4. Cardiomyopathies or myocarditis
5. Congenital heart disease
6. Coronary artery disease/ischemia
7. Genetic (familial) factors
8. Hypertensive heart disease
9. Idiopathic ("lone" atrial fibrillation)
10. Obstructive sleep apnea (OSA)
11. Paroxysmal supraventricular tachycardias
12. Pericardial disease (usually chronic)
13. Pulmonary disease (e.g., chronic obstructive pulmonary disease)
14. Pulmonary emboli (acute or chronic)
15. Sick sinus syndrome (tachy-brady variant)
16. Thyrotoxicosis (hyperthyroidism)
17. Valvular heart disease (particularly mitral valve disease)
18. Wolff–Parkinson–White (WPW) preexcitation

## Cardiac Arrest: Three Basic ECG Patterns

I. Ventricular tachyarrhythmia
   A. Ventricular fibrillation (or ventricular flutter)
   B. Sustained ventricular tachycardia (monomorphic or polymorphic)
II. Ventricular asystole (standstill)
III. Pulseless electrical activity (electromechanical dissociation)

## Digitalis Toxicity: Major Arrhythmias

I. Bradycardias
   A. Sinus bradycardia, including sinoatrial block
   B. Junctional (nodal) escape rhythms*
   C. Atrioventricular (AV) heart block,* including the following:
      1. Mobitz type I (Wenckebach) AV block
      2. Complete heart block*
II. Tachycardias
   A. Accelerated junctional rhythms and nonparoxysmal junctional tachycardia
   B. Atrial tachycardia with block
   C. Ventricular ectopy
      1. Premature ventricular complexes (Ventricular premature beats)
      2. Monomorphic ventricular tachycardia
      3. Bidirectional ventricular tachycardia
      4. Ventricular fibrillation

*Junctional rhythms may occur with underlying atrial fibrillation leading to slow or regularized ventricular response. Atrioventricular (AV) dissociation *without* complete heart block may also occur (i.e., with ventricular tachycardia).

# Select Bibliography

## BASIC CONCEPTS AND HISTORY

Fisch C. Centennial of the string galvanometer and the electrocardiogram. *J Am Coll Cardiol* 2000;26:1737-45.

Goldberger AL, Goldberger ZD. *Becoming a consummate clinician: what every student, house officer, and hospital practitioner needs to know.* Hoboken, NJ: Wiley–Blackwell; 2012.

Hurst JW. Naming of the waves in the ECG, with a brief account of their genesis. *Circulation* 1998;98:1937-42.

Kligfield P, et al. Recommendations for the standardization and interpretation of the electrocardiogram. Part I: The electrocardiogram and its standardization. *J Am Coll Cardiol* 2007;49:1109-27.

Pappano AJ, Weir GW. *Cardiovascular physiology.*10th ed. Philadelphia: Elsevier/ Mosby; 2013.

## NORMAL AND ABNORMAL P–QRS–T–U PATTERNS

Goldberger AL. *Myocardial infarction: Electrocardiographic differential diagnosis.* 4th ed. St. Louis: Mosby Year-Book; 1991.

Macfarlane PW, van Oosterom A, Pahlm O, Kligfield P, Janse M, Camm J, editors. *Comprehensive electrocardiology.* 2nd ed. London: Springer Verlag; 2010.

Mirvis D, Goldberger AL. Electrocardiography. In: Mann DL, Zipes DP, Libby P, Bonow RO, editors. *Braunwald's heart disease: A textbook of cardiovascular medicine.* 10th ed. Philadelphia: WB Saunders/Elsevier; 2015 (11th ed., editors Zipes D, Bonow R, Libby P, et al., forthcoming 2018).

Park MK, Guntheroth WG. *How to read pediatric ECGs.* 4th ed. Philadelphia: Mosby/Elsevier; 2006.

Surawicz B, Knilans TK. *Chou's electrocardiography in clinical practice.* 6th ed. Philadelphia: WB Saunders; 2008.

Wagner G, et al. AHA/ACC/HRS Recommendations for the standardization and interpretation of the electrocardiogram. Part VI: Acute myocardial ischemia. *J Am Coll Cardiol* 2009;53:1003-11.

## ARRHYTHMIAS, PACEMAKERS, IMPLANTABLE CARDIOVERTER–DEFIBRILLATORS, CARDIAC ARREST

Goldberger ZD, Rho RW, Page RL. Approach to the diagnosis and initial management of the stable adult patient with stable wide complex tachycardia: diagnosis and initial management. *Am J Cardiol* 2008;101:1456-66.

Goldberger ZD, Goldberger AL. Therapeutic ranges of serum digoxin concentrations in patients with heart failure. *Am J Cardiol* 2012;109:1818-21.

Klein G, Prystowsky EN. *Clinical electrophysiology review.* 2nd ed. New York: McGraw-Hill; 2013.

Kleinman ME, Brennan EE, Goldberger ZD, et al. 2015 American Heart Association guidelines update for cardiopulmonary resuscitation and emergency cardiovascular care. Part 5: Adult basic life support and cardiopulmonary resuscitation quality. *Circulation* 2015;132(Suppl 2):S414–S435.

Olshansky B, Chung MK, Poguizd SM, et al. *Arrhythmia essentials.* 2nd ed. Philadelphia: WB Saunders/Elsevier; 2017.

Page RL, Joglar JA, Caldwell, MA, et al. 2015 ACC/AHA/HRS guideline for the management of adult patients with supraventricular tachycardia: a report of the American College of Cardiology/American Heart Association Task Force on Clinical Practice Guidelines and the Heart Rhythm Society. *J Am Coll Cardiol* 2016;67:1575-623.

Spragg DD, et al. Disorders of rhythm. In: Kasper DL, et al., editors. *Harrison's principles of internal edicine.* 19th ed. New York: McGraw-Hill; 2015.

Zimetbaum PJ, Josephson ME. *Practical clinical electrophysiology*. Philadelphia: Lippincott, Williams & Wilkins; 2009.

Zipes D, editor. Arrhythmias, sudden death, and syncope. In: Mann DL, Zipes DP, Libby P, Bonow RO, editors. *Braunwald's heart disease: a textbook of cardiovascular medicine*. 10th ed. Philadelphia: WB Saunders/Elsevier; 2015 (11th ed., editors Zipes D, Bonow R, Libby P, et al., forthcoming 2018).

Zipes D, Jalife J. *Cardiac electrophysiology: From cell to bedside*. 5th ed. Philadelphia: WB Saunders; 2013.

## FREE WEB-BASED ECG/ARRHYTHMIA RESOURCES

American College of Cardiology (ACC): www.acc.org

American Heart Association (AHA): www.americanheart.org. Included here are the series of articles entitled AHA/ACC/HRS Recommendations for the Standardization and Interpretation of the Electrocardiogram: Parts I–VI. In addition, consensus guidelines for arrhythmia management, pacemaker and ICD indications, and resuscitation are available. See also ACC and HRS websites.

Heart Rhythm Society (HRS): www.hrsonline.org

Medical Multimedia Laboratories. SVT tutorial. http://www.blaufuss.org

Nathanson LA, McClennen S, Safran C, Goldberger AL. ECG wave-maven: self-assessment program for students and clinicians. http://ecg.bidmc.harvard.edu

# Index

Page numbers followed by "*f*" indicate figures, "*t*" indicate tables, and "*b*" indicate boxes.